D1259115

Movement System Variability

Editors

Keith Davids, PhD
University of Otago, New Zealand

Simon Bennett, PhD
*University of Manchester Institute of
Science and Technology, United Kingdom*

Karl Newell, PhD
The Pennsylvania State University, United States

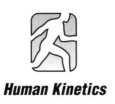

Human Kinetics

Library of Congress Cataloging-in-Publication Data

Movement system variability / Keith Davids, Simon Bennett, Karl Newell, editors.
    p. ; cm.
  Includes bibliographical references and index.
  ISBN 0-7360-4482-5 (hard cover)
  1. Human locomotion. 2. Musculoskeletal system--Variation. 3. Efferent pathways--Variation.
  [DNLM: 1. Movement--physiology. 2. Biomechanics. 3. Motor Skills--physiology. 4. Nonlinear Dynamics. WE 103 M9357 2006] I. Davids, K. (Keith), 1953- II. Bennett, Simon, 1970- III. Newell, Karl M., 1945-
  QP301.M698 2006
  612.7'6--dc22

                        2005006427

ISBN: 0-7360-4482-5

Acquisitions Editor: Judy Patterson Wright, PhD; **Managing Editor:** Lee Alexander; **Copyeditor:** Jocelyn Engman; **Proofreader:** Pam Johnson; **Indexer:** Marie Rizzo; **Permission Manager:** Dalene Reeder; **Graphic Designer:** Robert Reuther; **Graphic Artist:** Denise Lowry; **Cover Designer:** Robert Reuther; **Cover Art:** Robert Rein; **Art Manager:** Kelly Hendren; **Printer:** Sheridan Books

Printed in the United States of America   10 9 8 7 6 5 4 3 2 1

Human Kinetics
Web site: www.HumanKinetics.com

United States: Human Kinetics, P.O. Box 5076, Champaign, IL 61825-5076
800-747-4457
e-mail: humank@hkusa.com

Canada: Human Kinetics, 475 Devonshire Road Unit 100, Windsor, ON N8Y 2L5
800-465-7301 (in Canada only)
e-mail: orders@hkcanada.com

Europe: Human Kinetics, 107 Bradford Road, Stanningley, Leeds LS28 6AT
United Kingdom
+44 (0) 113 255 5665
e-mail: hk@hkeurope.com

Australia: Human Kinetics, 57A Price Avenue, Lower Mitcham, South Australia 5062
08 8277 1555
e-mail: liaw@hkaustralia.com

New Zealand: Human Kinetics, Division of Sports Distributors NZ Ltd.
P.O. Box 300 226 Albany, North Shore City, Auckland
0064 9 448 1207
e-mail: info@humankinetics.co.nz

Contents

Part II   Variability, Performance, and Excellence

Part III Issues in Measurement

Chapter 7 Coordination Profiling of Movement Systems 133
Chris Button, PhD, Keith Davids, PhD,
and Wolfgang Schöllhorn, PhD

Chapter 8 Clinical Relevance of Variability in Coordination . . 153
Joseph Hamill, PhD, Jeffrey M. Haddad, MS,
Bryan C. Heiderscheit, PhD, Richard E.A. Van Emmerik, PhD,
and Li Li, PhD

Chapter 9 Measuring Coordination and Variability in Coordination 167
Jonathan S. Wheat, PhD and Paul S. Glazier

Part IV Variability Across the Life Span

Chapter 10 Functional Variability in Perceptual Motor Development 185
Geert J.P. Savelsbergh, PhD, John van der Kamp, PhD,
and Karl S. Rosengren, PhD

Contributors

Joseph Baker, PhD
School of Kinesiology and Health Science,
York University, Canada

Benoît G. Bardy, PhD
Centre de Recherches en Sciences du Sport,
Université Paris Sud 11, Orsay, France

Roger M. Bartlett, PhD
The School of Physical Education,
University of Otago, New Zealand

Peter Beek, PhD
Institute for Fundamental
and Clinical Human Movement Sciences,
Vrije Universiteit of Amsterdam, the Netherlands

Simon Bennett, PhD
Faculty of Life Sciences,
University of Manchester, UK

Reinoud J. Bootsma, PhD
Laboratoire Mouvement et Perception,
CNRS-Université de la Méditerranée,
Marseille, France

Susan Bortolotto, PhD
University of Padova, Italy

Chris Button, PhD
University of Edinburgh, UK

Les G. Carlton, PhD
Department of Kinesiology,
University of Illinois at Urbana-Champaign, USA

John W. Chow, PhD
Department of Applied Physiology and Kinesiology,
University of Florida, USA

Evangelos A. Christou, PhD
Department of Integrative Physiology,
University of Colorado, Boulder, USA

Andreas Daffertshofer, PhD
Institute for Fundamental
and Clinical Human Movement Sciences,
Vrije Universiteit of Amsterdam, the Netherlands

Keith Davids, PhD
School of Physical Education,
University of Otago, New Zealand

Katherine Deutsch, PhD
Department of Kinesiology,
The Pennsylvania State University, USA

Till Frank, PhD
Institute for Theoretical Physics,
University of Muenster, Germany

Walter J. Freeman, MD
Department of Molecular and Cell Biology,
University of California at Berkeley, USA

Paul S. Glazier
School of Sport, Physical Education and Recreation,
University of Wales Institute, Cardiff, UK

Jeffrey M. Haddad, MS
Motor Control Laboratory,
University of Massachusetts at Amherst, USA

Joseph Hamill, PhD
Biomechanics Laboratory,
University of Massachusetts at Amherst, USA

Craig Handford, PhD
Department of Sport Science, Physical Education
and Recreation Management,
Loughborough University, UK

Bryan C. Heiderscheit, PhD
Department of Orthopedics and Rehabilitation,
University of Wisconsin at Madison, USA

Li Li, PhD
Department of Kinesiology,
Louisiana State University, USA

Ludovic Marin, PhD
Motor Efficiency and Motor Deficiency Laboratory,
Université de Montpellier I, Montpellier, France

Gottfried Mayer-Kress, PhD
Department of Kinesiology,
The Pennsylvania State University, USA

Alberto E. Minetti, MD
Institute for Biophysical and Clinical Research
into Human Movement,
Manchester Metropolitan University, UK

Karl M. Newell, PhD
Department of Kinesiology,
The Pennsylvania State University, USA

Olivier Oullier, PhD
Department of Neuroscience,
Université de Provence-CNRS, France

David L. Pease
School of Physical Education,
University of Otago, New Zealand

C.E. (Lieke) Peper, PhD
Institute for Fundamental
and Clinical Human Movement Sciences,
Vrije Universiteit of Amsterdam, the Netherlands

Carlo Reggiani, PhD
Department of Anatomy and Physiology,
University of Padova, Italy

Karl S. Rosengren, PhD
Department of Kinesiology
and Department of Psychology,
University of Illinois at Urbana-Champaign, USA

Geert J.P. Savelsbergh, PhD
Institute for Fundamental
and Clinical Human Movement Sciences,
Vrije Universiteit of Amsterdam, the Netherlands
Institute for Biophysical and Clinical Research
into Human Movement,
Manchester Metropolitan University, UK

Wolfgang Schöllhorn, PhD
Institut für Sportwissenschaft,
University of Muenster, Germany

Jaeho Shim, PhD
School of Education, Baylor University, USA

Jacob J. Sosnoff, PhD
Department of Kinesiology,
The Pennsylvania State University, USA

Thomas A. Stoffregen, PhD
Human Factors Research Laboratory,
University of Minnesota, USA

Brian L. Tracy, PhD
Department of Health and Exercise Science,
Colorado State University, Fort Collins, USA

John van der Kamp, PhD
Institute for Fundamental
and Clinical Human Movement Sciences,
Vrije Universiteit, Amsterdam, the Netherlands

Richard E. A. Van Emmerik, PhD
Motor Control Laboratory,
University of Massachusetts at Amherst, USA

Jonathan S. Wheat, PhD
The Centre for Sport and Exercise Science,
Sheffield Hallam University, UK

Preface

"Variability is inherent within and between all biological systems" (Newell & Corcos, 1993, p. 1). With that comment Newell and Corcos (1993) drew attention to the sustained research effort on variability in the human movement system. Their book gave due recognition to the need to reconsider the meaning of variability in movement systems. It was argued that the traditional study of motor behavior tended to operationalize variability with measurements of variance in motor output (e.g., measuring standard deviation around the distribution mean of a dependent variable measured over repeated trials). Within the past decade, a dynamic systems perspective has provided a backdrop for a theoretical reinterpretation of the role of variability in movement behavior. The alternative standpoint has been advanced that the inherent noisiness of the motor system results in variability being omnipresent, unavoidable, and an apparent problem of control for all high-dimensional and complex systems. However, it has become clear that variability is often functional, producing the adaptability in patterns of coordination needed to secure stable outcomes in dynamic performance.

The seminal text of Newell and Corcos (1993) built a solid platform for researching variability from a new perspective and was intentionally limited to the study of variability in processes of motor control, particularly from the perspectives of motor control and biomechanics. The emphasis on variability in dynamic systems theory has indicated that principles, concepts, and tools from nonlinear dynamics and chaos theory can provide insights into the role of variability at many different levels of analysis of movement system behavior. As many of the chapters of this book demonstrate, the study of variability need not be confined to the subdisciplines of motor control and biomechanics. New horizons are emerging, signaling the need for a multidisciplinary study of biological systems as physical systems. Future overviews and discussions need to include the analysis of variability in the perceptual subsystem as well as in the structure and function of microcomponents of the human body such as muscle synergies, muscle fiber types, motor unit populations, neuronal ensembles, and cell complexes. At this time, there is clearly a need to adopt an integrative perspective on the nature and role of variability and to take stock of current research at different levels of analysis. Such an approach will address the imbalance in the collated material on variability in different subsystems involved in human movement. Interestingly, an integrative approach is not new. Perhaps the most influential figure in the study of coordination in movement systems, Bernstein (1967) disliked the dichotomization of the theoretical field of movement science and sought to build a coherent explanation among different disciplines.

This book brings together established and emerging scientists from institutions across the world to review and discuss the nature and role of variability within and between individual systems of movement. This text represents a rich array of scientific disciplines including psychology, movement coordination, motor control and skill acquisition, perceptual-motor development, nonlinear dynamics, the sciences of chaos and complexity, biomechanics, molecular biology, physiology, philosophy, the neurosciences, pedagogy, and physical education. The book is targeted at readers working in many different subdisciplines, specifically those relating to the scientific study of human movement behavior. The authors have admirably discussed theory and data that offer insights into the nature and role of variability at different levels of analysis. Their aim was to thoroughly overview the work on variability in various disciplines and to relate the findings to research on other subsystems of the movement system. The main questions they address include: What is the nature and function of variability observed at specific subsystems of the human body? How can understanding variability enhance the practice of educators, teachers, coaches, physiotherapists, and developmental specialists? The editors would like to acknowledge the excellent work of the contributing authors in achieving these aims and addressing these and other relevant questions. They have done an admirable job in synthesizing the burgeoning literature on variability at different levels of the human movement system, providing an in-depth multidisciplinary analysis of the literature for researchers in the human movement sciences and related fields. We would also like to thank Judy Patterson Wright, the commissioning editor of Human Kinetics, for her advice and help in publishing this text.

Part I

Behavioral Analysis of Variability in the Movement System

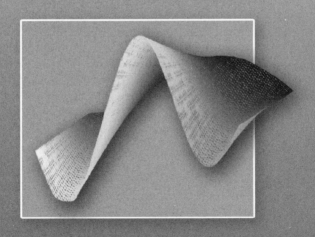

Chapter 1

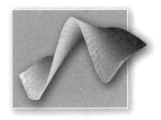

Variability in Motor Output As Noise

A Default and Erroneous Proposition?

Karl M. Newell, PhD, Katherine M. Deutsch, PhD,
Jacob J. Sosnoff, PhD, and Gottfried Mayer-Kress, PhD

Editors' Overview

Should variability in outputs of movement systems always be considered as unwanted noise? This chapter provides a very accessible and updated technical analysis of the difference between random variability and functional variability, highlighting the different types of noise in biological systems, and not merely focusing on white noise. The inherent noisiness of the motor system results in variability being omnipresent and unavoidable in all high dimensional and complex systems. The construct of noise (white or otherwise) in biological movement systems has never been fully developed and clarified in early accounts (based on information processing) of motor behavior. Numerous assumptions regarding noise in perceptual-motor systems are highlighted, the validity of which has rarely been evaluated over the years. The contexts of postural control and motor development illustrate some practical implications of the arguments discussed. In considering developments in nonlinear dynamics and chaos theory, a number of interesting questions are raised over the place of the so-called white noise hypothesis in motor learning and control. It seems that the color of noise in the motor system needs to be a strong consideration in understanding the nature and function of variability in motor behavior. Further research is needed for clarifying the proposed dissociation of the term *noise* as both cause *and* structure of variability in motor output if the "default and erroneous proposition" of variability as noise is to be corrected.

Variability is an inherent feature of motor output both between and within subjects in all categories of tasks. Yet traditionally this ubiquitous feature of motor behavior has been dismissed as insignificant in many theories of motor learning and control, and treated operationally as a standard deviation (SD) in distributional statistics (Newell & Corcos, 1993; Newell & Slifkin, 1998). In theories about the variability of motor output, the universal position has been that variability reflects noise (Fitts, 1951; Schmidt, Zelaznik, Hawkins, Frank, & Quinn, 1979; Welford, 1981; Harris & Wolpert, 1998).

In this chapter we examine the theoretical background and experimental veracity of the hypothesis that variability is noise, studying this hypothesis within the context of child development, aging, disease state, and individual skill. A central interest is whether this hypothesis is anything more than a long-standing default based on the natural appeal of its face validity. The following discussion proves that a clear view of the noise in the sensorimotor system is essential to evaluating the hypothesis that variability is noise.

The concept of noise can be applied to any analysis of the interaction between an organism and its environment and to any type of system construct (e.g., chemical, mechanical, electrical, thermal). In the discussion of motor behavior, noise has been primarily associated with the electrical transmission of information by the central and peripheral sensorimotor mechanisms of the neural system. This focus has even led to the use of the phrase *neural noise* in some emphases of motor behavior (Szafran, 1968; Welford, 1965). We use the general label *noise* while discussing motor output variability, though we also are focusing on neural noise in the transmission of sensorimotor information.

Noise and Movement Variability in Information Theory

The pervasive perspective of the role of noise in motor output variability is drawn from information theory in communication systems (Shannon & Weaver, 1949). In information theory, noise from the channels of the system adds to a signal during transmission so that the observed motor output is a result of signal and noise. In artificial systems where the properties of the input signal are known explicitly, one can take the difference of the input and output signals to estimate system noise. Of course, in biological systems, we do not directly know the properties of the input signal and thus have an inverse problem. As a consequence, the challenge of inferring properties of the input signal by analyzing properties of the output signal is a central focus of the experimental enterprise in motor control.

In experimental analysis of movement and posture, equipment and environmental noise also contaminate the output signal of the motor system. It is assumed that the amplitude of this noise is very small and that the frequency range is broadband, perhaps even reflecting white noise within the sampled range. The signal-to-noise ratio must be sufficiently large so that the equipment noise does not bias interpretations of the biological signal and the intrinsic dynamic noise. The contribution of equipment noise to signal output has rarely been reported in studies of movement variability. As a consequence, environmental noise is not pursued further here (see Newell & Slifkin, 1998) on the assumption (which may be erroneous in a number of cases) that experimental studies have met the standard guidelines regarding environmental noise.

In information theory, the noise of communication systems is taken to be white Gaussian noise (Pierce, 1963; Shannon & Weaver, 1949). White Gaussian noise has a Gaussian distribution of amplitudes, an equal representation of frequency contributions within the range measured, and independent successive values of the signal sampled. The white noise adds to the signal and interferes with the transmission of information through the system to a degree dependent on the ratio of signal to noise. Thus in this view noise is additive. The Gaussian distribution of the noise in the macroscopic output of the system of information transmission is explained by the central limit theorem and the law of large numbers. The distribution is the aggregation of broadband white noise that arises from various microscopic systems (see figure 1.1). In the information theory of system communications, noise is generally considered a nuisance that should be minimized and eliminated in the design of artificial systems when possible.

The information theory of Shannon and Weaver (1949) provided a foundation for numerous theories of information processing and models of human sensorimotor performance that were introduced in the 1950s and '60s (Attneave, 1959; Broadbent, 1958; Fitts & Posner, 1967) and subsequently developed (Kantowitz, 1974; Marteniuk, 1976; Wickens, 1984). This work provided the background for a wide-ranging application of constructs in information theory, including noise in both motor (Fitts, 1954; Kail, 1997; Schmidt et al., 1979; Welford, 1965) and sensory (Gregory, 1974; Pardhan, Gilchrist, Elliott, & Beh, 1996; Welford, 1981) experiments. The experimental studies arising from this theoretical perspective generally assumed that variability reflects noise, based on the tenets of information theory without directly testing the hypothesis of variability as noise.

Many experiments have been conducted on reaction time, movement time, psychological refractory period, decision time, sensory detection, and so on. All of these domains use time as the key dependent variable in order to reflect the speed of a particular mechanism in the channel of sensorimotor communication. It was assumed that higher noise levels impeded detection of the information content of signals and that therefore a longer segment of the signal and more time were required to detect and interpret the message of the signal. This interference of noise with the signal also increased the variability of the respective time measurement. Thus, noise was often used to explain the longer times and greater amplitudes of performance variability of some conditions or groups in a fashion consistent with the principles of the signal-to-noise ratio in information theory. As noted previously, the belief that the structure of variability matches that of white noise has rarely if ever been tested within this conceptual framework of motor control.

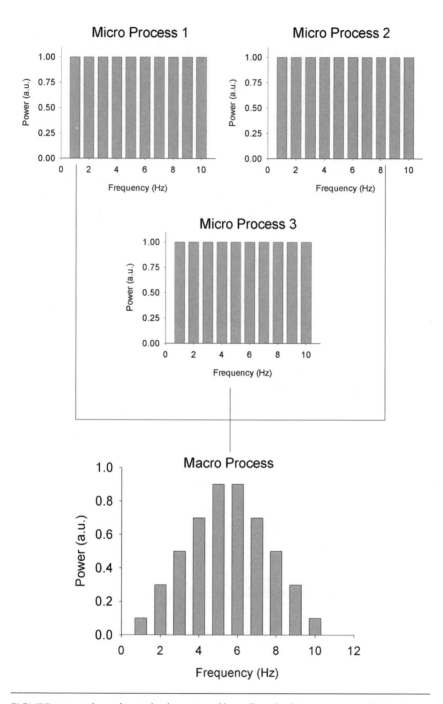

FIGURE 1.1 A hypothetical schematic of broadband white noise at individual microlevels that sum to a white Gaussian noise at the macrolevel.

The most well-known use of information theory in the motor domain is that of Fitts' law (Fitts, 1954; Fitts & Peterson, 1964) and the information processing interpretation of the movement relation between speed and accuracy. Fitts proposed that the channel capacity of the sensorimotor system is the rate at which it can transmit information. In tasks testing speed and accuracy, the channel capacity (*C*) can be estimated by

$$C = ID / MT, \tag{1.1}$$

where *MT* is movement time and *ID* is the index of difficulty.

$$ID = \log_2(2A / W), \tag{1.2}$$

where *A* is movement amplitude and *W* is target width. The target width can be manipulated as a marker of the outcome variation of the task-allowed movement. Fitts assumed that the capacity to transmit information is limited mainly by the amount of noise in the system. Several researchers have proposed theoretical modifications to Fitts' account of movement variability (Kvålseth, 1980; Welford, 1968), but these modifications retain the essential and original interpretation of the role of noise in the motor system.

In summary, information theory in communication systems provides a logical and formal framework for evaluating the information processing of the sensorimotor system. It outlines a direct theoretical role for noise that is assumed explicitly or implicitly in the many experimental studies motivated by the approach of information processing to motor control. The hypothesis that variability is noise is central to this approach, but this hypothesis was never directly investigated. For example, in the experimental work driven by information theory there are no sufficient tests of the notion that the variability of motor output is that of white Gaussian noise. Thus, when viewing the proposition of variability as noise from the perspective of information theory on human performance, it seems appropriate to conclude that this proposition has largely been a default argument. This default approach is, however, also inherent in more contemporary biological and psychological hypotheses about the role of noise in the variability of motor output.

Noise in Physiological Models of Motor Control

The approach using information theory to understand human performance and motor control is a systems viewpoint. It recognizes that noise can arise at any level of the system, but proponents of this view do not directly examine noise in particular physiological or general biological mechanisms. The appeal to neural noise is made primarily but implicitly in the terms of physiological mechanisms that supported information conduction such as neuronal increase, loss and refractoriness, inhibition and excitation of synaptic connections, and temporal coding of synaptic activity in the connections among neurons.

The systems approach focused its experiments to subprocesses of information input through output in a consideration of sensory systems and of information translation and subsequent organization into action planning and motor output. However, the strict isolation of the components of information processes is difficult to reconcile in its most literal interpretation, because as Sherrington (1906) articulated nearly a century ago, the motor neuron is the final common pathway of the motor system. As such, the variability of motor output is influenced by all neural processes before this point in the flow of behavior, and in many system perspectives, also by the anticipatory demands of the future states of the ongoing action.

We believe the 20th-century studies on the physiology of motor output largely undervalued the importance of variability, even the amount of variability, in posture and movement. Traditionally, experiments on the physiology of motor control have failed to report even a standard deviation (SD) for the dependent variable under study, we assume because variability was not an important part of the theoretical landscape (Brooks, 1986; Latash, 1998; Rothwell, 1994). Even if there had been an interest in variability (Gasteiger & Brust-Carmona, 1964; Matthews, 1972; Stein, 1965), experiments focusing on physiology tend to not generate enough repetitions or trials to accurately estimate a SD and the amount or structure of variability.

Noise as variability has been discussed (or more usually just mentioned) for a range of central and peripheral physiological mechanisms. Thus, noise in physiological mechanisms has been linked to the cause of the variability of motor output at the behavioral level, but relations to the sources of variability across levels have rarely been investigated. There have been a few exceptions to this trend which we mention so as to provide a perspective of the issues of variability and the physiology of motor control that have been addressed theoretically and experimentally. In principle, of course, noise and variability can exist in the output of any physiological mechanism of motor control.

Any questioning about variability and the physiology of motor control has probably been whether noise resides centrally in the motor command or peripherally in distinct sensorimotor processes. This question is another instance of the central versus peripheral debate that has pervaded theory and experiment in the field of motor control for many years (Brooks, 1986; Evarts, Wise, & Bousfield, 1985; Stelmach, 1975). There have been advocates of either side of this debate in addition to those who have juxtaposed these positions to form the logical extension that noise arises from *both* central and peripheral sources.

It has long been advocated without experiment that movement variability originates from central sources (Joseph, 1988; Wiesendanger, 1986). Harris and Wolpert (1998) have termed this variability *signal dependent noise,* although they recognize that noise can arise at all levels of the system. In this view, noise is a component of the central command signal and scales to the level (usually viewed as linear) of the force output or some other kinematic or kinetic property of the intended movement. This postulation is consistent with the notion of information processing of a central command signal becoming contaminated with noise as the information flows to the neuromuscular periphery. Although electroencephalography (EEG) studies were early biological advocates of nonlinear dynamic analyses (Basar, 1990; Mayer-Kress & Holzfuss, 1987; Mayer-Kress et al., 1988), these studies did not initially examine the variability of brain activity and central commands. Indeed, even today, most EEG analyses of brain activity use averaged data in order to distill the signal from background noise and variability.

A more prevalent position has been that peripheral neuromuscular processes drive the variability of motor output in posture and movement. For example, Schmidt and colleagues (1979) proposed that the variability of force output is proportional to the level of force (see Meyer, Abrams, Kornblum, Wright, & Smith, 1988). This model of impulse variability, however, did not specify the particular physiological processes that create noise. Van Galen and De Jong (1995) have proposed that inhibiting centrally driven neuromotor noise by using peripheral damping mechanisms is the key to specifying these physiological processes.

The study of peripheral influences on variability in motor output has centrally focused on the fluctuations in the firing rate of motor units and their relation to the variability of force control in the limb (De Luca, Foley, & Erim, 1996; De Luca, Le Fever, McCue, & Xenakis, 1982). Advances in recording several motor units simultaneously have facilitated the investigation of such questions. For example, De Luca (1988) explained the control of motor units using the hypothesis of common drive, whereby the central nervous system controls the motor units as a collective pool rather than as individual entities. The hypothesis is based in part on the finding that fluctuations in the firing rate of the pool of motor units are causally related to the fluctuations in force output at the behavioral level.

Several studies have provided additional evidence relating behavioral motor output and the variability of output across the levels of firing motor units. The heightened rate of discharge of motor units has been related to the greater variability of muscular contraction found in older adults (Laidlaw, Bilodeau, & Enoka, 2000). Indeed, it has been shown that up to 10% of the variance in finger tremor can be accounted for by motor unit activity in young healthy adults (Halliday, Conway, Farmer, & Rosenberg, 1999). However, variability in the firing rate of a single motor unit producing a constant force does not follow the distribution of white noise but demonstrates, as does the force output, time-dependent properties (Vaillancourt, Larsson, & Newell, 2002). The age-related increase in motor variability has also been linked to a high-to-low frequency shift in electromyograph (EMG) activity (Vaillancourt, Larsson, & Newell, 2003) and to a decrease in the low-frequency common drive applied to the pool of motor units (Erim, Beg, Burke, & De Luca, 1999).

The variability of motor output could arise from noise at both central and peripheral sources. Gilden, Thornton, and Mallon (1995) have modified the Wing and Kristofferson model (1973) for sequential timing behavior and have proposed that the variability of the central timer for action reflects a $1/f$ process (power is inversely proportional to frequency) whereas the variability in the motor program that drives the neuromuscular periphery reflects a process of white noise. These processes combine so that $1/f$ properties dominate the spectrum (of log power versus log frequency) of movement timing and spatial error data. However, this modeling approach is more in the spirit of information processing components rather than an examination of the roles of particular physiological mechanisms in motor output variability. A recent finding that the variability of force output is very different in an intentional muscular contraction than in a contraction arising from a cortical-electrical stimulation has been interpreted as support for the proposition that noise has both central and peripheral sources (Jones, Hamilton, & Wolpert, 2002).

In summary, there have been only isolated analyses of the relation between the variability of neurophysiological processes and the variability of effector output in posture and movement. Although a number of studies have examined how the fluctuations in the firing rates of motor units relate to the variability of force control, crucial testing of the amount, structure, and coherence of the variability of the motor units and force output remains undone. Nevertheless, the idea that noise in neurophysiological processes *causes* the observed variability in motor output prevails explicitly and implicitly in motor control. This position is consistent with the reductionist agenda describing the neurophysiology of motor control, but like the more behaviorally oriented perspectives of information processing, it has largely been a default argument.

Categories of Noise

There are many kinds of noise that are well documented in several domains including acoustics, physics, statistics, stochastics, and several branches of engineering (Gardner, 1983; Hartmann, 1997; Stark & Woods, 1994; van Vliet, 1981). It is useful to briefly look at certain categories of noise to assess the veridicality of the hypothesis of variability as noise in motor control. The issue of noise in biological systems has become a central topic in recent years (Bassingthwaighte, Liebovitch, & West, 1992; Schroeder, 1991; Ward, 2002), largely because of the increasing theoretical and empirical emphases of models of nonlinear dynamics, fractals, and chaos.

A major limitation in many of the previous studies on noise and motor control is the authors' failure to state explicitly what kind of noise, and hence distribution or system, they refer to in a study. The standard strategy has been to equate variability with noise without examining the type of noise and the structure of the variability. It is reasonable, given the tenets of communication theory outlined previously, to assume that the reports on movement variability that were based on information processing were considering white Gaussian noise, but it is also possible that in some cases another noise category was implicit.

The noise interpretation of variability typically refers to what in everyday language are called the random components of the observed signal. Thus, it is assumed that the sequential properties of discrete, sequential, or continuous motor output are independent. Certainly, many visual images of variability in motor output, such as tremors (Elble & Koller, 1990), impress that the fluctuations in the output, in this case in the limb acceleration from moment to moment, are independent and randomly distributed around some mean state.

The term *random* has several meanings and is a slippery term when used in a technical sense (Beltrami, 1999; Ruelle, 1991). However, a core belief underlying most everyday references to randomness is that the sequential properties of the time series are independent (as in a randomly shuffled deck of cards), or in other words, that there is no autocorrelation (one technical signature of white noise, as in delta correlated). The notion of randomness is typically not expressed in the context of whether or not there is variability (SD) that arises from repeated measurements.

In traditional nonfractal measurements, the smallest spatial feature of an object or measure of a process is its characteristic scale, and this observation is uninfluenced by measures that are finer than this scale. In contrast, with fractals, the resolution of the measurement influences the features the observation reveals. This leads to the self-similarity of observations made at one resolution of measurement to those taken at another level of resolution (Mandelbrot, 1983). The scaling relation defines what is observed relative to the resolution of measurement.

That measures can be fractal leads to the related idea that there may not be a single timescale or modal frequency in the time series of motor variability. The power spectrum of the time series can exhibit a scaling range in the log power versus log frequency plot showing that the data have no preferred timescale (Bassingthwaighte et al., 1994). The classic multiple timescale relation has more power at the low than at the high frequencies, and the slope of the log–log plot is taken to reflect the strength of the sequential dependence in the time series. The strength of the long-range correlations is denoted by the color assigned to the noise, ranging from white, where there is no time dependence, to black, where there is a highly structured, rhythmical time series. The $1/f$ spectrum, in which power is inversely proportional to frequency, has been shown to prevail in a range of natural phenomena (Bak, 1996; Schroeder, 1991) including variability in motor output (e.g., Duarte & Zatsiorsky, 2000; Gilden et al., 1995; Vaillancourt & Newell, 2003). This so-called colored noise could arise from numerous system models including deterministic chaotic systems, stochastic systems, and linear systems with filters.

A significant feature in considering categories of noise is that the central limit theorem so instrumental in Gaussian distributions and in considerations of white noise does not hold for certain fractal processes such as Lévy stable distributions (Bassingthwaighte et al., 1994; Liebovitch, 1998; West & Deering, 1995). In Lévy stable distributions, the mean and variance are infinite and do not settle on some central limit or average. Thus, the mean and variance of the distribution change as more data are collected, creating a scaling of the power law to elementary statistical properties. The extent to which this kind of fractal distribution exists in dynamic properties of movement behavior has not been determined.

A key feature of nonlinear dynamics is its focus on the time-evolutionary or sequential properties of the dynamic. In this view, the time-dependent properties of the signal or time series are central to understanding the organization of the system output and its variability. Thus, unlike in the experiments on human movement motivated by information theory, the successive samplings of the signal are not assumed to be white Gaussian noise or independent identically distributed (i.i.d.) samples of a white noise distribution.

The assumption that movement fluctuations are independent over time may have arisen from the view in a white noise model that noise is additive, where the noise at one moment is independent of the next. In an approach based on dynamic systems, however, the intrinsic dynamic noise may be multiplicative, in the sense that there is a time-evolutionary influence on noise that is dependent upon the state of the system. Most dynamic models of motor output variability invoke noise as an additive concept, and the implications of additive versus multiplicative noise have yet to be fully understood. Nevertheless, one clear finding in recent examinations of the structure of movement variability (experiments motivated by the tenets of nonlinear dynamics) is that intraindividual variability rarely shows the defining properties of white Gaussian noise and nearly always holds some time-dependent structure (for reviews covering a range of experimental applications in the movement domain see Newell & Slifkin, 1998; Riley & Turvey, 2002).

Thus, the prevailing theoretical approach to motor variability as noise has been that of additive white Gaussian noise rather than that of multiple timescales of variability and their multiplicative time-dependent influences. From the perspective of nonlinear dynamics, the multiple timescales of variability reflect the multiple control structures that influence motor output in a deterministic but probabilistic way (Mayer-Kress & Newell, 2003). These control structures can create variability that mimics aspects of the output of an additive noise model, but this capacity of the motor system should not be taken as a reflection of a white noise process per se. This theoretical perspective does not rule out a role for white noise as background in the system, even an adaptive role, but it postulates that the structure of motor variability is primarily due to the multiple timescale influences of the control structures of the sensorimotor system.

Variability and Noise in Motor Output

In this section we examine more contemporary views of variability in movement and posture. In particular, we address some central questions pertaining to the deterministic and stochastic structure of movement variability and to the role of white noise in the observed variability. The challenge is to reveal the contributions of different deterministic and stochastic processes to the variability of movement and posture through a detailed and coordinated analysis of the structure of the time and frequency domains of the motor output variability.

The operational approach is based on the traditional analysis of time series and the more recent theoretical influences of nonlinear dynamics, fractals, and chaos (Kaplan & Glass, 1995; Kantz & Schreiber, 1997). We do not address in detail the many technical assumptions and their relationships to the nuances in theoretical interpretation that pervade this domain. We do, however, raise certain key caveats because the adaptive nature of motor variability tends to challenge the technical assumptions of certain analyses. Moreover, the multiple timescales of motor output also lead to operational and theoretical challenges in understanding variability.

White Noise

The increasing application of nonlinear dynamics to motor control in the 1990s led to a number of direct investigations on the role of white Gaussian noise in the variability of motor output. In an early synthesis of this work, Newell and Slifkin (1998) concluded that if one thing could be said about the nature of motor variability at the effector level, it was that it did not tend to reflect the structure of white Gaussian noise (see also Slifkin & Newell, 1999a; Riley & Turvey, 2002). Indeed, it is difficult to find any experimental investigations of variability in posture and movement providing collective evidence for the three essential criteria of a normal Gaussian distribution, namely a Gaussian distribution of amplitudes, an equal contribution of frequencies, and an independence of the sequential properties of the time series.

Thus, one might say that the rule of thumb on variability in motor output is structure rather than randomness. Specifically, the empirical evidence shows that the essential assumption in applying the tenets of information processing to variability in motor output does not hold. Again, this is not to say that there is not random background noise in the time series of the motor output, but rather that the collective macroscopic structure of variability in movement and posture is not white noise, either broadband or Gaussian.

There is one caveat to this statement that pertains to all the subsequent analysis and interpretation we are presenting. Namely, analyzing the structure of the variability may depend on the time duration of data collection in each context. For example, analyzing the profile of postural center of pressure or the profile of finger tremor acceleration may lead to different interpretations when the profiles are considered over different timescales. Differing interpretations can arise because the time series is nonstationary or the sample length is not sufficient to determine the dynamic structure of the output.

A signal is nonstationary when the statistical properties of a time series differ in different segments of the series (Chatfield, 1984; Kantz & Schreiber, 1997). In many analyses of time series, stationarity is a prerequisite to the integrity of the analysis technique, so departures from stationarity present problems in analysis and interpretation, particularly of measures that depend on the average properties of a time series. This situation makes the more pointlike analysis procedures of wavelets and recurrence attractive for examining the structure of variability, as they are not based on averaging procedures over a trial length. In some fields, nonstationarity would lead to either discarding the data or attempting to detrend the nonstationarity of the data so as to conform with the assumptions of the analysis technique. However, nonstationarity is a hallmark of biological systems even when observations are made over a relatively short time such as 10 s in a standing posture (Newell, Slobounov, Slobounova, & Molenaar, 1997b). Of course, the characterization of time as short or long needs to be interpreted in relation to the natural timescales of the time series.

Nonstationarity reflects additional timescales that are introduced into the dynamic because of the changing contributions of processes that could relate to boredom, fatigue, attentional shifts, and so on. In a task performance, nonstationarity could also arise from an intentional shift of the performer to pursue different task goals, such as thinking about future events while performing the primary task. If the variation of a given motor output is measured over a long enough time, the variability will depart from white noise, even if the time series briefly exhibits properties consistent with white noise. Thus, the timescale of observation needs to be longer than the natural timescale of the movement or posture dynamic, but the natural dynamic inevitably changes its stable state given enough time. Nonstationarity is a pervasive natural element of movement and posture, and analyses of variability need to use the proper timescale rather than follow the engineering approach in artificial systems of massaging the data to fit the technical confines of the analysis.

Although the structure of variability in motor output is not that of white noise, spectral analysis shows that in some frequency bands there is an equal proportion of power (a trademark of white noise). Thus, motor output can show $1/f$-like characteristics (discussed in a later section) over most of the frequency range examined (Gilden et al., 1995; Deutsch & Newell, 2003), but the higher frequency band might show properties of white noise within the limits of the high-frequency cutoff (see the 5% maximal voluntary contraction (MVC) conditions in figure 1.2). This pattern of motor output is consistent with white noise being present as background in the time series, even if this noise does not capture the essence of the time series.

Deutsch and Newell (2003) have shown that this kind of background noise contributes a very small percentage (<0.01%) of the variance in isometric force

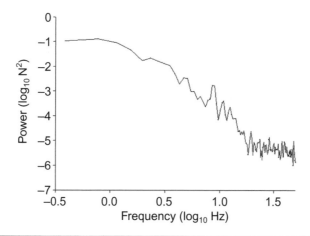

FIGURE 1.2   Simulated example of log normalized power versus log frequency for isometric force output as a function of visual feedback (present or absent) and force level (5% and 35% MVC).

variability and that it is not age dependent over the range of age 6 y to young adulthood. This finding counters the account of information processing (Kail, 1997; Prechtl, 1970) of the declining role of noise in the growing child's motor output variability (for a review see Deutsch & Newell, in press). Thus, age-related differences in the variability of motor output are not due to changes in the level of noise but rather to differences in the deterministic and probabilistic structures of the multiple timescales of colored noise. The changing and multiple time delays of feedback loops can contribute to age-related differences in 1/*f* behavior (Mayer-Kress & Newell, 2003).

Humans are not very adept at producing random streams of output in a variety of behavioral domains (Rosenberg, Weber, Crocq, Duval, & Macher, 1990; Wagenaar, 1972; Ward, 2002). It has been shown that subjects cannot approximate white noise in the output of finger oscillations and that the facility to generate unstructured output was poorer in the larger effector systems as measured in finger, hand, and arm motions (Newell, Challis, & Morrison, 2000). Our estimate of the dimension of an intended random motor output of a single effector system was approximately 6. Furthermore, practice over 5 d did not increase the dimensionality of the motor output (Newell, Deutsch, & Morrison, 2000), suggesting that there is considerable structural and functional constraint on the dynamic degrees of freedom of the system (Newell & Vaillancourt, 2001). In short, an intention to move randomly does not generate highly dimensional behavior.

In discrete movements, the distribution of the outcomes has been shown to hold properties similar to white noise (Spray & Newell, 1986; Newell, Liu, & Mayer-Kress, 1997). Newell, Liu, and Mayer-Kress (1997) showed that in a discrete-timing task repeated in 200 trials, the time series approximated the distribution of white Gaussian noise in about 50% of the trials, whereas in the other 50% of the trial sequences some local structure or dependence was observed in trial n to $n + 1$ and to a lesser extent in trial n to $n + 2$. There was a weak tendency for the more skilled subjects to show stronger trial-to-trial correlations. Clearly, though, as Gilden et al. (1995) have shown, the trial-to-trial structure becomes $1/f$-like when there are many more trials and the experiment is run over a longer time. These contrasting findings regarding the degree of sequential structure in motor output nicely demonstrate the differences that may arise in assessing the structure of movement variability as a function of different timescales of observation.

Structure of 1/f

Noise in time series is usually estimated using spectral analysis and the properties of the power spectrum (Hartmann, 1997). White noise has an equal power in the frequency range examined that in principle, although not in practice, should extend to infinity. However, there are many other patterns to the density in the power spectrum that can arise in motor output, including those that exhibit a scaling range in the power over a frequency bandwidth. These patterns are known as colored noise (labeled as a parallel to the filter properties that produce colored light) and more technically as $1/f$ processes. In $1/f$ processes, the power is inversely proportional to the frequency. The spectral power falls off as a power function with a particular exponent from a range of lower to higher frequencies. These $1/f$ processes are highly prevalent in living and nonliving systems (Bak, 1996; Mandelbrot, 1983; Schroeder, 1991), but interpreting these power functions is still controversial given the range of models that can produce them.

As noted previously, $1/f$ processes reflect multiple timescales expressed in the scaling of the log–log relation of the power spectrum. The larger the exponent and the steeper the slope of the log–log function, the darker is the colored noise and the stronger are the long-range correlations in the time series. This is because the slower frequencies have longer timescales and hence longer durations of relations in the data given the nature of oscillatory processes. Thus, using the term *noise* to capture these timescales of influence can be very misleading as there is deterministic although probabilistic structure in the range of scaling frequency. Certainly, however, this is not the kind of noise that theoretical and experimental analyses of movement variability have been referring to all these years.

An increasing amount of experimental data in motor control show that the structure of variability in motor output is consistent with that of a $1/f$ process. This includes data on postural control (Duarte & Zatsiorsky, 2000), isometric force output (Vaillancourt & Newell, 2003), repetitive discrete movements (Gilden et al., 1995), tapping movements (Chen, Ding, & Kelso, 2001), motor units (Vaillancourt et al., 2002), ECG (Kobayahi & Musha, 1982), EMG (Gitter & Czerniecki, 1995), and EEG (Musha, 1981; Pritchard, 1992). Interestingly, the total duration of the data sampling in these experiments reflects the product of different central and peripheral mechanisms and a wide range of timescales, but $1/f$-like processes in the power spectrum hold nonetheless.

It is conventional to speak of particular colored noises that have distinct integer exponents, such as pink noise (exponent = 1), brown noise (exponent = 2), and black noise (exponent > 3), but the range of actual exponents in log–log power spectra is not confined to these low integers. Also, there is not necessarily a single scaling region in a spectrum. For example, there might be two scaling regions with different exponents that capture the influence of a different organization of deterministic processes in a different bandwidth of the frequency spectrum (Bassingthwaighte et al., 1994). There are other systematic ways in which a $1/f$-like process may depart from a single scaling (for examples, see the contrasting $1/f$-like profiles for 6-year-olds versus adults and 5% versus 35% MVC in figure 1.2).

One common feature of colored noise is that the spectrum is strong at low frequencies (long timescales) and weak at high frequencies (short timescales). On the one hand, this pattern implies strong long-term correlations and on the other hand, it implies the reduction of high-frequency fluctuations. The former can be induced under appropriate conditions by using time delays in the dynamics of systems whose current states are directly influenced by earlier states (Mayer-Kress & Newell, 2003). Of course, single time delays do not automatically guarantee $1/f$ spectra that indicate the absence of specific timescales.

The high-frequency decay of the spectrum is also a signature of the smoothness of the time series or trajectory. For close enough inspection, in other words, for small enough timescales, the signal appears smooth. The asymptotic smoothness of the trajectories for timescales that are short enough corresponding to frequencies that are high enough is also one of the main characteristics of chaotic (as opposed to stochastic) systems. These distinguishing characteristics have still to be investigated in the variability of motor control.

The particular bandwidth properties in the power spectrum need to be cautiously interpreted, usually in conjunction with other measurements of the time series that agree in the description of the multiple timescales of the data. Limitations in the properties of the data set can compromise analyses, but motor output data tend to have fewer problems in this regard than data from other domains. Nevertheless, analysis of $1/f$ processes can reveal properties of the background noise and the deterministic and stochastic structure of variability. An advantage of $1/f$ analysis is that the scaling range of the frequency spectrum of motor output may often directly link to the timescales of particular physiological mechanisms (such as when brain activity is reflected in EEG bands).

Time-Dependent Structure

One of the criteria for white Gaussian noise is that the sample points in the time series are independent.[1] This criterion has been examined by spectral analysis and the finding of a null slope across the log–log spectrum. Given the structured oscillatory output in most motor tasks (e.g., preferred rhythms or highly reproducible space-time patterns of movement), it seems intuitively unlikely that any movement or postural time series would approximate white noise. Even in a repetition of discrete movements, the outcomes are likely to be influenced by a range of factors that only increases their potential for impact, and hence structure is introduced into the time series as the time course for the observation of performance increases.

Another approach to examining the independence of samples in the time series is to determine the degree to which an analyst can predict a later segment of the time series using information from earlier segments. There are several techniques for determining time-domain dependence in a data set (e.g., mutual information or autocorrelation), but approximate entropy (ApEn) (Pincus, 1991) has many useful features (see Richman & Moorman, 1999). ApEn is a measure of the regularity or irregularity of a time series. Unlike many other nonlinear techniques, it can be used with relatively short data sets.

Figure 1.3 shows ApEn from the postural acceleration tremors of different arm links under conditions of vision or no vision (Morrison & Newell, 1996). There is a similar pattern to the mean ApEn across arms even though the value of the right hand was noticeably lower than that of the left hand. The figure shows more regularity at the shoulder and wrist joints, suggesting that arm posture is controlled by coordinated motion at these joints.

ApEn has been shown to be very sensitive to change in the time-dependent structure of variability in motor output in a range of posture and movement tasks (for arm posture, see Morrison & Newell, 1996; for isometric force control, see Slifkin & Newell, 1999b; for postural finger tremor, see Vaillancourt & Newell, 2000). A prevalent finding is that as variability (standard deviation) increases, the structure of the time series shifts to lower dimensions and the ApEn index of regularity and predictability in the time domain strengthens. There is not a universal trend of an inverse pattern in the amount and structure of variability in motor output, although many tasks reveal the increased SD and reduced ApEn relation. For example, when the task requires a reduction in the dimension of the intrinsic dynamic, the relationship between the amount and structure of variability can be reversed (Newell, Broderick, Deutsch, & Slifkin, 2003; Vaillancourt & Newell, 2003).

Our analyses have also revealed that changes in the time-dependent structure of the variability of motor output can occur even when there is no apparent change in the amplitude, SD of the amplitude, and modal frequency of the data

---

[1]Some domains use the terms *time dependent* and *time independent* to reflect whether the data are nonstationary or stationary, respectively. We use the terms to describe whether the sequential properties of the time series are independent or dependent.

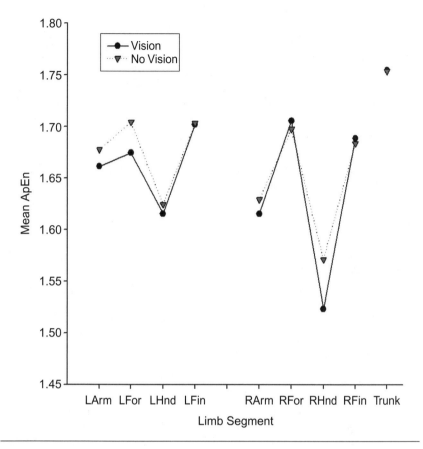

FIGURE 1.3   Mean ApEn for postural arm tremor (left and right) as a function of vision (present or absent) and arm segment (Fin = finger, Hnd = hand, For = forearm, Arm = upper arm).

Reprinted, by permission, from S. Morrison and K.M. Newell, 1996, "Inter and intra-limb coordination in arm tremor," *Experimental Brain Research* 110: 455-464. With kind permission of Springer Science and Business Media.

set. In a study of postural finger tremor in Parkinson's disease (Vaillancourt & Newell, 2000), ApEn revealed differences in the time-dependent structure of tremor in age-matched healthy controls, even though there was no difference in the modal frequency and amplitude of tremor. ApEn was lower in the Parkinson's group, and it also systematically changed as a function of the severity of Parkinson's disease (as indexed by the Unified Parkinson's Rating Scale). This finding nicely illustrates the significance and relative sensitivity of an analysis of the time-dependent structure of motor output and reveals that the disease state reduces the adaptability of the postural control. The regularity in the time domain across two streams of data, such as the force outputs of the finger and thumb in precision grasping, can also be determined by using cross ApEn (Vaillancourt, Slifkin, & Newell, 2002).

There are some limitations to ApEn, the significance of which varies with the questions a study addresses and the properties of the data set. ApEn is a kind of average statistic in that it is determined over the entire time series. As a consequence, assessing dependence in the time domain through action is influenced by the nonstationarity of the time series. Nevertheless, ApEn is very useful in many situations, particularly those where the goal is to discriminate (test for differences) among conditions or population groups. If the primary interest is modeling the data, ApEn provides some preliminary background about the relative structure of the time series.

The pattern of changes in ApEn as a function of movement condition or population group tends to be theoretically consistent with the pattern of changes found in correlation dimension, exponents of the $1/f$ log–log slope, and other measurements. This is expected given the structure of the ApEn statistic (Pincus, 1991) and its relation to other measures of dynamic structures in a time series. Nevertheless, ApEn has fewer limitations than many other measurements on the properties of the data, and thus is a very useful index of time dependence in a data set. ApEn also provides a ready test of one important property of white Gaussian noise and has helped confirm that most movement and posture data sets do not display sequential independence in the time series.

Multiple Timescales of Variability

Applying the theory of dynamic systems to human movement has been appealing because the theory provides a way to characterize many of the basic phenomena of movement, including change, stability, variability, and the emergence of new structure and function. The concepts of nonlinear dynamics have provided the stimulus to consider the variability of movement and posture not merely as noise in the system, but as a reflection of nonlinear deterministic and stochastic processes. For example, the developmental progression in the rates of change to the confluence of constraints in children's action (Kugler, Kelso, & Turvey, 1980; Newell, 1986; Thelen, 1986) leads to multiple timescales in behavioral output that in and of themselves vary over developmental time (Newell, Liu, & Mayer-Kress, 2001).

The changing, age-related level and structure of variability may be viewed as indexes of the changing timescales and dimensions of feedback control loops (Mayer-Kress & Newell, 2003). Indeed, the structure of the variability of the output indicates what in dynamic terms are the degrees of freedom being regulated (Lipsitz & Goldberger, 1992; Newell, 1998; Newell & Vaillancourt, 2001) and the change in adaptation and complexity over the life span. These active degrees of freedom may relate to feedback loops that each have different timescales (loop times) that converge in the control system to influence the structure and amount of movement variability (Kaplan & Glass, 1995). However, there may be no obvious correspondence between the dynamic degrees of freedom (dimension) and the physical mechanical degrees of freedom of human movement that were emphasized by Bernstein (1967) (see Eubank & Farmer, 1997; Newell & Vaillancourt, 2001).

The role of variability in coordination transitions (Haken, Kelso, & Bunz, 1985) and the emergence of new movement forms (Thelen & Smith, 1994) have been particular theoretical contributions of dynamic systems to development in bifurcation analysis and the theory of phase transitions. However, we have emphasized the roles of noise and variability in steady states of postural and movement behaviors. These steady states of behaviors are examined in terms of the deterministic and stochastic properties of the dynamics of fixed points or other attractors that arise from the fixed points through bifurcations (Kaplan & Glass, 1995; Strogatz, 1994).

The fluctuation or variability of fixed-point dynamics provides the most fundamental examination of the deterministic and stochastic properties of movement variability, as it is determined by the attractor-basin dynamics. Furthermore, fluctuations are minimally influenced by the changing long-term timescales of the evolving dynamics as long as the system is not close to a critical point or bifurcation. The condition of attractor-basin dynamics near a fixed point essentially provides the cleanest (uncontaminated) test of the role of noise in movement variability in the sense that the irregularities of output are either not or less likely due to nonstationary dynamics associated with changing fixed points (as in learning) (Newell et al., 2001). Thus, the level of noise at a fixed point can be taken as an index of the stability of the system.

A classic example of a task that reflects a steady state of dynamics is upright postural standing, where there is variability in the motion of the torso and limbs of the body. Indeed, although many postures may be viewed as stable or even defined (on occasion) as not moving, they still exhibit variability of motion. The amount and structure of the postural motion indexes the stability and instability of the system output and the roles of deterministic and stochastic processes in system control. The structure of this random motion of postural behavior has been shown to change with age both in young children (Newell, Slobounov, Sobounova, & Molenaar, 1997a; Newell, 1998) and in the elderly (Lipsitz & Goldberger, 1992; Newell, 1998).

Liu, Mayer-Kress, and Newell (1999) introduced a generalized Ornstein-Uhlenbeck process with a threshold as nonlinear extension that can model the deterministic as well as stochastic components of dynamics close to a stationary target (fixed point). The model has two parameters (threshold value and feedback timescales) that can be estimated from the observed data. This map of deterministic threshold is perturbed by adding Gaussian noise of a given level. The model also permits a constructive algorithm to estimate the magnitude of the stochastic or noise component. For deviations above the threshold that originate from the target, a linear feedback mechanism dominates with a characteristic timescale (eigenvalue) that can be estimated from the experimental data. It is assumed that this characteristic threshold depends on developmental and learning parameters and captures the participant's decision for active control (as in signal detection theory) (Green & Swets, 1966). Therefore, we model the dynamics within the threshold distance from the target as a purely stochastic random walk. Within the framework of this model, with increasing age we would expect an increasing sensitivity corresponding to a reduced threshold value and shorter feedback time delays.

In Mayer-Kress, Deutsch, and Newell (2002) and Mayer-Kress and Newell (2003), we have developed a multidimensional generalization of our basic model (Liu et al., 1999). In this model we now include the activation of additional degrees of freedom in the form of new feedback terms with their own delayed timescales. These could be implemented in a directly observable manner by, for example, introducing independent sensory (acoustic or tactile) feedback loops. Our preliminary simulations of isometric force production have shown that the model generates the basic inverse relation between the amount of variability and the increased dynamic complexity of the output found in children (Deutsch & Newell, 2001, 2002; Newell, 1998). In our model, all parameters and variables have direct experimental interpretations. For example, developmentally relevant manipulations of noise level, information feedback gain, intermittency (degree of discontinuous display of information), and delay all directly relate to the model parameters.

Finally, it should be emphasized that background biological noise in the motor output is not necessarily a problem as has been implied implicitly and explicitly by the views of systems information on noise and variability. The very low level of noise in the system could still adaptively facilitate task-relevant changes in motor output (Gasteiger & Brust-Carmona, 1964). The work on stochastic resonance in human performance (Collins, Imhoff, & Grigg, 1966; Cordo et al., 1996; Wiesenfeld & Moss, 1995) has provided direct evidence for this viewpoint by showing that noise can enhance the detection of weak signals. Nevertheless, further work is clearly required to more directly examine the adaptive role of white noise in the multiple timescales of motor control.

Concluding Comments

A significant part of the problem in considering movement and posture variability is that the word *noise* has been used both as an observation of the structure of variability in motor output and as a construct for the cause of the structure of the output. This dual use of the term assumes the face validity of the output reflecting the construct without using the appropriate considerations for establishing the principles of theory construction. It might be useful to preserve *noise* to denote the construct, but the use of the term for describing the observation of irregularity is so ingrained in the literature that a shift to restricted usage is unlikely. Furthermore, Van Vliet (1981) has suggested that systematically classifying noises as causes or manifestations is impossible.

It also could be argued that it is unfortunate that the 1/*f* scaling in bandwidths of the power spectrum is labeled as *colored noise*. *Noise* clearly has a different meaning when used with white noise than when used with any of the colored noises. Colored noise has dynamic properties that *noise* is not typically meant to refer to when used in everyday language. As Bak (1996, p. 22) remarked, it might be misleading to call the 1/*f* scaling *noise* rather than *signal*. The ranges of 1/*f* scaling reveal interesting mixes of deterministic and stochastic processes that need to be examined more directly in movement and posture variability. Our working hypothesis is that these scaling phenomena are driven by feedback processes that have multiple timescales of influence on the dynamic (Mayer-Kress & Newell, 2003).

Variability in movement and posture is not synonymous with noise and, moreover, white Gaussian noise is a very small background component in the structure of variability. The variability of motor output is dominated by deterministic but probabilistic structures that we are now in a better position to formally model, given the theoretical and experimental work of the last 10 years or so. It seems reasonable that the hypothesis that variability is noise is not only a default proposition based on untested assumptions but also an erroneous assumption.

Chapter 2

Variability in Postural Coordination Dynamics

Olivier Oullier, PhD, Ludovic Marin, PhD,
Thomas A. Stoffregen, PhD, Reinoud J. Boostma, PhD,
and Benoît G. Bardy, PhD

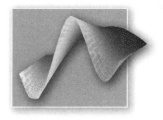

Editors' Overview

Research on the use of vision for controlling posture is examined, showing how it has focused on (1) neurophysiological processes underlying the intrinsic coordination in posture and (2) the importance of informational coupling in achieving the control of stance. This chapter aims to overview recent research in this area, particularly emphasizing the relationship between intentionality and variability in shaping the dynamics of intersegmental coordination during stance. It is argued that data on modulating a pattern of coordination for postural control reveal the influence of local constraints such as intentions and forces, whereas transitions between patterns reveal self-organization processes at work. Focusing on the small number of postural control strategies identified in previous work, the ankle and hip strategies, it is proposed that there is a need to examine the coordination between these two key joints in maintaining upright postural control. In particular, variability in coordination between the ankles and hips is proposed as a functional relationship designed to maintain upright posture during suprapostural tasks. The findings discussed in this chapter support a new perspective on the dynamics of whole-body coordination during postural control, signaling that there is no primary role solely for neural, mechanical, or muscular mechanisms, as has been espoused in previous research. Many constraints interact to shape postural behavior in humans, and variability in the postural system plays a functional role in adapting to perturbations.

The experiments reported in this chapter were supported by the *Ministère de l'Education Nationale de la Recherche et de la Technologie* (France) and by the *National Science Foundation* (USA). The authors would like to thank the *Laboratoire Mouvement et Perception* (CNRS-Université de la Méditerranée, Marseille, France), the *Postural Stability Laboratory* (University of Cincinnati, Cincinnati, USA), and the *Département de Psychologie Expérimentale* (Université de Genève, Genève, Suisse) for allowing to conduct the experiments reported in this chapter in their facilities. Olivier Oullier is very grateful to Gonzalo de Guzman, Idell Weise, Unk L. Woody, Daniel Kukolj and Audrey Di Caro for their help and J.A. Scott Kelso for critical discussions and support.

One of the major problems that movement scientists have to face is how humans (and animals) coordinate the multiple degrees of freedom of their bodies, constraining them to act as a single unit in accomplishing behavioral tasks (Kelso, Southard & Goodman, 1979). To achieve control, the high dimensionality of the body must be reduced to a system exhibiting order, that is, stable and flexible patterns of coordination (Bernstein, 1967). In research on the control of standing posture, many neuro-physiological (e.g., Nashner & McCollum, 1985) and biomechanical studies (e.g., Winter, 1990) have demonstrated the role of local constraints (e.g., forces, central command signals) in shaping patterns of whole-body coordination. These local constraints play a key role in the emergence of preferred postural coordination patterns. They operate in the context of self-organization principles governing coordination, postural pattern formation being no exception. Until recently, this more general level of organization remained largely unstudied in the field of postural coordination (however, see Saltzman & Kelso, 1985, for early suggestions). Typically, the influence of local constraints is assessed through the modulation of a behavioral pattern, while self-organization is revealed in changes between patterns (Haken, 1977). In the present chapter, we discuss recent studies that have focused on the dynamics of human postural coordination. Based on these studies, we argue that multi-joint control of standing posture exhibits typical signatures of self-organized systems.

Maintainance of upright stance depends upon stable control of the posture of the head and body. On earth this implies that the support surface, that is, the surface on which one is standing, can support the body mass. From a purely mechanical point of view, there is balance when the sum of the gravito-inertial forces acting on a body is compensated by an opposite and equal reaction force applied from the support surface. Such a rule would apply to the postural system if it were static, but this is not the case. The human body is a multi-joint system that offers a (potentially) unlimited number of combinations of motion at different joints spontaneously and continuously oscillating at low frequency and low amplitude (Yoneda & Tokumasu, 1986). The spontaneous oscillations are centered around the direction of balance (Riccio & Stoffregen, 1988; Stoffregen & Riccio, 1988). The high order of complexity defining the postural system and the constraints that are applied to it, such as ground reaction and gravity, generate a large amount of variability at different levels of observation (Newell & Corcos, 1993). Controlling such a system is therefore difficult and requires reduction of its dimensionality (Kay, 1988).

Ambiguity of the Neurophysiological Approach to Postural Coordination

Nashner and McCollum (1985) proposed that amongst the many possible relations between joints or muscles, the maintenance of stance commonly relies on a small number of *postural strategies*. These strategies are muscular synergies that reduce the high dimensionality of the postural system mainly involving relationships between the muscles recruited in movements of the ankles and hips. Nashner and McCollum proposed that in most situations humans use one of two postural strategies. In the *ankle strategy*, control of balance is achieved by producing muscular torques around the ankle joint to counterbalance gravito-inertial torques acting on the body. The ankle strategy is thought to be chosen to regulate perturbations at low frequencies (under 0.2 Hz; Nashner, Shupert, Horak & Black, 1989) or at low sway amplitudes (under 20°; McCollum & Leen, 1989). In the *hip strategy*, gravito-inertial torques are counteracted by rotations of the hips (these are generally accompanied by rotations of the ankles in the opposite directions). Nashner and McCollum argued that the hip strategy would be used to counter perturbations at higher frequencies (>2.5 Hz) and/or amplitudes (>20°).

The concept of ankle and hip strategies has met with wide acceptance. One reason for this may be that Nashner and McCollum's (1985) approach succeeds at (conceptually) reducing the dimensionality of the postural system (cf. Kay, 1988). At the muscular and joint levels, hip and ankle strategies compress a high-dimensional postural space with many degrees of freedom requiring coordination into a low-dimensional space with only a few degrees of freedom to be mastered (cf. Bernstein, 1967; Turvey, 1990). The strategies permit mini-mization of behavioral variability arising from the large amount of movement created by combinations between limbs and joints. Postural synergies might be used to reduce the number of degrees of freedom of the body, in which case the system would become less variable and easier to control. Another reason for the appeal of hip and ankle strategies may be experience of the use of the hips for postural control. Most people are familiar with the sudden fore-aft motion of the hips that can occur when the body is perturbed. Common examples include a sudden lurch in a subway train or stance on a balance beam, each of which commonly produces noticeable bending at the hips.

Despite its widespread acceptance, the concept of hip and ankle strategies (Nashner & McCollum, 1985) presents some ambiguities. For the purpose of this chapter, the emphasis will be put on one of these ambiguities (for a more extensive discussion on this topic see Bardy, 2004 and Bardy, Marin, Stoffregen & Bootsma, 1999). It is often assumed that in an ankle strategy there is no rota-tion at the hips. This idea is accepted and reported in many areas of postural research including sensorimotor control (Gurfinkel, 1973; Horak & Nashner, 1986; Nashner et al., 1989), pathology (Horak, Nashner & Diener, 1990), and biomechanics (McCollum & Leen, 1989). This assumption contrasts with the original description of postural strategies by Nashner and McCollum (1985, p. 140), who stated that the ankle strategy rotation takes place "primarily" rather than exclusively about the ankle joint. For instance, hip rotation is evident in their graphical example of an ankle strategy (Nashner & McCollum, 1985, figure 5*a*, p. 141). In addition, empirical studies have consistently shown some degree of rotation at both ankles and hips (Bardy et al., 1999; Horak & Nashner, 1986, figure 7; Horak et al., 1990, figure 4; Marin, Bardy, Baumberger, Flückiger & Stoffregen, 1999; Oullier, Bardy, Bootsma & Stoffregen, 1999; Stoffregen, Adolph, Thelen, Gorday & Sheng, 1997). This suggests that in most cases there is motion at both joints. Given this empirical fact, why do researchers and theoretical models (e.g., Kuo, 1995) assume that in the ankle strategy there is no rotation at the hips?

One way to answer this question is to assume that in the ankle strategy, rotation around the hips is uncontrolled noise, having no specific function in postural control (e.g., Horak & Nashner, 1986; Nashner & McCollum, 1985). Such an assumption may be influenced by the ambiguity that exists in the operational definition of both ankle and hip strategies. In empirical studies, ankle and hip strategies have been differentiated on the basis of their respective muscle activity, joint movements (e.g., Buchanan & Horak, 1999; Horak & Nashner, 1986; Nashner & McCollum, 1985), and forces generated by postural activity with respect to the support surface (e.g., Buchanan & Horak, 2001; Horak & Nashner, 1986; Horak et al., 1990; Ko, Challis & Newell, 2001). Definitions of the ankle and hip strategies at these three levels of behavioral analysis are not equivalent, resulting in ambiguity about whether ankle and hip strategies are defined in terms of muscle activity, kinematics, or kinetics. When there is a strong correlation between activities at the different levels of analysis, the definitional ambiguity is not a problem. However, under many normal circumstances the relations between these levels are equivocal, nonlinear and therefore extremely complex (see Bernstein, 1967; Tuller, Fitch & Turvey, 1982 for theoretical discussions and Bonnard, Pailhous & Danion, 1997 for an experimental illustration). For instance, authors observe some hip muscle activities in an ankle strategy (Nashner & McCollum, 1985) while there is no hip motion if the ankle strategy is defined in terms of forces (nonsignificant shear forces can be detected in an ankle strategy; cf. Horak et al., 1990).

Kinematic Analysis of Dynamic Patterns in Postural Coordination

Mixing levels of behavioral analysis when trying to understand movement coordination can lead to misunderstanding (Bernstein, 1967). Following early analyses (Saltzman & Kelso, 1985; Woollacott & Jensen, 1996), Bardy and colleagues have focused on the kinematics of postural coordination (Bardy et al., 1999; Marin et al., 1999a; Oullier et al., 1999). This analysis of multi-segment postural coordination is consistent with the dynamical systems approach (Beek, Peper & Stegeman, 1995; Kelso, 1995; Kugler, 1986; Riccio, 1993; Turvey, 1990). Bardy and colleagues assume that if ankle and hip movements are involved in the control of upright stance, then it is appropriate to analyze coordination (i.e., relative displacement) between these two joints. It would not be so much the degree of involvement that determines the type of postural organization adopted, rather the way in which the movements of the different joints are coordinated. In this case, their respective movements might not be a simple random motion that can be neglected but could be sensible and coordinated movements. Hence, variability in behavior can be a source of information that helps in understanding the underlying dynamics of a system (see Fuchs & Kelso, 1994). The variability between coordination of the (ankle and hip) joints should therefore be considered to be useful and functional for the scientist (and possibly for the standing person). A natural variable for characterizing modes of coordination in postural coordination dynamics is the relative phase ϕ_{rel} between movements of the hips and of the ankles. The phase of one joint captures both its position and its velocity. This means that the relative phase ϕ_{rel} of two joints reduces four degrees of freedom to one. The coordination between the hip and the ankle can therefore be summarized in ϕ_{rel}. Hence, with a single value of this (collective) variable, the organizational state of the system can be known at any time. Such a variable has been used in a variety of studies involving coordination to an external event (Jantzen, Steinberg & Kelso, 2004; Kelso, DelColle & Schöner, 1990; Lagarde & Kelso, 2004; Oullier, Jantzen, Steinberg & Kelso, in press), inter- and intra-limb coordination (de Guzman, Kelso & Buchanan, 1997; Diedrich & Warren, 1995; Kelso, 1984, 1995; Kelso, Buchanan & Wallace, 1991; Kelso & Zanone, 2002; Salesse, Oullier & Temprado, in press) as well as interpersonal coordination (Oullier, de Guzman, Janzten & Kelso, 2003; Richardson, Marsh & Schmidt, 2005; Schmidt, Carello & Turvey, 1990; Temprado, Swinnen, Carson, Tourment, & Laurent, 2003). In recent studies, Bardy and colleagues have identified two basic patterns (modes) of coordination between hips and ankles (Bardy et al., 1999; Marin et al., 1999a; Marin, Bardy & Bootsma, 1999; Oullier et al., 1999): an *antiphase* mode characterized by a relative phase close to 180°, in which the hips and ankles move in opposite directions, and an *in-phase* mode of coordination characterized by a relative phase around 20°, in which the hips and ankles move in the same direction. In the next section, we describe several experiments that illustrate these findings.

Postural Coordination Emerges from the Interplay of Different Constraints

Riccio and Stoffregen (1988; see also Newell, 1986) suggested that postural organization emerges from the interaction of constraints operating, respectively, at the level of the participant, the environment, and the task. This contrasts with researchers who have argued that the adoption of postural strategies solely depends upon the effects of a single constraint. For example, it has been proposed that the effect of environmental properties alone can influence the organization strategy (Horak & Nashner, 1986; McCollum & Leen, 1989). At the surface of support, an ankle strategy produces mostly torque while a hip strategy produces mostly shear forces. For this reason, Horak and Nash-ner (1986) as well as McCollum and Leen (1989) suggested that all surfaces that have low resistance to shear, such as slippery surfaces, require the use of the ankle strategy for maintaining upright stance. In contrast, a hip strategy should be used on surfaces that have low resistance to torque, such as foam or a narrow beam (Nashner & McCollum, 1985). These assertions are consistent with the findings of some studies previously mentioned, but several other studies have produced counterexamples. For instance, Stoffregen et al. (1997) found that some fourteen-month-old children maintained stance on a soft surface (foam rubber) without detectable rotation at the hips. Conversely, in some children, hip rotation was observed during stance on a low friction surface. These examples suggest that a single constraint (in this case, environmental) is not sufficient to explain the adoption of a given postural strategy. This is true also for constraints imposed by properties of the participant. For example, according to Horak and Nashner (1986), the effective length of the feet can be the main constraint that influences the selection of postural strategies. When standing on a narrow beam, a person's toes and heels are unsupported, reduc-ing the effective length of his/her feet. Horak and Nashner (1986) found that the coordination between hips and ankles was affected by varying the length of the support surface. Marin et al. (1999*a*), however, found that, thanks to their expertise, gymnasts can sway about the ankles while standing on a beam when moving at low frequency. Thus, reduction in effective foot length does not always mandate a reliance on hip rotations for postural control.

Classical analyses of multi-segment control (e.g., Nashner & McCollum, 1985) have concentrated on properties of the environment and the person, such as forces (torque and shear), surfaces (soft, slippery, and short, etc.), bio-mechanics (foot length and height of the center of mass, etc.), and joints (ankle, hip). Marin et al. (1999*a*) considered an additional category of constraints: the goal of the task in which participants were engaged. Indeed, posture is often analyzed in the context of quiet stance, that is, when postural control is the primary or sole activity. However, from an ecological point of view, quiet stance does not represent ordinary posture (Stoffregen, Smart, Bardy & Pagulayan, 1999). Outside the laboratory, upright posture is rarely maintained for its own sake, but rather it facilitates the achievement of *supra-postural* tasks such as looking, walking, and manual manipulation (Balasubramaniam, Riley & Turvey, 2000; Balasubramaniam & Wing, 2002; Bardy & Laurent, 1998; Bardy, Warren & Kay, 1996; Danion, Duarte & Grosjean, 1999; Riccio & Stoffregen, 1988). Accordingly, the research conducted by Bardy and colleagues examines postural control in the context of an explicit supra-postural task.

Bardy et al. (1999) and Marin et al. (1999*a*) claimed that the emergence of hip-ankle coordination cannot be the result of only one of these types of constraint (body properties, support surface, and task) but instead a function of the interactions between them. In studies that we discuss in the following sections (Bardy et al., 1999; Marin et al., 1999*a,b*; Oullier et al., 1999), participants were instructed to move their heads so as to track the back-and-forth oscillations of a computer-generated target moving in the anterior–posterior axis; the aim of the task was for the participants to maintain a constant distance between their head and the target. In their first experiment, Bardy et al. (1999) added mass at different body locations in order to manipulate the height of the body's center of mass (creating *normal, high,* and *low* conditions of center of mass height). For each height of the center of mass, participants were asked to follow four different amplitudes of target oscillations that simulated 5, 14, 18, and 35 cm peak-to-peak displacements of the object (see figure 2.1a). There were three main results. First, for each condition only two stable values of ϕ_{rel} were observed: $\approx 20°$ and $\approx 180°$. This result confirmed that there was rotation about the hips in all conditions. The observation that hip movements were coordinated with ankle movements militates against interpreting the hip movements as noise. Second, as figure 2.1a illustrates, under similar conditions increasing target amplitude (across conditions) was associated with a change in the value of ϕ_{rel} from 20° to 180°. Third, the selection of in-phase ($\phi_{rel} \approx 20°$) or antiphase ($\phi_{rel} \approx 180°$) coordination emerged from the interaction of the location of the center of mass and the target amplitude. These results confirmed the hypothesis that the emergence of a coordination mode depends on the interaction between tasks and body properties.

In their second experiment, Bardy et al. (1999) varied the effective length of feet (creating conditions of *normal, short,* and *long* feet). For the *long* condition, participants wore a pair of shoes similar to skis, whereas for the *short* condition participants' feet were tied to a beam 40% shorter than the length of their feet. As in the previous experiment, there were three main results. First, in each condition only two coordination modes were found ($\phi_{rel} \approx 20°$, $\phi_{rel} \approx 180°$) (see figure 2.1b). This indicated that there was functional hip movement in all conditions. Second, for the normal and long foot length conditions, increasing the target amplitude produced a shift from in-phase to antiphase coordination. In the short foot length condition, antiphase coordination was observed for all values of target motion amplitude. These findings were consistent with the results of Horak and Nashner (1986). Third, shifts between coordination modes depended on the interaction between the target amplitude and the length of feet (see figure 2.1b).

Marin et al. (1999a) varied the friction and rigidity of the support surface, and crossed these variations with changes in the amplitude of the target motion (see figure 2.2). In the *standard* condition, participants stood barefoot on a flat, rigid floor. In the *foam* condition, they stood on a gymnastic mat (23 cm thick), and in the *roller* condition, they wore roller skates (ankle motion was not restricted). The results showed once again that 20° and 180° of ϕ_{rel} were found (see figure 2.2), suggesting that hip and ankle moves were not nonfunctional noise. On the *standard* surface, ϕ_{rel} of 20° was observed with target amplitude below 30 cm, with ϕ_{rel} of 180° for target amplitudes greater than 35 cm. For the two other surfaces, the amplitude of target oscillation did not influence

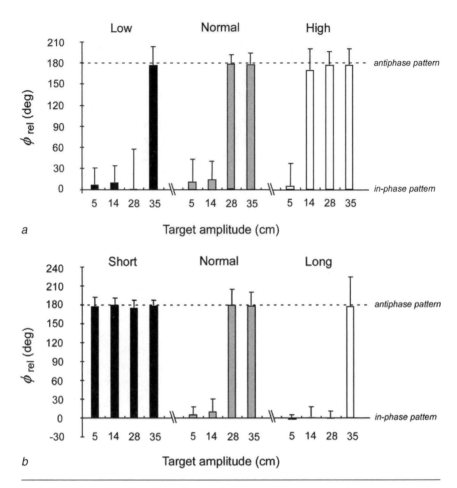

FIGURE 2.1   *(a)* Effects of cross-manipulating the height of the center of mass (low, normal, and high) and the amplitude of sway (5, 14, 28 & 35 cm) on the circular mean of ϕ_{rel}; *(b)* Effects of cross-manipulating the length of the support surface (short, normal, and long feet) and the amplitude of sway (5, 14, 28 & 35 cm) on the circular mean of ϕ_{rel}.

From B.G. Bardy et al., 1999 "Postural coordination modes considered as emergent phenomena," *Journal of Experimental Psychology: Human Perception and Performance* 25: 1284-1301. Copyright © 1999 by the American Psychological Association. Adapted with permission.

coordination. In the *roller* condition, participants always adopted the in-phase coordination, while in the *foam* condition, the antiphase pattern was always observed (figure 2.2). Taken together, the results of Marin et al. (1999a) and Bardy et al. (1999) clearly reveal that postural coordination emerges from the interaction of different constraints.

These studies confirm that the ankles and the hips are coordinated and that the hip-ankle coordination is functional in the control of stance. Only

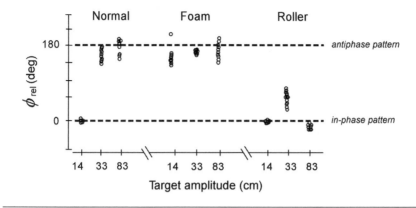

FIGURE 2.2   Effects of varying the surface of support (*normal, foam,* and *roller*) on the circular mean of ϕ_{rel} as a function of target amplitude (14, 33, and 83 cm) and the surface of support.

Reprinted from *Human Movement Science* Vol 18, L. Marin et al., Interaction between task demands and surface properties in the control of goal-oriented stance, pgs. 31-47, Copyright 1999, with permission from Elsevier.

two modes of coordination (in-phase or antiphase) were observed, and the emergence of these modes depended on the interaction of task-, and environment-based constraints. In their experiments, Bardy et al. (1999), Marin et al. (1999a) and Oullier et al. (1999) have either manipulated the nature of the surface of support and the amplitude or frequency of target movements to investigate the emergence of the postural coordination modes and their stability. For each trial, participants were asked to oscillate their heads back and forth at constant values of the control parameter (amplitude or frequency of target movements). The different values of the control parameter that were tested enabled the researchers to show that the stability of each mode depended on the coalition of constraints applied to the standing human similarly to what has been reported in other studies on coordination between a limb and an external event (e.g., Kelso, Fink, DeLaplain & Carson, 2001; Lagarde & Kelso, 2004) and interpersonal coordination (e.g., Oullier et al., 2003). This stability can be quantified in terms of the variability of the relative phase between the hips and the ankles, ϕ_{rel}. The variability of ϕ_{rel} was low for extreme values of the control parameter, in other words, for very large or very low amplitudes (Bardy et al., 1999) and very high or very low frequencies (Oullier et al., 1999). When the values of the control parameter were in between these extremes, an increase of variability could be observed. According to the dynamical systems theory (Kelso, 1995), Bardy and colleagues assumed that this increase of variability was due to being in the vicinity of the region of transition from one coordination pattern to another. The variability of the relative phase between the ankle and the hip therefore provided information about the organization of the system. Nevertheless, this remained an assumption since the design of these experiments (Bardy et al., 1999; Marin et al., 1999a) did not directly address this point. Indeed, control parameters remained constant within a trial and were varied only on a between-trials basis. One other point in common among these experiments is that participants were always asked to intentionally track the target with their heads. The possible question of the influence of intention on modulating the dynamics of postural coordination had never been addressed. This is why Oullier, Bardy, Stoffregen, and Bootsma (2002) tested the stability of the coordination modes while continuously varying the control parameter within a trial and having participants perform two different tasks involving intentional and nonintentional sway in the experiment. The question behind Oullier et al.'s (2002) study was to know whether intention (to sway) could affect the variability of the relative phase between the ankles and the hips. These results are summarized and discussed in the following section.

Intention (to Sway) Modulates the Stability of Postural Coordination

Oullier et al. (2002) asked participants either to track the back-and-forth oscillations of a target (e.g., Bardy et al., 1999; Marin et al., 1999a; Oullier et al., 1999) or merely to look at it as it moved (Stoffregen, 1985; Stoffregen et al. 1999; Oullier, Bardy & Boostma, 2001). In controlling stance, looking at the target favors rotation of the body about the ankles (Stoffregen et al., 1999), whereas tracking it favors in-phase or antiphase coordination between the ankles and hips depending on the frequency of the target (e.g., Marin et al., 1999b). Both looking and tracking, however, require an adaptive intrinsic (ankle and hip) coupling between the segments of the postural system, and both require an adaptive visual coupling between the body and the target (Oullier, Bardy & Bootsma, 2001). Research relating vision to stance has repeatedly demonstrated the importance of visual coupling for the achievement of stance (e.g., Schöner, 1991), however little is known regarding how intention modulates the dynamics of both the visual coupling and the postural coordination. A hypothesis to explain postural sway that has enjoyed a wide acceptance in the literature on postural control is that humans control body sway by attempting to minimize retinal slip (e.g., Lee & Lishman, 1975). However this is not sufficient to understand the dynamics of the underlying coordination. The dynamic coupling of vision and intrinsic coordination in the postural system must be taken into account (Dijkstra, Schöner, Giese & Gielen, 1994). This is why studying the relative influences of the postural and the visual systems is useful to understand the coupling between postural coordination and the nature of the task. Standing in order to look at a target or in order to track it with the head are tasks that impose different constraints on the postural system. In contrasting by using looking and tracking tasks, the goal was to understand how intention to move could influence postural coordination and modulate its variability. Results revealed that the visually based coupling between motion of the head and of the target (attached to the front wall of a moving room in which participants were standing to perform the tasks) was influenced by the frequency of target motion and by intention to move or not (tracking versus looking). Frequency and intention had a significant effect on all of the dependent variables that were used to assess head-room coupling[1]. The influence of intention was consistently greater than the influence of frequency. The results illustrate the role of supra-postural tasks in modulating motion of the body as indicated by the effects of the type of task on several dependent variables. Even when the amplitude of the target matched the amplitude of natural oscillations of the body, tracking induced larger amplitudes of head movement than merely looking at it. Consistent with this, both target-head and ankle-hip couplings were stronger in the tracking task. Changes in these couplings were observed as functions of the type of task and the oscillation frequency of the target. Increasing target frequency was accompanied by decreasing visual coupling during both looking and tracking tasks, although coupling remained stronger during tracking. The looking task was associated with reductions in target-head and ankle-hip couplings. In this context, the task effect (i.e., the effect of differences in intention) is regarded as illustrating the relative weakness of coupling in the task of looking.[2]

Bardy et al. (1999) documented the emergence of two preferred modes of postural coordination when participants used voluntary movements of the head to track motion of a target in the anterior–posterior axis. Oullier et al. (2002) found that similar modes emerge whether participants track the target, or merely look at it. Thus, the ankle-hip coordination underlying the maintenance of upright stance was found to be qualitatively similar whether performing a looking or a tracking task. This result is illustrated by the emergence of in-phase and antiphase modes of postural coordination, as shown in figure 2.3 by the bimodal distribution of ϕ_{rel} values for each task. Thus, coordination dynamics underlying the maintenance of upright stance appears similar with or without the intention to sway. This result raises doubts about the widely accepted distinction between quiet stance and deliberate sway (e.g., Creath, Kiemel, Horak, Peterka & Jeka, 2005).

Oullier et al.'s (2002) results also have clear implications for research on the visual control of stance. Implicitly or explicitly, the body is often considered as a simple inverted pendulum oscillating about the ankles and actively matching

---

[1] Oullier et al. (2002) computed and analyzed the movement amplitude, cross-correlation, frequency overlap and the relative phase between the target and the head and between the ankle and the hip.

[2] Some of the results relating to coupling between target and head differ from previous research relating vision and stance. For instance, the tracking task Oullier et al. (2002) studied closely resembled the one used by Bardy et al. (1999). However, in the findings of Oullier et al. (2001, 2002) the coupling between stimulus and head was stronger and the relative phase between target and head was lower than the values reported by Bardy et al. (1999). The differences across studies might have arisen from a difference in the means used to generate optical flow. Oullier et al. (2001, 2002) used a moving room to generate flow while Bardy et al. (1999), Marin et al. (1999a, b) and Oullier et al. (1999) generated flow using tri-dimensional computer graphics and video projection. The different results are consistent with the hypothesis of Stoffregen, Bardy, Merhi and Oullier (2004) that coupling of body sway with optical flow imposed by the experimenter may vary with the technology used to generate the flow (see also Faugloire, Bardy, Merhi & Stoffregen, 2005).

the optical flow created by body sway (Schöner, 1991) or passively driven by this flow. Results of Oullier et al. (2002) indicate that the inverted pendulum analogy may not be correct, for adaptive patterns of postural coordination underlie the simple act of looking. Whether changes in ankle-hip coordination may influence the coupling of head movement to the visual environment remains an open question. The fact that in-phase coordination between ankle and hip emerged under conditions of slow motion of the visual surrounds and antiphase coordination under conditions of rapid motion may or may not be related to the finding reported in this experiment and in earlier studies that the strength of coupling between motion of the room and head decreases with increasing frequency (e.g., Dijkstra, Gielen & Melis, 1992; Dijkstra et al., 1994; Lestienne, Soechting & Berthoz, 1977).

Interestingly, the looking and tracking tasks seemed to exhibit differences in stability, as suggested by the smaller number of in-phase peaks in figure 2.3 and the systematically larger circular deviation of relative phase in the *looking* condition (Oullier et al., 2002). These results suggest the variability of the relative phase is modulated by the intention to sway. Such a result corroborates the assumption that intention should be considered as a modulating factor of the intrinsic dynamics of the postural system similarly to the way it modulates bimanual coordination (Kelso, 1995; Scholz & Kelso, 1990). In the results reported by Oullier et al. (2002), the variability of the coupling between the ankle and the hip also provided information about the nature of visual coupling.

Another important aspect of the data presented in figure 2.3 is the deep valley between the two distribution peaks. This valley represents the absence of transient modes of coordination between the in-phase and the antiphase patterns. This valley (visible separately on figures 2.3a and b) suggests that there must have been a sudden change in coordination mode in each of the (looking and tracking) tasks. Once again (see figure 2.1 and Bardy et al., 1999), when a control parameter was increased, the variability of the ankle-hip relative phase increased, announcing the imminent transition. The higher the variability of ϕ_{rel}, the closer the transition. It is clear from figure 2.3 that the observed bi-modal distribution of relative phase is congruent with a phase transition between postural patterns. However, the methods used by Bardy et al. (1999), Marin et al. (1999a) and Oullier et al. (2002) did not allow the researchers to determine the nature of the transition or the role of the variability of the order parameter in the phase transition. This is because transitions occurred between rather than within trials and so were neither observed nor manipulated as such.

Dynamics of Postural Transitions

The sharply bi-modal distribution of relative phase into two values (figure 2.3) suggests that there is no transient mode of coordination between the in-phase and the antiphase patterns. The values of the relative phase reported by

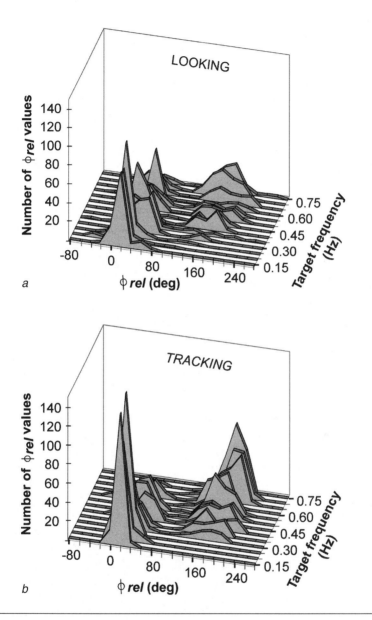

FIGURE 2.3 Distribution of values (in 20° frequency bins) for the ankle-hip relative phase ϕ_{rel} as a function of the target oscillation frequency. Depending on the
experimental condition, participants were asked to (a) simply watch the target
oscillating in the anterior–posterior plane (*looking* condition) or (b) track it with the
head (*tracking* condition). In both conditions, two modes of coordination emerged
for the peak distribution: in-phase (about 20°) and antiphase (about 180°).

Reprinted from *Human Movement Science* Vol 21, O. Oullier et al., Postural coordination in looking and tracking tasks, pgs.
147-167, Copyright 1999, with permission from Elsevier.

Oullier et al. (2002) suggest that a transition should occur but do not indicate why the system changes from one postural pattern to the other. A direct study of postural transitions was still necessary. In this section we review previous attempts to understand how the postural system changes from one mode of coordination to the other. We then report recent research in which this question is directly addressed.

In their research, Bardy and colleagues have examined the existence of postural patterns, focusing on the number and type of patterns, and on the conditions under which each pattern occurs. While this approach has yielded much information about postural patterns, it has provided little knowledge about the dynamic, real-time shift from one coordination mode to another (for recent reviews see Horak & MacPherson, 1996; Woollacott & Jensen, 1996). For example, Horak and Nashner (1986) observed that different control strategies were used on different support surfaces, but they limited their study to situations in which the pattern of multi-segmental coordination was stable. They did not attempt to document the process by which the postural control system dynamically reorganized itself within trials. This may be because transitions between states have often been considered to derive from the states themselves (Bardy, 2004). In other words, it was assumed that changes between states could be understood in terms of the characteristics of stable states. Bardy, Oullier, Bootsma and Stoffregen (2002) argued that four general perspectives of change between postural patterns occur in the context of controlling upright stance.[3] We discuss each of these perspectives next.

First, postural transitions can be considered as a way to minimize the metabolic cost associated with controlling stance. Hoyt and Taylor (1981) argued that preferred locomotory states are characterized by the minimization of energy expenditure. If such an observation is transposed to posture, shifts from one postural pattern to another might occur when, as conditions change, the current pattern becomes less efficient than some other pattern, where the efficiency is defined in terms of the amount of energy expended in achieving the goal (Sparrow & Newell, 1998). Corna, Tarantola, Nardone, Giordano and Schieppati (1999) reported that participants standing on an oscillating platform switched from a single to a double inverted pendulum pattern as platform frequency increased and that this switch reduced the effort required to maintain stability. Minimization of effort may help shape postural patterns, but it is not sufficient to trigger changes between patterns. This is because there are many situations in which maintenance of upright stance is not the sole goal of postural control. Stance is not maintained solely for its own sake but, often, it aids in the achievement of supra-postural tasks such as lifting, throwing, or looking (Stoffregen et al., 1999). The argument is that when controlling stance, people aim to minimize energy expenditure, as is consistent with efficiently

---

[3] In this section, we present different accounts of postural control separately. This is done solely for clarity. The reader should not regard the different accounts as being mutually exclusive.

performing suprapostural tasks. It is believed that there is a trade-off between achieving the lowest metabolic cost and achieving the goals of suprapostural tasks (Newell, 1986; Riccio & Stoffregen, 1988; Sparrow & Newell, 1998). Diedrich and Warren (1995) demonstrated that walk-run transitions are not governed solely by energetic considerations; in the vicinity of the transition region there is not a one-to-one correspondence between the different gait patterns adopted and their metabolic costs. Thus, explaining the transition between coordination modes exclusively in terms of energy minimization would be incomplete.

The second possibility is that the switch from one postural state to another is determined by mechanical limits on the states involved. Mechanical limits may be characterized in a variety of ways, such as limits on the forces and torques applied at the support surface (Horak & Nashner, 1986; Marin, 1997; Pai & Patton, 1997) or at the joints (Yang, Winter & Wells, 1990), limits on the intrinsic frequency of postural patterns (Buchanan & Horak, 1999; McCollum & Leen, 1989), or limits on the amplitude of body movements tolerated by these patterns (McCollum & Leen, 1989; Riccio & Stoffregen, 1988). There is evidence that mechanical properties of the body and/or the environment constrain the appropriateness of particular postural patterns. Nevertheless, a theory of postural transitions based solely on mechanical factors would be inadequate. This is because there is not a one-to-one correspondence between mechanical conditions and patterns of postural control. A given set of mechanical properties can give rise to more than one coordination mode (Bardy et al., 1999; Krizkova, Hlavacka & Gatev, 1993; Marin et al., 1999*a*; Stoffregen et al., 1997). Conversely, different types of mechanical properties can give rise to a single coordination mode. These effects occur because posture is not constrained solely by mechanical properties of the individual and its environment, but is simultaneously constrained by additional factors (e.g., Oullier, Bardy, Stoffregen & Bootsma, 2004). Thus, the question of postural coordination modes and the transitions between them cannot only be assessed with Newtonian mechanics (Beek et al., 1995).

A third possibility is that transitions between postural patterns may result from changes in the information available to the central nervous system. A large body of research on sensory loss, or sensory deficit, has been interpreted as indicating that a change in postural coordination can be caused by changes in the information available for the actor (Allum, Honegger & Schicks, 1993; Buchanan & Horak, 1999; Corna et al., 1999; Horak, et al., 1990; Horstmann & Dietz, 1988; Kuo, Speers, Peterka & Horak, 1998; Nashner et al., 1989). Other researchers have examined the relationship between postural control, a response, and the optical consequences of body sway, considered as a stimulus to the postural control system. Simulation of the optical consequences of body sway leads to direction-specific postural responses during stance (van Asten, Gielen & Denier van der Gon, 1988), postural oscillations (Mégrot, Bardy & Dietrich, 2002; Oullier et al., 2002, 2004), walking (Bardy et al., 1996; de Rugy,

Taga, Montagne, Buekers & Laurent, 2002; Warren, Kay & Yilmaz, 1996), and running (Young, 1988). Again, however, the methodology used in these studies was designed to test for the existence of functionally specific postural adjustments and not for characterizing transitions between different types of adjustments. Thus, while perceptual information certainly influences the organization of posture, its exact role in the organizational processes underlying the formation of postural patterns is not clear at present. The study of postural transitions requires different methodologies.

Fourth and last, postural transitions may be understood within the broader context of the dynamical systems theory (Kelso, 1995; Turvey, 1990). This approach has motivated strong interest in phenomena that occur in the vicinity of the regions of transition from one coordination mode to another. These regions may reveal general principles governing pattern formation that are not directly accessible via the study of the patterns themselves (Fuchs & Kelso, 1994). This does not, of course, imply that biomechanical, metabolic, or informational properties have no influence on the emergence of postural coordination modes (Bardy et al., 1999; Buchanan & Horak, 1999) or on transitions between modes. Rather, the causes of transitions are not to be sought in each of these properties alone (Diedrich & Warren, 1995).

Bardy et al. (2002) argued that modes of postural coordination may function as attractors in the postural state space and that changes between these different modes may be characterized as nonequilibrium phase transitions between attractors (e.g., Saltzman & Kelso, 1985; Woollacott & Jensen, 1996). The neurophysiological and biomechanical studies described above are consistent with the idea that local constraints participate in shaping patterns of whole-body coordination. However, these local constraints operate in the context of general principles governing postural pattern formation that remain largely unknown (Saltzman & Kelso, 1985). Whereas the influence of local constraints is typically assessed through the modulation of a behavioral pattern, self-organization is revealed in changes between patterns (Haken, 1977). The macroscopic variables, the order parameters, that emerge from the (nonlinear) interaction between the various degrees of freedom reveal interesting features. The collective variable that has been used by Bardy and colleagues to describe the behavior of the postural system is the ankle-hip relative phase, ϕ_{rel}. The behavior of ϕ_{rel} in the vicinity of phase transitions can reveal whether or not ϕ_{rel} is an order parameter for postural coordination. In studying transitions between postural coordination modes, Bardy et al. (2002) used the tracking task in which participants were instructed to use head movements to track the oscillations of a visible target along the fore-aft axis of the body. Using preliminary results (Oullier et al., 1999), a method was developed for observing transitions from one postural mode of coordination to another. The heart of this method was varying the frequency of target oscillations within trials (e.g., Kelso, Scholz & Schöner, 1986).[4] Studies of bimanual coordination have characterized coordination modes (in-phase and antiphase) as attractors in the phase space. Given this characterization, Bardy et al. (2002) hypothesized that postural transitions occur when one attractor (i.e., coordination pattern) becomes less stable than the other. Bardy et al. (2002) sought to identify five typical hallmarks of dynamical systems (Kelso, 1995; Kelso, Scholz & Schöner, 1988; Turvey, 1990): (i) at least two stable attractors defined by two different values of the order parameter ϕ_{rel}. When a non-specific control parameter (here, the oscillating frequency of the target) is continuously varied, a sudden shift from one attractor to the other should occur. This shift is called (ii) a *phase transition* (see Kelso, Schöner, Scholz & Haken, 1987). In the vicinity of the phase transition, a loss of stability expressed in (iii) *critical fluctuations* (an increase of variability in the order parameter ϕ_{rel}) should be observed (Scholz, Kelso & Schöner, 1987). The value of the control parameter at which transitions occur should be different for transitions from antiphase to in-phase than for transitions from in-phase to antiphase (if any). This is called (iv) *hysteresis* and reveals the tendency of the (postural) system to remain in its current state as long as possible before switching to a different pattern. Hysteresis therefore reveals the sensitivity of the system to initial conditions, i.e., to its own history. Finally, the best way to test the stability of a system is to perturb it (Kelso, 1995), and for this reason Bardy et al. (2002) designed a second experiment that permitted us to analyze the relaxation time (i.e., the time the system needs to return to its initial state after perturbation). If the increase in variability of ϕ_{rel} when approaching the transition region indeed denotes loss of stability, then the relaxation time should be smaller when the system is far from the transition and larger when it is near the transition. This effect is called the (v) *critical slowing down*, i.e., an increase of the relaxation time in the vicinity of the phase transition (Scholz et al., 1987).

Bardy et al.'s (2002) results revealed two values of ϕ_{rel}, each of which tended to predominate in a certain region of the control parameter space (figure 2.4). At low frequencies of target oscillation the ankles and hips moved in-phase, while at higher frequencies of target motion antiphase oscillations were observed. The interesting feature here is that not only do these results corroborate Bardy et al.'s (1999) results on the identification of two coordination modes, but the fact that these modes emerge even when the control parameter is varied on a within-trial basis.

---

[4] Bardy et al. (2002) varied the frequency of target oscillation in a stepwise manner and in two conditions. In the *up* condition, frequency increased from 0.05 Hz to 0.80 Hz in steps of 0.05 Hz. In the *down* condition, it decreased from 0.80 Hz to 0.05 Hz in similar steps. Each frequency step lasted for 10 oscillation cycles, for a total of 160 cycles per trial. In the procedure Bardy et al. (2002) used before computing dependent variables, 18 segments were defined for each trial: nine before and nine after the transition. Each segment included the mean values of the dependent variables for four cycles, with an overlap of two cycles (see Kelso et al., 1986, for a similar analysis). The use of 18 segments was imposed by the large variability among participants in the frequency at which transitions occurred, and the 18 segments corresponded to the maximal range including data points from all participants at all frequencies. Second, segments were aligned across each participant on the first cycle following the transition. Overall, this procedure resulted in the analysis of a limited portion of the ascendant or descendant run corresponding to 5 to 6 frequency steps. At the same time, the procedure promoted a detailed analysis of the behavioral organization (and its changes) in the transition region.

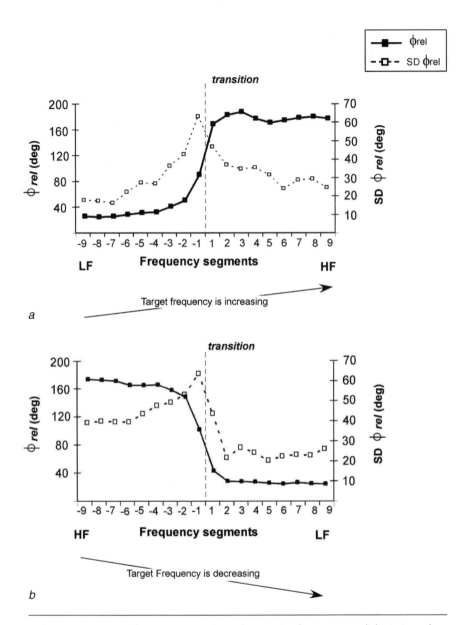

FIGURE 2.4 Postural transitions, point estimate circular mean, and deviation of ϕ_{rel} in the *(a) up* (frequency increasing) and *(b) down* (frequency decreasing) conditions. Each segment includes a temporal average of ϕ_{rel} over four cycles of oscillation, with an overlap of two cycles. *LF* and *HF* refer to low frequency and high frequency, respectively.

From B.G. Bardy et al., 1999 "Postural coordination modes considered as emergent phenomena," *Journal of Experimental Psychology: Human Perception and Performance* 25: 1284-1301. Copyright © 1999 by the American Psychological Association. Adapted with permission.

The second dynamical hallmark that Bardy et al. (2002) observed was that small, stepwise changes in the frequency of target oscillation lead to sudden shifts between coordination modes. The data illustrate the rapid nature of this transition. Eighty percent of the transitions occurred within a single cycle (overall mean = 1.2 cycles). This was true despite the fact that there was high inter-subject variability of the control parameter value at which transitions occurred (Oullier et al., 1999). When the frequency of the target was increased the system switched from in-phase to an antiphase coordination and, conversely, when the control parameter was decreased transitions from antiphase to in-phase were observed systematically. The variability of ϕ_{rel} was small when the system was far from transition, but as the system approached transition variability markedly increased (see figure 2.4). This progressive increase of the variability of ϕ_{rel} reached a peak in the region of transition. The variability data reveal the loss of stability in the current mode of coordination. After the transition the variability of ϕ_{rel} returned to lower values (Bardy et al., 2002). This is the phenomenon referred to as critical fluctuations.

The fourth hallmark observed was hysteresis, that is, the fact that transitions from in-phase to antiphase (figures 2.4a) and from antiphase to in-phase (figure 2.4b) did not occur at the same value of the control parameter. Hysteresis was found in 80% of the transitions, revealing the tendency of the system to remain in its current state by delaying the switch from the mode of coordination losing stability to a more stable one. As noted earlier, Bardy et al. (2002) found that increasing the frequency of target oscillation lead to a switch from in-phase to antiphase and that decreasing target frequency lead to a switch from antiphase to in-phase. This result differs from studies of unimanual (e.g., Kelso et al., 1990) and bimanual coordination (e.g., Kelso et al., 1986, 1988), in which transitions have been found only with increasing frequency. The stability of the in-phase mode in bimanual coordination explains why there is no switch to the antiphase mode, which is less stable. Bardy et al.'s results therefore suggest that the stability of the two modes of postural coordination is sufficiently similar for the transition to occur in both directions (in-phase to antiphase and antiphase to in-phase).

In a separate experiment, Bardy et al. (2002) investigated the stability of postural coordination both close to and far away from the region in which transitions between coordination patterns occurred. The authors did this by introducing a perturbation in the motion of the target to be tracked and by varying the location of the perturbation relative to the transition region.[5] Then, the relaxation time was calculated. Relaxation time was found to be shorter for

---

[5] The transition frequency *TF* was determined separately for each participant. In four experimental conditions, the frequency of target oscillation was set at a constant value, either far from the participant's *TF* (*TF* − 0.30 Hz, *TF* + 0.30 Hz) or close to it (*TF* − 0.15 Hz, *TF* + 0.15 Hz). Thus, in the two conditions of low frequency (*TF* − 0.30 Hz, *TF* − 0.15 Hz), participants were expected to exhibit in-phase coordination, while in the conditions of high frequency (*TF* + 0.15 Hz, *TF* + 0.30 Hz), participants were expected to exhibit antiphase coordination.

perturbations that occurred when the system was far away from the transition region. This finding is consistent with the concept of critical slowing down. Relaxation times were also compared for the in-phase and antiphase patterns. The relaxation time was found to be shorter for the in-phase pattern which appeared to be more stable than the antiphase one.

Nature of the Transitions Between Postural Coordination Patterns

In two experiments, Bardy et al. (2002) examined self-organized properties of postural coordination. Two postural coordination modes (in-phase and antiphase) were observed and changes between modes exhibited character-istics of nonequilibrium phase transitions, including differential stability, critical fluctuation, bifurcation, hysteresis, and critical slowing down. One implication of these results is that the ankle-hip relative phase ϕ_{rel} can serve as the order parameter of the postural system. The results are consistent with a dynamical systems approach of the multisegment control of stance, in which postural states behave like attractors in the postural space and changes between states behave like self-organized, nonequilibrium phase transitions between attractors. This transition appears to be from a mono-stable (fixed point) state to another mono-stable state, with a marginal bi-stable region in between. The bi-stable region appears when the control parameter reaches a critical value, that is, when the system can adopt either of the two modes of coordination. It appears that the variability of the order parameter is high before the transition, and it determines if the system switches to another mode. The bi-stable region is also the hysteresis region. Observation of these hallmarks leads to the hypothesis that the transition was a saddle-node type of bifurcation (Kelso, Ding & Schöner, 1992) rather than a Hopf bifurcation (Buchanan & Horak, 2001). The phase transition observed in postural coordination contrasts with that reported in studies of bi-manual coordination (Haken, Kelso & Bunz, 1985; Schöner & Kelso, 1988) that have reported transitions from bi-stable states (two fixed points) to mono-stable states (one fixed point). The dynamics of transitions between coordination modes seem specific to the properties of the system and the level at which the system is analyzed.

Variability in Self-Organization of Postural Coordination

Bernstein (1967) pointed out that there is not a one-to-one correspondence between movement and muscular, mechanical, or neural activity; this state-ment is known as the *equivocality principle*. This is why Bardy and colleagues have concentrated on a higher-order collective variable (ϕ_{rel}) defined at the kinematic level. Hip-ankle relative phase captures the order of the postural system in the space of a low dimensional state (Bardy, 2004; Bardy et al., 1999). At any time, a single (order) parameter, ϕ_{rel}, provides information about how the upper body moves relative to the lower body. One of the consequences of Bernstein's equivocality principle is that abrupt changes at the level of the movement trajectory may not exist at different levels of observation of the postural system, such as the muscular activity. Recent research reports that under diverse environmental, task, and body constraints, postural movements serving goal-directed supra-postural behavior exhibit typical signatures of self-organization (see Bardy, 2004 for a review). Bardy et al. (2002) used two indices of postural stability to investigate the dynamics of postural coordination. In their first experiment, changes in the variability of the ankle-hip relative phase (during a trial) showed a decrease in stability as the transition point was approached. This result was confirmed in their second experiment by analyzing local relaxation time following perturbations of the visual target. As predicted, the relaxation time was greater near the region of transition. Hence, changes in postural coordination were accompanied by a loss of stability in the order parameter (expressed by critical fluctuations and critical slowing down).

In all the studies presented in this chapter, variability was considered to be functional, and its analysis provided a better understanding of the behavior of the postural system. When focusing on the postural coordination modes *per se*, differences of variability between the two patterns were found, also variability of ϕ_{rel} increased when approaching the region of transition. Interestingly, under minimal constraints, for many values of the control parameter either of the two coordination modes could be adopted, depending on the situation (Bardy et al., 2002; Oullier et al., 2002). This result suggests that a general theory of postural transitions cannot be solely rooted in central mechanisms, such as motor programs, nor, for that matter, in mechanical, energetic, or perceptual mechanisms. If that were the case, then for each value of each parameter (or combination of parameters) there would be one specific postural state to be adopted by the system. But as Fuchs and Kelso (1994) pointed out, self-organization is expressed in the vicinity of the region of phase transition. By definition, when the system is in the marginal region of bi-stability it can adopt either one of the two coordination patterns. The marginal region is where the variability of the order parameter plays its most important role, since what was considered in previous studies as noise is the factor that causes the system to switch to another mode of coordination. Depending on the increase or decrease of the control parameter (Bardy et al., 2002), the change in the surface of support (Marin et al., 1999b; Oullier et al., 2004), body properties (Bardy et al., 1999), or the intention to sway (Oullier et al., 2002, 2004), the variability of the relation between the hips and the ankles is changing and will be determining the organization of the postural system.

Unique Aspects of Postural Coordination

In line with previous studies of bimanual coordination (Haken et al., 1985; Schöner & Kelso, 1988), and locomotion (Diedrich & Warren, 1995, 1998), two preferred stable pattern were observed in the experiments on postural coordination dynamics: an in-phase mode ($\phi_{rel} \approx 20°$) and an antiphase mode ($\phi_{rel} \approx 180°$). Like the bi-manual and locomotor systems, the postural system is multi-stable. Multi-stability refers to the existence of multiple qualitatively distinct patterns in a state space, each of which is stable over a coalition of constraints that shapes its dynamics (Kelso et al., 2001; Lagarde & Kelso, 2004; Oullier et al., 2003). Despite the many similarities in the coordination of the manual, locomotor, and postural systems, there are differences. The most obvious are the values for the coordination patterns that were found by Bardy and colleagues, which differ from the usual 0° and 180° of non-postural coordination (Kelso, 1995). In their studies of postural coordination dynamics, the in-phase mode exhibited a value close to 20° (i.e., the hip is lagging). This difference in the order parameter may arise from the nature of the oscillators involved in postural control. While both hands of a person are primarily coupled at the neural and perceptual level (Kelso, 1995), movements of the trunk and legs have a reciprocal mechanical effect on each other. This coupling might be one of the reasons why there is a 20° relative phase in the in-phase mode (see Fourcade, Bardy & Bonnet, 2003).

Conclusion

Many areas that can modulate the stability of postural coordination remain to be explored, such as the effect of learning (e.g., Faugloire, Bardy & Stoffregen, submitted; Kelso & Zanone, 2002; Ko, Challis & Newell, 2003), development (e.g., Marin & Oullier, 2001), attention (e.g., Monno, Chardenon, Temprado, Zanone & Laurent, 2000), expertise (Bardy, Faugloire & Fourcade, in press) or the interaction with another person (e.g., Oullier et al., 2003). Taken together the studies reported in this chapter support an interpretation of the organization of multi-segmental postural control that does not rely exclusively and primarily on neural, mechanical or muscular mechanisms, but rather a perspective where postural coordination dynamics emerge from a coalition of constraints of different nature (Oullier et al., 2004).

Although many researchers still consider variability in postural sway as only stochastic noise (e.g., Kiemel, Oie, & Jeka, 2002), the experiments reported in the present chapter suggest that variability often serves as a functional component of the postural system rather than noise, at least at the kinematics level. The self-organized features of the postural system are highly associated with variability of the order parameter. The resemblance of human postural phase transitions to self-organizational phenomena found in other biological and nonbiological systems (Kelso, 1995) raises questions about the necessity of appealing primarily to local constraints in understanding whole-body movement, and reinforces the hypothesis of general and common self-organization principles governing pattern formation in complex systems in which variability (modulated by a coalition of constraints) plays a key functional role.

Chapter 3

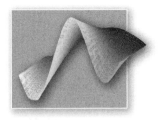

The Interface of Biomechanics and Motor Control

Dynamic Systems Theory and the Functional Role of Movement Variability

Paul S. Glazier, Jonathan S. Wheat, PhD, David L. Pease, and Roger M. Bartlett, PhD

Editors' Overview

An integrative perspective provided by the link between biomechanics and motor control is developed in this chapter, and the implications for biomechanical modeling and measurement are discussed in detail. Running and swimming are used to examine the measurement of variability in gait under the different environmental constraints of with and without gravitational forces (swimming is viewed as an aquatic gait). The classic biomechanical method of hierarchical modeling is outlined, and components of the functional pattern of coordination used to achieve locomotion are placed in this integrated schematic to facilitate motion analysis. In analyzing the literature on running gait and overuse injuries, it is shown that variability in coordination during the interval between the initial foot contact and the neutral position of the stance phase is an important feature of normal, healthy running.

The emergence of dynamic systems theory as a viable multidisciplinary framework for modeling the sensorimotor system stimulated a radical reassessment of the concept of movement variability. Traditionally, movement variability has been considered a dysfunctional aspect of human motor behavior directly related to the amount of noise—random fluctuations that compromise the deterministic relation between input and output at different levels of analysis—in the sensorimotor system (Newell and Corcos, 1993; Slifkin and Newell, 1998). However, the introduction of nonlinear dynamics and chaos theory into the study of biological systems (see Glass and Mackey, 1988; Thompson and Stewart, 2002) has prompted motor control theorists to suggest that movement variability may occupy a functional role in human motor behavior. Indeed, recent evidence from research based on dynamic systems theory strongly supports the notion that movement variability is an essential feature of human motor behavior that affords the sensorimotor system the necessary flexibility and adaptability to operate proficiently in a variety of performance, development and learning contexts (see van Emmerik & Wagenaar, 1995; Newell & Slifkin, 1998; van Emmerik & van Wegen, 2000, 2002; Latash, Scholz, & Schöner, 2002; Piek, 2002; Riley & Turvey, 2002; Davids, Glazier, Araújo, & Bartlett, 2003 for comprehensive reviews).

Movement Variability: Traditional and Contemporary Approaches

One of the main reasons for this change of ethos is the shift in the experimental paradigms motor control theorists use to study motor behavior. In cognitive science, empirical studies have been dominated by outcome measures obtained from sensorimotor tasks requiring the use of a single biomechanical degree of freedom (Newell, 1985). These artificial tasks have typically been favored by proponents of information processing because they enable theoretical inferences about underlying hierarchical control structures such as schemas, programs, and representations (Davids, Handford, & Williams, 1994). As movement variability cannot be directly determined from these tasks, it has often been inferred from the variability of outcome measures such as accuracy or error scores (Schmidt & Lee, 1998). The general assumption is that the variability of outcome measures is accompanied by a similar amount of variability in the movement patterns that produced the outcome measures (Newell & Corcos, 1993). As skilled motor performance is often characterized by low variability of outcome measures (e.g., Anderson & Pitcairn, 1986), it follows that skilled motor performance is also characterized by highly consistent patterns of movement. Therefore, movement variability has been considered as a problem in the sensorimotor system that should be minimized or eliminated.

It has become apparent, however, that these experimental paradigms may have contributed to the negative connotations of movement variability in human motor behavior. As sensorimotor tasks requiring the use of a single biomechanical degree of freedom eliminate the problem of coordination at the behavioral level of analysis (Newell, 1985, 1986), it is reasonable to assume that the variability of outcome measures directly relates to the variability of the accompanying patterns of movement. However, under different task constraints such as those encountered in tasks requiring the use of multiple biomechanical degrees of freedom, it has been found that the variability of outcome measures does not necessarily relate to the variability of the accompanying patterns of movement. For example, in the frequently cited studies by Arutyunyan, Gurfinkel, and Mirskii (1968, 1969) investigating the accuracy of aiming in pistol shooting, it was found that compensatory movements of the arms enabled skilled marksmen to reduce the variability in the spatial orientation of the pistol barrel. In contrast, novice marksmen were unable to demonstrate such compensatory movements and therefore exhibited greater variability in the spatial orientation of the pistol barrel. Under these task constraints, movement variability needs to be interpreted carefully in relation to specific task goals rather than be dismissed as random fluctuations that lead to variability in the performance outcome.

In contrast to the experimental paradigms used in cognitive science, the theoretical approach of dynamic systems to motor behavior places greater emphasis on the space-time characteristics of coordination patterns in tasks requiring the use of multiple biomechanical degrees of freedom. In dynamic systems theory, patterns of coordination emerge through generic processes of physical self-organization rather than being prescribed by some sort of executive regulating agent (Kelso, 1995). A central tenet of this theoretical approach is the spontaneous formation and dissipation of coordinative structures or functional synergies in response to changes in energy surrounding the sensorimotor system (Kugler, Kelso, and Turvey, 1980, 1982). Kay (1988) has defined these task-specific units as "an assemblage of many micro-components . . . assembled temporarily and flexibly, so that a single micro-component may participate in many different coordinative structures on different occasions" (p. 344). As the morphology of these coordinative structures entirely depends on the internal and external constraints acting on the sensorimotor system (Higgins, 1977; Kugler, 1986; Newell, 1986; Clark, 1995), the space-time characteristics of the ensuing patterns of coordination not only provide insight into these constraints, but also into the state of the dynamics of the sensorimotor system at that specific moment (McGinnis & Newell, 1982).

A research strategy for proponents of dynamic systems theory has, therefore, been to identify observable low-dimensional macroscopic variables—the so-called order parameters (Haken, 1983)—that define stable and reproducible relationships occurring among the components of the sensorimotor system as it searches for and adopts functionally preferred states of coordination or attractor states (e.g., Kelso & Schöner, 1988; Kelso & Ding, 1993). At the behavioral level of analysis, these order parameters are typically kinematic measurements such as displacements, velocities, and accelerations or are electromyographic measurements and other variables, such as relative timing, that are derived from these biomechanical measurements (e.g., Scholz, 1990). It has been shown that when the sensorimotor system adopts a functionally preferred state of coordination, the dynamics of order parameters are highly ordered and stable, reflecting the capacity of the sensorimotor system to produce consistent patterns of coordination (Kelso, 1984; Haken, Kelso, & Bunz, 1985). It has also been shown that variability in the dynamics of the order parameters, exemplified by fluctuations in stability, reflects the capacity for flexible and adaptive sensorimotor system behavior, thus enabling patterns of coordination, to be tailored to specific environmental and task demands. As the internal and external constraints—acting as the so-called control parameters (Haken, 1983)—increase toward a critical value, fluctuations in stability increase until stability is lost, leading to a non-equilibrium phase transition or bifurcation and the adoption of a new attractor state. Clearly, these empirically-derived findings suggest that movement variability is a functional entity that facilitates the discovery and adoption of optimal states of coordination.

Biomechanics and Motor Control

It would appear from the literature that the integration of biomechanical measurement tools and data collection techniques has substantially contributed to the discovery and monitoring of order parameters, the subsequent mapping of attractor states in different control spaces, and the redefinition of movement variability as a functional entity rather than simply noise in the sensorimotor system. In addition to describing the motion of the components of the sensorimotor system, biomechanical modeling techniques have also been used to investigate the mechanisms that physically cause this motion (see Zernicke & Schneider, 1993; Kamm, Thelen, & Jensen, 1990 for comprehensive overviews). For example, Thelen and colleagues (e.g., Schneider, Zernicke, Ulrich, Jensen, & Thelen, 1990; Thelen, Zernicke, Schneider, Jensen, Kamm, & Corbetta, 1992; Thelen, Corbetta, Kamm, Spencer, Schneider, & Zernicke, 1993; Thelen, Corbetta, & Spencer, 1996; Thelen, 1998) used the inverse dynamics[1] approach to examine the influences of active and passive joint torques and forces on the reaching and grasping of young infants during their first year of life. Active joint torques and forces were considered to be those that were generated primarily by muscle action, whereas passive joint torques and forces included gravitational force, frictional forces and torques within the joint, and inertial forces and torques transferred from other body segments. Thelen and colleagues found that the infants became more adept at managing the complex interplay between active and passive joint torques and forces with skill acquisition. Furthermore, they found that passive joint torques and forces were used more effectively as skill was acquired, and thus the dependence on active joint torques and forces decreased. Similarly, Schneider and Zernicke (1989) and Schneider, Zernicke, Schmidt, and Hart (1989) used the inverse dynamics

---

[1] The term *dynamics* has two very different meanings in dynamic systems theory and biomechanics. In dynamic systems theory, *dynamics* refers to the time evolution of a system at any level of analysis whereas in biomechanics, *dynamics* refers to the forces and torques that physically cause motion (Beek, Peper, & Stegeman, 1995).

approach to examine the relative influences of active and passive torques and forces in the learning of a task requiring rapid arm movement. They found that with practice, active torques and forces complimented and counteracted passive torques and forces more effectively, particularly during movement reversals. The increased effectiveness helped hand velocities and accelerations to increase, hand trajectories to become smoother and more parabolic, and total movement times to decrease. Both of these studies empirically support Bernstein's (1967) hypothesis regarding the exploitation and utilization of reactive phenomena as an advanced feature of skill learning (e.g., Newell and Vaillancourt, 2001).

Despite the important contributions of biomechanics to the study of motor behavior, development, and learning, biomechanics has not experienced the same degree of reciprocity, particularly in sport biomechanics. Although the theoretical concepts and methods of the study of dynamic systems were extensively covered in the scientific literature over the past decade, their huge scope and potential have yet to be fully realized by sport biomechanists and have rarely been integrated into research on sport biomechanics. It could be argued that sport biomechanists have so far missed an important opportunity, especially considering recent criticisms of applied sport biomechanics for (i) being too descriptive (Vaughan, 1984; Norman, 1985; Baumann, 1987; Cavanagh, 1990; Yeadon & Challis, 1994; Elliott, 1999), and (ii), for lacking a sound theoretical rationale (Hay, 1983; Bartlett, 1997; Hatze, 1998). Furthermore, it has frequently been suggested that in order to make significant scientific progress, sport biomechanists need to collaborate with experts from other disciplines of sport science (Nelson, 1971; Cavanagh & Hinrichs, 1981; Cavanagh, 1989; Dillman, 1989; Gregor, 1989; Norman, 1989; Winter, 1989; Gregor, Broker & Ryan, 1992; Nigg, 1993; Zatsiorsky & Fortney, 1993; Coleman, 2002; Elliott, 2002; Enoka, 2004). From this perspective, there is a unique opportunity for sport biomechanists to form a mutually beneficial partnership with motor control theorists. Indeed of all the potential interdisciplinary partnerships, this collaboration could be the most fruitful in satisfying the two main goals of sport biomechanics—reducing injury and improving performance (e.g., Baumann, 1987; Nelson, 1989; Elliott, 1997; Nigg, 1998; Bartlett, 1999; Zatsiorsky, 2000).

In this chapter, we explore some of the potential implications of dynamic systems theory and this new view of movement variability for applied sport biomechanics. We have previously argued that this theory provides a relevant framework for performance-related research in sport biomechanics, as it emphasizes an interdisciplinary approach to the processes of coordination and control in the human sensorimotor system (Glazier, Davids, & Bartlett, 2003). Here, we consolidate our previous assertions and extend our analysis to injury-related research in sport biomechanics, using running and swimming—which has been described as the aquatic equivalent of running (Alexander, 1984, 1989)—as vehicles for our analysis. We begin, however, with a critical overview of the philosophical and theoretical paradigms used in performance-related and injury-related research in sport biomechanics.

Sport Biomechanics: A Critical Overview

The main goals of performance-related and injury-related research in sport biomechanics are to identify the characteristics of technique that contribute to successful motor performance or that predispose to injury (Bartlett, 1999). In performance-related research, a combination of theoretical and statistical modeling techniques is often used to identify key biomechanical variables known as performance parameters (Bartlett, 1999; Lees, 1999). The initial development of a deterministic or 'hierarchical' model (Hay & Reid, 1988; Lees, 2002), based on the theoretical principles of biomechanics and the fundamental laws of physics and biology that govern biomechanics (Bunn, 1972; Cooper & Glassow, 1976; Bober, 1981; Hochmuth, 1984), can greatly assist in identifying relationships between the performance criterion (the task goal or outcome) and the underlying performance parameters. A 'hierarchical' model can also be instrumental in helping to establish the causative mechanisms underpinning these relationships.

In the hierarchical model for swimming shown in figure 3.1, the performance criterion (the official swimming time) is identified at the top of the model. As the performance criterion is a temporal measurement, it can be divided into a series of constituents—starting time, stroking time, and turning time—that form the second tier of the model. The final stage of model development is to identify the performance parameters that underpin each of the constituents of the performance criterion. As stroking time is the most important of these constituents, we have only included its underpinning performance parameters for the sake of brevity. There are two main rules for constructing a hierarchical model. First, where possible, the performance parameters included in the model should be mechanical quantities, and second, each of the performance parameters should be completely determined by those performance parameters that appear directly below it (Hay & Reid, 1988). By employing this systematic approach to model development, no performance parameter that influences the outcome is overlooked and no performance parameter is included more than once.

Once a hierarchical model has been constructed, the most important performance parameters and their relative contribution to successful motor performance need to be empirically verified. Typically, two basic experimental research designs are used for verification—the correlation approach and the contrast approach (Hay, Vaughan, & Woodworth, 1981). In the correlation approach, relationships between the performance criterion and the underlying performance parameters for a single homogenous group are formally examined using multiple or partial correlation statistics. Conversely, in the contrast approach, differences in the mean values of key performance parameters for two or more heterogeneous groups are formally examined using mean difference statistics. An advantage of having a rigorously developed hierarchical model at this stage of an investigation is that performance parameters can be

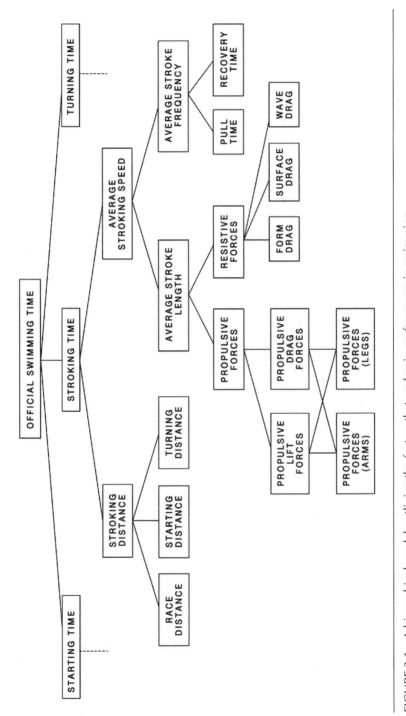

FIGURE 3.1   A hierarchical model outlining the factors that underpin performance in swimming.

Fig. 14.4, p. 358 from *The Biomechanics of Sports Techniques*, 4th ed. By James G. Hay. Copyright © 1993 by Prentice-Hall, Inc. Reprinted by permission of Pearson Education, Inc.

selected and justified on the basis of a sound theoretical rationale. Using the hierarchical modeling approach can, therefore, be considered superior to the arbitrary shotgun approach in which performance parameters tend to be randomly selected, as the model helps ensure that all the truly important variables are included and all the trivial ones are omitted.

Although hierarchical models have been used predominantly in performance-related research, they have also been adapted for use in injury-related research to identify possible injury mechanisms (e.g., Dixon & Kerwin, 1998). More specifically, hierarchical models can be useful for determining the characteristics of technique that might cause excessive loading or stress and lead to injury by exceeding the critical stress limits of the biomaterials (Nigg, 1985; Whiting & Zernicke, 1998; Zernicke & Whiting, 2000). As in performance-related research, once potentially harmful mechanical factors are identified, the relationships between kinematic or kinetic variables and injury can be formally evaluated using correlation statistics. This approach, which was termed the *empirical approach* by Nigg and Bobbert (1990), ideally incorporates a prospective research design in which individuals are monitored over time and analyzed on a post hoc basis when identifying the source of the injury, as it is inherently difficult to ascertain cause and effect with retrospective designs. Moreover, prospective designs provide the scope to subsequently manipulate population samples and implement alternative statistical analyses that might be more effective at identifying 'offending' characteristics of movement (see Foster, John, Elliott, Ackland, & Fitch, 1989; Elliott, Hardcastle, Burnett, & Foster, 1992).

Interpretations of Movement Variability

In the past, sport biomechanists have rarely considered movement variability to be an important topic worthy of research attention in its own right. There appears to be a number of interrelated reasons why researchers have ignored this aspect of human motor performance. First, biomechanical analyses examining the kinematics of human motion have typically been inhibited by the design of equipment for motion analysis and the inefficiency of techniques for data reduction. A main problem is the laborious nature of manual coordinate digitizing, which has typically restricted kinematic analyses to a single performance trial and has, therefore, precluded analysis of any trial-to-trial variability. Second, an implicit assumption held by many sport biomechanists is that human motor performance is characterized by invariance in the motor system (Schmidt, 1985) and, therefore, trial-to-trial variability has typically been deemed to have negligible practical significance. This assumption appears to have been perpetuated by the concept of motor programming that has dominated the movement sciences for the past three decades (e.g., Keele, 1968; Schmidt, 1982). On the premise that patterns of movement are highly consistent over repeated trials, the analysis of a single performance trial has been justified on the grounds that it represents a performer's normal technique. Third, the frequent use of hierarchical models has encouraged sport biomechanists to adopt a reductionist approach in searching for performance parameters that contribute most to the performance criterion. However, these performance parameters do not provide any information about the underlying patterns of coordination that generate these performance parameters (see figure 3.1). In principle, a multitude of different movement patterns could be used to produce the same set of performance parameter values. The emphasis is very much outcome-oriented rather than process-oriented, and in this respect, shares many of the problems that have dogged traditional research in motor behavior. Fourth, sport biomechanists often make the significant assumption that people share a common optimal pattern of movement. In other words, they believe there is a single most efficient and effective way of performing a movement in the majority of the population (Brisson & Alain, 1996). On the basis that highly skilled performers are likely to have 'more optimal' techniques than their lesser skilled counterparts, pooled group data are typically analyzed using inferential statistics to establish 'normative' values for specific performance parameters. Any group-based differences can then be used to develop generalizable laws of action that may be used to characterize a hypothetical ideal technique or motor template. However, when pooling group data, any performer-to-performer variability tends to get masked as sport biomechanist focus on the 'big picture' to the detriment of understanding the emergence of individualized movement solutions. Literally, biomechanists cannot see the 'trees for the forest.' Fifth, any observed moment-to-moment variability in kinematic time series data has invariably been treated as random measurement errors and has either been disregarded or removed using recognized data filtering and smoothing techniques (for example, see Wood, 1982). In chapter 1, Newell and colleagues discuss the inadequacies of treating all observed movement variability as random variability.

Dynamic Systems Theory Applied to Sport Biomechanics

So far in this chapter, we have critically analyzed the philosophical and theoretical paradigms used in applied research in sport biomechanics. It is clear from the literature that if significant progress is to be made in both performance-related and injury-related sport biomechanics, more complex research questions based on the sound theoretical rationale of dynamic systems need to be formulated. In turn, these questions require more innovative research designs and methods of analysis (see Stergiou, 2003 for a review). Wherever possible, a combination of group and single-individual designs should be incorporated so that both intra- and inter-individual differences can be analyzed. Moreover, greater emphasis should be directed towards analyzing actual patterns of movement, instead of discrete kinematic measurements, as they provide a window into the underlying dynamics of the sensorimotor system. The use of more innovative research designs and methods of analysis will also enable sport biomechanists to more thoroughly examine the role of movement variability in human motor performance. In the following sections, we discuss the potential applications of dynamic systems theory to performance-related research in sport biomechanics, focusing on movement models of terrestrial and aquatic gait, and we examine how this new view of movement variability could be, and has been, used to enhance injury-related research in sport biomechanics.

Performance-Related Research in Sport Biomechanics

Perhaps the most pertinent example of how biomechanics has improved sport performance is the work of Counsilman (1968, 1969, 1971), Brown (Brown & Counsilman, 1971), Schleihauf (1974, 1979), and others (Hay, Liu, & Andrews, 1993; Liu, Hay, & Andrews, 1993) on the generation of propulsive forces in freestyle swimming. Before this research, the general consensus among swimming practitioners was that propulsive forces were generated predominantly by hydrodynamic drag created by moving the hand directly backwards during the pull phase of the swimming stroke (Cureton, 1930; Kiphut, 1942; Armbruster & Morehouse, 1950). However, using underwater photography, Brown and Counsilman (1971) observed that world-class freestyle swimmers use other techniques involving complex curvilinear hand paths. This observation led the authors to suggest that propulsive forces in freestyle swimming are generated predominantly by hydrodynamic lift created by medial and lateral sculling movements of the hand during the pull phase of the swimming stroke. Further research by Schleihauf (1979) and Schleihauf, Gray, and De Rose (1983) has since provided empirical evidence that propulsive forces in freestyle swimming are generated by both hydrodynamic lift and drag.

Although more recent computer simulation and experimental research by Hay et al. (1993) and Liu et al. (1993) has shown that much of the lateral movement of the hand during freestyle swimming is caused by body roll[2] rather than by horizontal movements of the arms relative to the swimmer's body, there can be no mistaking the contribution of the original work by Counsilman and others to the understanding of how propulsive forces are generated in freestyle swimming. Despite recent suggestions that the original work of Counsilman and others was, in fact, flawed (see Sanders, 1998), this series of investigations has not only provided a solid foundation for scientific endeavour in this area of study, but it has also profoundly influenced the teaching and coaching of freestyle swimming techniques over the past three decades. Indeed, their contribution has been widely acknowledged as one of the most significant made by sport biomechanists to the enhancement of knowledge and performance of sports techniques since biomechanics emerged as an academic discipline in the 1960s (Hay, 1983; Bartlett, 1997).

---

[2] Body roll can be defined as the angular displacement along the longitudinal axis of the swimmer's body.

Although maximizing propulsive forces in freestyle swimming is an important factor in proficient performance, it is equally important to minimize resistive drag forces, which act on the swimmer to inhibit forward motion (see figure 3.1). As with many other sports techniques, an 'optimal' freestyle swimming technique can be described as one that is both highly efficient and effective. In general, efficiency refers to the relationship between energy input and energy output in the athlete-environment system. To optimize efficiency in swimming, it is necessary for a swimmer to maximize the utilization of biochemical energy generated by the anaerobic and aerobic metabolic energy systems (energy input) by using techniques that most effectively generate mechanical energy (energy output) to maximize propulsive forces. To optimize effectiveness, however, it is necessary for these techniques to maximize propulsive forces while minimizing resistive drag forces, which are influenced by, among other factors, the size and shape of the swimmer and swimming speed. As these resistive drag forces are constantly fluctuating, an effective freestyle swimming technique must be sufficiently flexible and adaptable to enable emerging patterns of coordination to be modified according to these and other constraints impinging on the swimmer.

In this section, to exemplify the functional role of movement variability, we examine the different strategies that might be used by swimmers to maintain optimum efficiency and effectiveness in relation to key performance constraints. We specifically focus on the effect of swimming speed on emerging patterns of coordination. It is important to note, however, that although swimming speed is likely to be one of the most important constraints acting on the swimmer, it is the interaction of all the different types of organismic, environmental, and task constraints that ultimately determines the morphology of the ensuing patterns of coordination (Newell, 1986; Newell, van Emmerik and McDonald, 1989). From the perspective of dynamic systems theory, any variability in movement patterns could be interpreted as reflecting the conscious or unconscious attempt to satisfy, in the best way possible, the unique confluence of constraints impinging on the swimmer—a process referred to as self-organizing optimality by Newell (1986).

Although success in most sports activities is governed by the efficiency and effectiveness of the techniques used by the individuals participating in those activities, swimming is unique in that swimmers during aquatic gait must satisfy the task constraint of moving their bodies through the medium of water while virtually all other athletes move through air. Owing to the increased density of water, which is approximately 800 times greater than air, the magnitude of resistive drag forces is increased dramatically. Consequently, swimming has been calculated to be less than 9% mechanically efficient (Toussaint, Knops, DeGroot & Hollander, 1990), whereas other forms of terrestrial gait, such as walking and running, have been estimated to be between 20% and 80% mechanically efficient depending on the method used to calculate mechanical efficiency (see Williams, 1985).

A further important task constraint influencing the magnitude of resistive drag forces in swimming is the relative speed of the swimmer to the oncoming flow of water. Indeed, according to the equations used to calculate resistive drag, there is a quadratic relationship between drag and swimming speed. One of the artifacts of increasing swimming speed is that the point of boundary layer[3] separation moves farther upstream towards the head of the swimmer, leading to the generation of high-energy eddies or vortices and a large low-pressure area of water farther downstream from the swimmer. As there is also a concurrent high-pressure build-up of water in front of the swimmer, a large pressure gradient is created, which significantly increases the magnitude of resistive drag forces experienced by the swimmer. To maintain optimum efficiency and effectiveness under these changeable environmental constraints, swimmers need to be able to readily adjust their swimming techniques and the patterns of propulsive forces produced within the task constraints imposed by the rules governing the specific swimming stroke.

As we briefly mentioned at the beginning of this section, another important characteristic of an effective freestyle swimming technique is body roll because it facilitates lateral movements of the arm during the pull phase of the swimming stroke, enabling the hand to interact with 'new' water or water that has not already had kinetic energy imparted to it by the swimmer's hand (Hay et al., 1993). With the hand pulling against stationary water, 'slippage' is reduced and larger reaction forces can be generated. One of the effects of increasing swimming speed, however, is that body roll invariably decreases, which causes lateral movements of the arm to decrease and the hand path to become more linear during the pull phase (Hay et al., 1993). As the hand is pushing against water that has already had kinetic energy imparted to it, 'slippage' is increased and smaller reaction forces are generated, which consequently causes a change in the pressure distribution exerted by the water on the swimmer's hand. On the basis of this change in the water's 'feel'—acting as an important informational constraint on performance—the patterns of movement produced by the swimmer's arm and the orientation of the hand during the pull phase need to be modified to increase the propulsive forces generated by the hand.

The preceding analysis of aquatic gait exemplifies how interacting organismic, environmental, and task constraints shape the relatively unique patterns of coordination that emerge during performance for individual swimmers. Despite the clear need to understand how patterns of coordination are modified during performance, this aspect of performance has rarely been examined in the literature. The main reason for the lack of research attention appears to originate from the fact that most scientific investigations (e.g., Craig and Pen-

---

[3] The boundary layer is the layer of water across which the relative velocity between the swimmer and the water adjusts from zero at the surface of the swimmer's body to the free stream velocity, which, in the present example, is the velocity of the swimmer.

dergast, 1979; Hay & Guimaraes, 1983; Grimston and Hay, 1986; Keskinen, Tilli and Komi, 1989; Arellano and Pardillo, 1992; McArdle and Reilly, 1992; Keskinen, 1993) have tended to adopt a reductionist approach and examine those descriptive stroke characteristics that are more readily observable from the pool deck such as swimming speed, stroke length, and stroke frequency, rather than the actual patterns of coordination that produce them. Moreover, the selection of these stroke characteristics has been justified on the basis that they represent important performance parameters, which are strongly related to the performance criterion (see figure 3.1). Although the vast majority of studies have focused on stroke characteristics, there have been a few studies that have examined, with varying degrees of success, patterns of coordination in swimming. A major limitation of these studies, however, was that they tended to analyze either spatial (Ringer and Adrian, 1969) or temporal characteristics (Vaday and Nemessuri, 1971; Chollet, Chalies and Chatard, 2000) separately and not together. Clearly, future empirical studies on this aspect of swimming performance need to examine the space-time characteristics of patterns of coordination using analytical techniques such as those outlined in chapter 7 by Button, Davids & Schöllhorn, and chapter 9 by Wheat & Glazier.

How swimmers actually adjust their coordination patterns as swimming speed increases is, therefore, of great importance to practitioners and sport scientists. Small-scale adjustments to the orientation of the hand, based on changes in the 'feel' of the water, may be made prospectively in skilled swimmers because of the tight coupling between the perception and movement sub-systems. However, large-scale changes in whole body patterns of coordination may be necessary to maintain optimal efficiency and effectiveness, particularly with the concurrent increase in resistive drag forces experienced by the swimmer. It is feasible that a non-equilibrium phase transition or bifurcation, characterized by a shift from one state of coordination to another by the swimmer, may occur (e.g., Kelso, Southard and Goodman, 1979; Kelso, Holt, Rubin and Kugler, 1981; Beuter, Flashner and Arabyan, 1986; Kelso, Scholz and Schöner, 1986; Scholz and Kelso, 1989; Kelso and Jeka, 1992). As we discussed earlier, bifurcations are characterized by increased variability of a relevant order parameter (e.g., relative phase) and are brought about by a systematic change in a relevant control parameter (e.g., swimming speed). These bifurcations have been observed in many different types of motion such as finger waggling (e.g., Kelso, 1984), human gait (e.g., Diedrich and Warren, 1995), equine gait (e.g., Hoyt and Taylor, 1981), and the swimming motion of marine animals (e.g., Alexander, 1989; Drucker, 1996) and have been suggested to occur for a variety of reasons, including optimizing mechanical efficiency (Grillner, Halbertsma, Nilsson and Thorstensson, 1979; Hoyt and Taylor, 1981; Alexander, 1984, 1989; Taylor, 1985) and decreasing muscular contraction velocity and the associated muscular and joint forces (Hreljac, 1995). Despite these different explanations, and the greatly varied physical and physiological make-up of humans, the speed at which adults change from a walking gait to a running gait has been consistently shown to be approximately 2.5 m/s (Alexander, 1984). Owing to the apparent ubiquity of phase transitions in human and animal movement, it is likely that such a phase transition would be evident during aquatic gait among swimmers of a similar size and ability.

A possible factor influencing the speed at which phase transitions might occur is the training methods used by many of today's leading swimmers, which typically consist of large volumes of relatively slow swimming (approximately 1.2 m/s). According to the principle of specificity of training, combined with the empirical findings of Zanone and Kelso (1992), only the patterns of coordination used by the swimmer at these lower speeds are likely to be developed. However, since competition swimming speeds are typically much higher (approximately 2 m/s) than the typical training pace, swimmers are likely to adopt a different pattern of coordination when swimming at these higher speeds. Owing to their lack of training at these higher speeds, swimmers are unlikely to maintain stability of alternative patterns of coordination and hence their speed would decrease after a relatively short period of time. At that point, swimmers are likely to transit back to the more stable patterns of coordination established during training.

With the theoretical possibility of phase transitions and new attractor states emerging during swimming, and with the lack of previous research, it is unclear whether swimmers are training under appropriate task constraints by swimming at speeds lower than those habitually used in competition. The principle of specificity of training dictates that task constraints between training and competition conditions (e.g., swimming speed) should remain consistent to enhance the stability of coordination patterns used at high swimming speeds. However, sport scientists and practitioners should remain tolerant of functional variability shown by swimmers in the emergent adaptations to basic coordination of patterns of aquatic gait owing to the interaction of organismic, environmental, and task constraints. Clearly, further investigations based on dynamic systems theory are necessary to establish whether separate walking- and running-type strokes exist and, if so, how appropriate current training and conditioning programs of top freestyle swimmers are in terms of developing stable running-type strokes.

Injury-Related Research in Sport Biomechanics

Recently, a dynamic systems approach has been used in injury-related research in sport biomechanics to examine lower-extremity running injuries (Hamill, van Emmerik, Heiderscheit, & Li, 1999; Heiderscheit, Hamill, & van Emmerik, 1999; Heiderscheit, 2000a, 2000b; Heiderscheit, Hamill, & van Emmerik, 2002). A criticism of previous research on lower-extremity running injuries is that kinematic analyses have almost exclusively focused on time-discrete variables obtained from isolated joints or segments, such as maximum rearfoot pronation, maximum velocity of rearfoot pronation, and maximum tibial internal rotation (e.g., Clarke, Frederick, & Hamill, 1984; Messier & Pittala,

1988; Duffey, Martin, Cannon, Craven, & Messier, 2000). A major problem with this approach is that it fails to take into account the relative motions of various lower-extremity segments or joints, such as the subtalar and knee joints, which have frequently been implicated in the etiology of overuse injuries to the knee (Bates, James, & Osternig, 1978; Lafortune, Cavanagh, Sommer, & Kalenak, 1994; McClay & Manal, 1997; Stergiou & Bates, 1997; Hintermann & Nigg, 1998; Nawoczenski, Saltzman, & Cook, 1998; Stergiou, Bates, & James, 1999). A dynamic systems approach overcomes this problem, as it focuses on the coordination or coupling among segments or joints (Hamill et al., 1999). In this section, we briefly review the research by Hamill, Heiderscheit, and colleagues on lower-extremity running injuries, highlighting the utility of this relatively new approach and specifically focusing on variability in coordination and its relationship to injury.

Previously, the quadriceps angle (Q-angle) has been proposed as an important factor in the etiology of patellofemoral pain[4] (Subotnick, 1975; Cox, 1985; Messier & Pittala, 1988; Messier, Davis, Curl, Lowery, & Pack, 1991). The Q-angle is formed by the intersection of a line projected through the center of the patella from the tibial tuberosity and a line connecting the center of the patella to the anterior superior iliac spine of the pelvis (see figure 3.2). Subotnick (1975) hypothesized that a large Q-angle may cause excessive foot pronation or rearfoot eversion, increasing tibial internal rotation and altering tracking of the patella if accompanied by external femoral rotation. Furthermore, Cox (1985) suggested that altering the tracking of the patella changes the contact regions and pressure distributions in the patellofemoral joint, thus predisposing patellofemoral pain.

In their first reported study, Hamill et al. (1999) examined the influence of the Q-angle on the coordination and variability in the coordination of lower-extremity body segments during over-ground running. Healthy individuals with Q-angles greater than 15° were compared to healthy individuals with Q-angles less than 15°, as it has been suggested that the former might be more susceptible to lower-extremity injury (Messier et al., 1991). The assigned task was to run repeatedly over a force platform (used to identify initial foot contact) at speeds between 3.60 and 3.83 m/s—the range typically used by most noncompetitive runners (Cavanagh, 1987). Standard three-dimensional filming and reconstruction techniques were used to obtain kinematic data describing the space-time characteristics of lower-extremity body segments. Coordination among lower-extremity body segments was assessed using the continuous relative phase (CRP) technique (see chapter 9 by Wheat & Glazier). CRP profiles for the following couplings were calculated: thigh flexion and extension and tibial rotation, thigh abduction and adduction and tibial rotation, and tibial rotation and foot eversion and inversion. Each of these CRP profiles was interpolated and normalized to 100 data points and an ensemble average CRP profile for

---

[4] Patellofemoral pain is a term used to describe generalized pain in the anterior knee (Winter and Bishop, 1992).

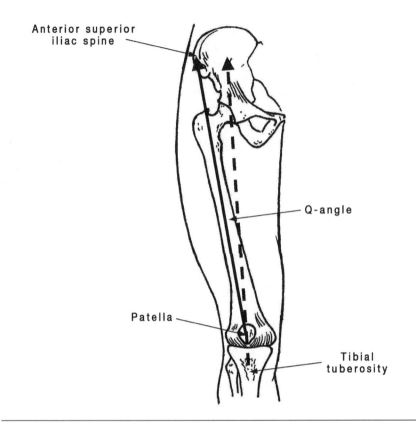

FIGURE 3.2   The quadriceps angle (Q-angle).

each coupling was constructed from ten trials performed by each individual. To quantify variability in coordination, the CRP standard deviation (CRP_{SD}) was calculated at each of the 100 data points. In addition to calculating the average CRP and average CRP_{SD} over the entire stance phase, average CRP and average CRP_{SD} over the following intervals of the stance phase—determined by key events in rearfoot inversion-eversion—were calculated: from initial foot contact to the neutral position, from the neutral position to maximum eversion, from maximum eversion to the neutral position, and from the neutral position to toe-off.

The main finding of this study was that despite the differences in Q-angle, there were no statistically significant differences between the two groups for all three couplings during the entire stance phase, both in terms of the average CRP and the average CRP_{SD}. However, among the four intervals of the stance phase, there were systematic differences in the average CRP and average CRP_{SD} for all three couplings. Generally, all three couplings were out of phase between initial foot contact and the neutral position but, as the stance phase progressed, the tibial rotation and foot eversion and inversion coupling became increasingly in phase, and the thigh flexion and extension and tibial rotation coupling and, more particularly, the thigh abduction and adduction and tibial rotation coupling, became increasingly out of phase. Perhaps more importantly, the average CRP_{SD} of all three couplings during the period between initial foot contact and the neutral position was considerably greater than the average CRP_{SD} during any other interval of the stance phase.

In a follow-up study, Heiderscheit et al. (1999) used a similar research design and method to examine the influence of the Q-angle on variability in coordination. Again, no statistically significant differences in average CRP_{SD} were found between the low Q-angle group and the high Q-angle group for all three couplings over the entire stance phase. However, among the four intervals of the stance phase, statistically significant differences in average CRP_{SD} were found for all three couplings. During the period between initial foot contact and the neutral position, both the thigh flexion and extension and tibial rotation coupling, and the thigh abduction and adduction and tibial rotation coupling, displayed significantly greater average CRP_{SD} than during any other interval of the stance phase. Moreover, the average CRP_{SD} for the tibial rotation and foot eversion and inversion coupling during the period between initial foot contact to the neutral position was significantly greater than during the period between the neutral position to maximum eversion. Overall, the average CRP_{SD} for all couplings was greatest during the period between initial foot contact to the neutral position, and it generally decreased throughout the remainder of the stance phase.

From the results of these two studies, it appears that variability in coordination during the period between initial foot contact and the neutral position of the stance phase is an important feature of normal, healthy running. Holt, Jeng, Ratcliffe, & Hamill (1995) reported similar findings for walking, which led them to suggest that variability in coordination during this period of the gait cycle could have important implications for injury prevention and performance enhancement. First, by constantly varying the point of force application, different anatomical surfaces are exposed over repeated trials, thereby preventing the overloading of the same anatomical surface and limiting overuse injuries (see Nigg, 1985). Second, variability in coordination during this interval could provide the flexibility necessary to adapt to environmental perturbations such as uneven terrain or irregular surfaces and thus reduce the risk of injury through falling.

In their second reported study, Hamill et al. (1999) examined the influence of patellofemoral pain on the coordination and variability in the coordination of lower-extremity body segments during motorized treadmill running. In this study, individuals with patellofemoral pain were compared to those with no history of patellofemoral pain. As in their first study, Hamill et al. (1999) used standard three-dimensional filming and reconstruction techniques to obtain kinematic data describing the space-time characteristics of lower-extremity body segments. However, in this study, subjects were recorded throughout the entire stride cycle and at three different running speeds (2.5, 3.0, and 3.5 m/s). CRP and CRP_{SD} for the three body segment couplings described in the first study were calculated, and an additional femoral rotation and tibial rotation coupling was also included to examine the possible influence of antagonistic rotations of these segments on patellofemoral pain. In addition to calculating average CRP and average CRP_{SD} over the swing phase, the stance phase, and the entire stride cycle of each trial, average CRP and average CRP_{SD} were calculated for each of the four intervals of the stance phase we previously described for the first study by Hamill et al. (1999).

As the results obtained from the three different running speeds were similar, only data for the trials ran at 2.5 m/s were reported. Although slight differences between the two groups were found in the average CRP for all four couplings throughout the entire stride cycle, the greatest differences were apparent during the interval between neutral position and maximum eversion and the interval between maximum eversion and the neutral position, in which the individuals with patellofemoral pain were more in phase for the thigh abduction and adduction and tibial rotation coupling. However, the main finding of this study was that the average CRP_{SD} of each of the four couplings was consistently less in the individuals with patellofemoral pain than in those with no history of patellofemoral pain, particularly during the transition from stance to swing, throughout the swing phase, and during the transition from swing to stance. This finding appears to contradict traditional clinical and biomechanical wisdom, which generally assumes that the amount of variability directly relates to the degree of pathology. Although Hamill et al. (1999) suggested that this lack of variability could relate to a loss of complexity through the development of patellofemoral pain, it is difficult to prove cause and effect with this type of retrospective research design. In other words, it is unclear whether the lack of variability is the cause or the effect of patellofemoral pain. As we discussed earlier, a prospective design (Nigg and Bobbert, 1990) could help overcome this problem. Despite the design limitation, however, subsequent research by Heiderscheit (2000a) appears to empirically support the original hypothesis postulated by Hamill et al. (1999) regarding the relationship between variability in coordination and patellofemoral pain. By monitoring changes in variability in coordination during treatment, Heiderscheit (2000a) found that the reduction of patellofemoral pain coincided with an increase in variability. These findings provide some support for the notion that patellofemoral pain may be the cause rather than the effect of reduced variability.

In another study, Heiderscheit et al. (2002) examined the influence of patellofemoral pain on the variability of joint coordination and of stride characteristics (e.g., stride duration and stride length). As we just discussed, increased variability of body segment coordination has been reported in healthy individuals as compared to individuals with patellofemoral pain (Hamill et al.,

1999). However, no information is available regarding the influence of patellofemoral pain on the variability of stride characteristics. Previously, it has been shown that variability of stride characteristics increases the risk of falling in elderly individuals (Gabell & Nayak, 1984; Nakamura, Meguro, & Sasaki, 1996; Hausdorff, Edelberg, Mitchell, Goldberger, & Wei, 1997) and that it is related to neuromuscular diseases such as Huntington's disease and Parkinson's disease (Hausdorff, Cudkowicz, Firtion, Wei, & Goldberger, 1998). Therefore, whereas variability of joint coordination might be considered functional because it appears to protect against overuse injuries and aid adaptation to environmental perturbations, variability of stride characteristics might be considered dysfunctional, as it appears to be associated with postural instability and an increased likelihood of injury through falling.

In the study by Heiderscheit et al. (2002), the variability of stride characteristics was compared to the variability of joint coordination in individuals with symptoms of unilateral patellofemoral pain and nonimpaired individuals. The task of each individual was to run on a motorized treadmill at two different speeds—a preferred running speed and a fixed running speed. Each individual was able to select a preferred running speed between 0.5 and 8.0 m/s by manually adjusting the speed of the motorized treadmill. A fixed running speed of 2.68 m/s for all individuals was selected to avoid coinciding with the transition between walking and running or between running and walking (which occurs between 1.8 and 2.2 m/s). A system for automated motion analysis was used to capture and reconstruct 15 consecutive strides at both the preferred and fixed running speeds for each of the individuals. Bilateral three-dimensional kinematic data describing the space-time characteristics of lower-extremity segments were generated and relative motion plots were constructed for the following joint couplings: femoral rotation and tibial rotation, hip flexion and knee flexion, knee rotation and ankle inversion, knee flexion and ankle inversion, and knee flexion and ankle dorsiflexion. As the data were predominantly nonsinusoidal, a modified vector coding technique (Sparrow, Donovan, van Emmerik, & Barry, 1987) was used to quantify joint coordination (see chapter 9 by Wheat & Glazier). As in the studies we previously described, the stride cycle was divided into five intervals, with each interval containing a functional event (i.e., midstance, toe-off, swing acceleration, swing deceleration, and heel strike). The variability of joint coordination was quantified by calculating the average standard deviation within each of these periods as well as over the entire stride cycle. Kinematic data describing stride length and stride duration were also obtained for the 15 strides at each running speed. The mean and standard deviation of each of these parameters were then used to calculate the coefficient of variation (CV), which was used to quantify the variability of stride characteristics for each of the individuals.

Several important findings emerged from this study. First, the average CV for stride length obtained from the individuals with unilateral patellofemoral pain was significantly greater than that obtained for nonimpaired individuals at the preferred running speed. This finding appears to concur with previous research reporting an increased variability of stride length in individuals at risk of falling (Gabell et al., 1996; Hausdorff et al., 1997) and in individuals with various neurological diseases (Hausdorff et al., 1998). However, as there was no significant difference in the average CV for stride length between the groups at the fixed running speed, Heiderscheit et al. (2002) remained skeptical about the generalizability of these results. Second, no significant differences in variability of joint coordination existed between the injured and noninjured limbs of the individuals with patellofemoral pain when variability was analyzed over the entire stride cycle. Moreover, no significant difference in variability existed between the individuals with unilateral patellofemoral pain and the nonimpaired individuals when variability was analyzed over the entire stride cycle. However, in the coupling between thigh rotation and leg rotation, a significant difference in variability of joint coordination existed between the injured and noninjured limbs of the individuals with patellofemoral pain among the five intervals of the stride cycle. Although Heiderscheit et al. (2002) suggested that this difference could simply be an error in measurement, the decreased variability in the injured limb during the interval containing heel strike at the preferred running speed appears to concur with previous research by Hamill et al. (1999). Heiderscheit et al. (2002) found that the injured limbs of individuals with patellofemoral pain exhibited less variability than either limb of the nonimpaired individuals, but neither limb of the nonimpaired individuals exhibited as much variability in coordination as the noninjured limbs of the individuals with patellofemoral pain. The concurrent increase in the variability of the noninjured limb with the decrease in the variability of the injured limb implies a compensatory mechanism. Similar findings have been reported in children with spastic hemiplegic cerebral palsy (see Jeng, Holt, Fetters, & Certo, 1996).

Despite the limitations of the studies outlined in this section, it appears that a dynamic systems approach could greatly assist in the detection, treatment, and rehabilitation of running injuries (see also chapter 8 by Hamill, Haddad, Heiderscheit, van Emmerik & Li). For example, by examining the variability in coordination of lower-extremity body segments, sport biomechanist and clinicians might be able to detect the gradual deterioration of sensorimotor functioning and predict the onset of overuse injuries, as variability in coordination appears to inversely relate to the degree of pathology. Likewise, by examining variability in coordination during treatment and rehabilitation, scientists in sport biomechanics and clinicians can monitor the effectiveness of treatment modalities and estimate the extent of recovery, which could help prevent a premature return to physical activity and avoid compounding the original injury. Furthermore, by examining the coordination between lower-extremity body segments it may be possible to ascertain the cause of injury. Although Hamill et al. (1999) failed to identify any significant differences in the coordination of lower-extremity components between injured and noninjured individuals, it is hard to dispute the plethora of anecdotal evidence that implicates a disruption to the relative motions of the segments comprising the knee joint as a major factor in the etiology of overuse injuries. Only further research using a dynamic systems approach can verify the accuracy of these claims.

Clearly, the emphasis on the coordination and the variability in coordination of body segments and joints has arguably provided more useful information about lower-extremity running injuries than conventional research designs in sport biomechanics, which have generally failed to provide empirical evidence relating the mechanics of the lower-extremity body segments to knee injury (McClay, 2000; DeLeo, Dierks, Ferber & Davis, 2004). The emergence of a dynamic systems approach appears to be particularly timely in this respect, as an increasing number of individuals from the medical profession have begun to question whether biomechanics has made a meaningful contribution to the diagnosis, treatment, and prevention of running injuries. From the evidence presented in this section, it appears that adopting a dynamic systems approach and using variability in coordination as a clinical measurement (see Heiderscheit, 2000b) may enhance the richness and improve the productivity of injury-related research in sport biomechanics. Although we have focused predominantly on running injuries in the lower extremity, it is likely that this relatively new approach is equally applicable to the general study of orthopedic injuries.

Concluding Remarks

In this chapter, we have used examples from the literature to demonstrate the utility of dynamic systems theory in performance-related and injury-related research in sport biomechanics. We have shown that dynamic systems theory not only provides the scope for alternative research designs, but also provides a scientifically rigorous theoretical rationale that some individuals from other disciplines of sport science might argue, albeit incorrectly, does not presently exist in applied research in sport biomechanics. Although this relatively new approach has yet to become routine in sport biomechanics, some of the examples outlined in this chapter suggest that it could provide more important information for performance enhancement and injury prevention than other research designs currently being used. Importantly, dynamic systems theory provides the scope, rationale, and methods to examine more thoroughly the functional role of movement variability, which has, to date, been rarely investigated by sport biomechanists.

Part II

Variability, Performance, and Excellence

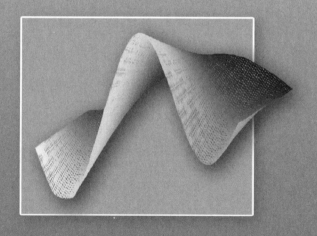

Chapter 4

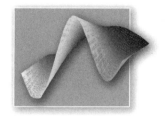

Serving Up Variability and Stability

Craig Handford, PhD

Editors' Overview

This chapter suggests that traditionally accepted approaches to breaking down complex tasks into components for practice may or may not be correct approaches. These approaches actually have few rigorously tested underpinning principles. A reconceptualization of variability in the movement system has significant implications for the process of practice in sport, particularly for part-practice conditions and transfer of learning. Recently, applications of the theory of complex systems to coaching has suggested that the Newtonian reductionist ideas of simplification and abstraction, although successful in physical investigations, have not had the same influence in the study of human behavior. The revelation of universal properties of complex, nonlinear systems is likely to facilitate the development of fundamental theories of coaching. For example, the concept of quantum entanglement, which signifies that states do not have equivalents in classical systems, when applied to coaching theory indicates that the role of the coach is to help each individual athlete search the fitness landscape and find an optimal performance solution. It is argued that the implicit influence of the theory of linear systems on coaching theory has resulted in an overemphasis on consistent, repeatable, almost stereotyped movements. The idea that consistency in motor patterns should be the prime goal of practice organization and structure is rejected. Rather, when the dynamic relationship between a performer and the environment is considered, variability clearly plays a key role in attaining consistent outcomes.

Many teachers, coaches, and performers have long considered stability and consistency in movement to be essential characteristics of skilled performance. For some, practice has become almost obsessive in its pursuit of this holy grail of skill acquisition. Popular opinion suggests that such an approach has been largely influenced by traditional views that movements are programmed and there can be little doubt that concepts such as memory representations have provided sport with a foundation upon which a user-friendly model of human performance can be formulated. However, a somewhat inflexible interpretation of movement programming has resulted in countless 'textbook' approaches toward developing sport technique. The method of "one size fits all" is commonplace, along with the suggestion that technical elements can be delivered in a generic way and across individuals. In a similar vein, numerous methods for manipulating practice conditions have permeated popular coaching literature with the intention of facilitating the learning process. The common practice of separating parts of a movement for isolated development is one well-established example.

While these lines of thought have an intuitive appeal and appear largely appropriate in promoting successful performance, a more detailed examination reveals potentially important addendums, most notably the need to distinguish exactly what features of a movement pattern should be held stable and consistent. Should the goal of deliberate practice simply be consistency in all aspects of a movement, or are some elements of movement organization more critical to stability than others? Indeed, certain elements of movement may best be left free to vary, and in many cases such variability could be viewed as a necessary and functional aspect of satisfying the task demands. The question of generalizability across both individuals and tasks is equally worthy of some qualification. For example, are the patterns of movement developed by or for a particular individual applicable to another learner attempting the same task? Are these patterns specific to the particular task, and if not, are there particular elements that transfer better than others? Pursuit of such distinctions is surely worthwhile when considering the acquisition of effective movement and the efficient use of often limited practice time.

Recent examinations of this area have been increasingly concerned with these questions and have been largely committed to uncovering the so-called dynamics of movement. In contrast to traditional views, these ecological approaches strive to explain movement behavior and to understand the relationships between the environment and the underlying mechanics of action. Within this particular theoretical context, variability and stability in movement are central concepts for the practitioner to understand (Handford, Davids, Bennett, & Button, 1997). This chapter attempts to illuminate several pertinent and practical observations on these concepts and presents the findings from a study that examined skilled serving in volleyball from an ecological perspective. Experimental data from a group of skilled servers are offered in support of three basic statements, and the implications for future practice are discussed.

Deliberate Practice Is Not Always About Movement Consistency

In serving, consistency in ball placement during the toss phase is widely believed to be a prerequisite for successful performance in a number of sports including squash, racquetball, badminton, and table tennis. In particular, tennis and volleyball focus on this topic, with coaching texts repeatedly highlighting the importance of invariant positioning in the vertical, forward-backward, and side-to-side dimensions (see McGehee, 1997 and Neville, 1994). To confirm this belief, the serves of senior international female volleyball players were analyzed using three-dimensional video and kinematic analysis techniques (see Davids, Bennett, Handford, & Jones, 1999 for a detailed description of procedures). Figure 4.1 illustrates the group data and shows the three-dimensional displacement of the ball for one particular server, which was sampled at key points in its trajectory and over a number of trials. For all points in the trajectory of the ball, greater trial-to-trial variability in the frontal (side-to-side) and sagittal (back-to-front) dimensions is indicated by a larger degree of scatter as compared to the vertical dimension, which is significantly less variable.

These general observations of variability in ball positioning are further corroborated by a more precise examination of the variability in key points on the trajectory as the toss unfolds. Figure 4.2 shows changes in measurements of variance of ball position for the group mean data as the ball travels from its initial starting point to the peak (zenith) of its trajectory and finally to the point of contact with the striking hand. Clearly, for both the side-to-side (x) and front-to-back (y) dimensions, variability actually increases as contact between ball and hand is approached. This finding substantiates the conclusion that, contrary to dominant coaching theory, stability in these particular parameters is perhaps not critical for success. On the other hand, the inverse is true for variability in the vertical (z) position, with it becoming significantly reduced as both zenith and contact are approached. A degree of inconsistency in initial conditions seems tolerable, but trial-to-trial stability in the vertical plane of the later part of the trajectory appears to be one element of technique that successful servers are unwilling to concede. These findings show the complementary nature of stability and variability in motor performance.

Such a simple finding has potentially profound practical implications. Existing coaching methods that have performers (and coaches) devoting untold hours of practice toward perfecting elements of a skill that are not necessary for success seem misplaced. Given the results of the study on serves, it appears that practice of ball tosses should emphasize the development of a stable peak height in favor of consistency in the other directions. In fact, over-constraining particular parameters may be undesirable and even detrimental to acquiring certain skills. Coaches, teachers, and therapists should consider the possibility that consistency at one point in a movement actually relies on the freedom of another point to vary. In this way, variability can be viewed as a necessary and natural part of the solution to any particular movement problem. The additional negative consequences of increased anxiety and decreased motivation that accompany over-restrictive practice are also worthy of consideration in this context. The findings outlined earlier clearly demonstrate the need for practitioners to precisely understand skills in terms of exactly which aspects of a skill should be consistent. Moreover, those of an inquisitive nature could

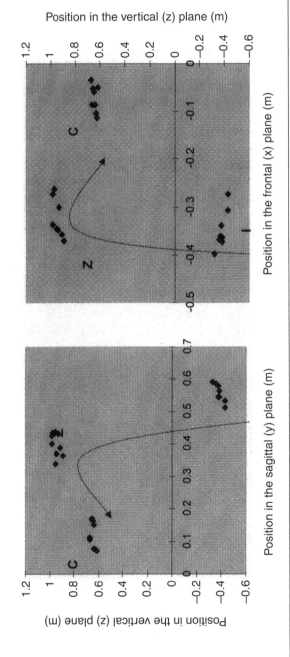

FIGURE 4.1 Typical trial-by-trial displacements at key points in the trajectory of the ball. The key points are initial (I), zenith (Z), and contact (C).

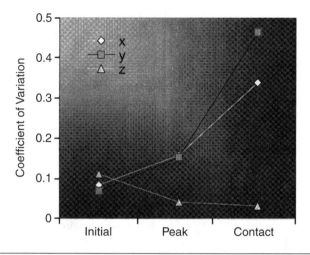

FIGURE 4.2 Group mean measurements of variation in three dimensions at key points along the trajectory of the ball.

be forgiven for questioning why, in a sea of inconsistency, is it important that particular aspects be stable? Presumably, in the case of serving, there is something about a consistent vertical peak that is significant to successfully solving the movement problem, i.e., coordinating the ball toss and the movement of the striking arm. It is to this something that we now direct attention.

Solutions to Movement Problems Can Be Generic and Yet Individual

Exclamations such as "Agassi's execution of that forehand was absolutely textbook!" are not uncommon and many sport observers (and coaches) would have us believe that a blueprint for technical perfection has been established that performers should follow. Likewise, comments such as "Agassi hits the backhand like no one else" suggest that a degree of individualism is also present in technical performance. Contradiction in sports commentary is nothing new, but is it unreasonable to suggest that there are aspects of effective movement that are relatively fixed but also allow for individual differences? In seeking to explain the significance of a consistent vertical peak of ball placement in volleyball serving, numerous findings came to light that support this apparent paradox.

Closer examination of the inter-subject and inter-trial values for vertical ball position revealed some important features that were otherwise masked in the group data. Most notably, servers demonstrated a wide range of differences at each of the key phases of the trajectory when the mean displacements were compared across individuals. In fact, individual differences of more than 25 cm were present at both the zenith and contact points. This result was the first indication that any solution to the problem of coordinating the serve would need to account for these differences, which may ultimately reflect anatomical variability. Table 4.1 shows the mean times at which the peak point of the ball flight *(Tz)* occurred for each server. Predictably, the findings related to the spatial analysis previously discussed were translated in the temporal analysis. Considering the data in this way highlights the great stability in individual performances, particularly when standard deviations of as little as 20 to 40 ms (1-2 frames) are demonstrated.

TABLE 4.1   Time of Peak Point *(Tz)* and Time of Foreswing *(Th)* for Each Server

Subject	Tz (s) Mean (SD)	Th (s) Mean (SD)	Difference *(Tz – Th)* Mean (SD)
1	0.624 (0.018)	0.610 (0.028)	0.014 (0.011)
2	0.689 (0.054)	0.691 (0.056)	-0.003 (0.016)
3	0.496 (0.029)	0.485 (0.045)	0.010 (0.023)
4	0.638 (0.024)	0.638 (0.031)	0.000 (0.010)
5	0.657 (0.022)	0.640 (0.034)	0.021 (0.018)
6	0.730 (0.041)	0.725 (0.049)	0.005 (0.010)
Mean	0.639	0.631	0.008
(SD)	(0.073)	(0.076)	(0.008)

It appears that by ensuring spatial stability in the peak point, skilled servers introduce temporal stability to the action. The significance of such a strategy becomes apparent when questioning how successful servers coordinate the timing of the striking action with the descending ball. Findings from a previous analysis of coordination in volleyball serving showed relatively small intra-subject variations in total movement time, with average deviations ranging from 12 to 39 ms (see Davids, Bennett, Handford, & Jones, 1999). In particular, the timing of the directional change of the center of the hip joint from backswing to foreswing *(Th)* was more stable than any other kinematic event in the serving action (Mean = 79% of total movement time, SD = ± 0.5). Evidently the servers prefer to initiate force production at a specific moment during the sequence of movement regardless of the absolute time of movement. An analysis of the relationship between the temporal characteristics of ball flight and the initiation of forward hip movement showed that the timing of ball peak (a perceptual event) was strongly related to this action event. Table 4.1 shows the mean differences $(Tz - Th)$ for each server, which ranged from an impressive 0 to a maximum of 21 ms.

In summary, it seems that servers were attempting to stabilize the height of ball peak to ensure that if the initiation of the foreswing coincided with this event, the time remaining before contact would be equivalent to the time required for the unfolding of the striking action, and so successful contact would be guaranteed. The equation describing the displacement of a descending ball shows how servers using this strategy of timing would need to develop a sensitivity to personal anatomical characteristics and movement times in order to ensure appropriate peak height.

According to the proposed strategy,

peak height = contact height + displacement of descending ball *(d)*, (4.1)

where

$$d = V_i t + 1/2gt^2 \qquad (4.2)$$

and V_i, initial velocity = 0 m/s; *g*, acceleration due to gravity = 9.8 m/s; and *t*, time from peak to contact = foreswing time.

Therefore,

$$d = 1/2gt^2 = 4.99(\text{foreswing time})^2, \qquad (4.3)$$

and so

peak height = contact height + 4.99(foreswing time)^2. (4.4)

From this equation it seems that coordination in serving could be defined by information that resides in both the organism and the environment. In other words, ball toss could be parameterized with an intrinsic metric measured in units that are relative to the performer's body parts and capacity for movement, which is so-called body-scaled information (Konczak, 1990). Such an approach links dimensions of the task and the environment to anatomical properties of the performer so that the key (generic) relationships that describe successful coordination are expressed across persons of different body sizes and dimensions (Davis & Burton, 1991). With this in mind, Newell's (1986) commentary on the consequences of child growth and the implications of changing body size on moments of inertia in body segments becomes pertinent (see also Corbetta and Vereijken, 1999). In the case of serving, changes in the absolute peak height of ball placement can be predicted as contact height increases due to physical growth. Furthermore, as learners improve the intralimb coordination of the striking action, the time required for the sequencing of the various limb segments during foreswing is likely to decrease and influence ball placement accordingly.

These explanations may account for many of the discrepancies in the coaching literature in recommendations for the height of ball placement in serving. In fact, if peak height relates to contact height and foreswing time, then practical advice should encourage a more hands-off approach to ball placement, with fewer prescriptions for movement. Coaches would be wise to teach the key perception–action relationship (i.e., coincidence of ball peak and start of foreswing) that suits all performers. However, a little freedom should be built into skill acquisition so that servers can discover and develop a custom solution to the problem of movement that is uniquely scaled to their personal (anatomical) attributes and stage of learning. In serving, it is clear how movement variability from one individual to the next can be viewed as both a functional and a necessary characteristic of performance. Furthermore, since peak height is so closely linked to the serving movement, traditional practice that breaks down movement into its components should be re-examined in the light of this new understanding of coordination in serving.

Variability Can Provide a Basis for Practice in Parts

The dilemma of whether complex motor skills should be broken into smaller parts or left as a whole for the purpose of practice has been one of the most enduring for those studying the acquisition of movement skills. Unfortunately, meaningful theoretical guidance has not been forthcoming and there have been few direct examinations of the topic with little support for the prediction that part practice regimes have positive transfer qualities. This lack of information has resulted in somewhat arbitrary and unsystematic approaches to the dilemma, with traditional pedagogy focusing on the subjective assessment of skills in terms of "appropriate units of action" and their perceived relationships with one another (see Chamberlin & Lee, 1993; Burton & Davis, 1996). Magill (1998) adds to the ambiguity, suggesting that "the critical part to making the decision about whether certain parts can be practiced separately or together with other parts is dependent on the instructor's knowledge of the skill itself" (p. 299). Clearly the success of this approach rests on the assumption that the key factors that influence the dynamics of the skill are known a priori. Lintern (1991) casts serious doubt on this assumption, suggesting that significant limitations in current knowledge restrict the development of practical guidelines. The result is that many practices in sport are presently implementing methods that are at best based on unprincipled and tentative foundations. The problems with this area are neatly summarized by Newell (1981), who suggests that current practices are "not founded on strong evidence and theoretical interpretations of their effects are even more hazardous" (p. 218).

The description of timing in the volleyball serve provides the detailed understanding necessary for assessing a commonly used part-practice regime in acquiring the skill of serving. It has been proposed that separating the toss and strike phases in the part practice of serving would disrupt the relationship shown to be essential to successfully coordinating the action. The contention was that such a disruption would manifest itself in measurements of key variables previously identified for the task of serving. Specifically, comparing the magnitude and variability of ball zenith would usefully estimate transferability from part to whole. The performance of expert servers was filmed and analyzed for conditions of ball placement and full serve. In the part-practice condition of ball placement, servers were instructed to toss the ball without striking, stopping short of contact and allowing the ball to drop. Comparing the trajectory profiles of the ball under this condition with profiles from the condition of full serve revealed two key differences: i) the variability in peak height was greater for the condition of ball placement, and ii) the mean value of peak height was also greater for the condition of ball placement (see figure 4.3).

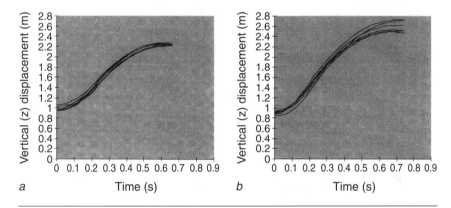

FIGURE 4.3   Profiles of displacement times for vertical ball trajectory for one typical server in the conditions of *(a)* full serve and *(b)* toss only.

The differences in the profiles suggested that manipulating task constraints for part practice leads to an adaptation in the spatial pattern of ball placement. That is, the constraints imposed on ball placement when the ball is tossed in isolation are quantitatively different from those present in the serve. Not only were servers less consistent when tossing the ball in isolation, but they seemed to overshoot the ball placement because of the absence of actual contact. The explanation is that manipulating task conditions in order to focus on a key element decouples the critical perception–action relationship that governs coordination in serving. Differences between whole and part conditions were not limited to only the all-important vertical positioning of the ball. A comparison of variability in the front-to-back and side-to-side dimensions revealed other substantial differences between the conditions. Figure 4.4 shows variance in three dimensions for two typical subjects. Notably, variability in the x and y

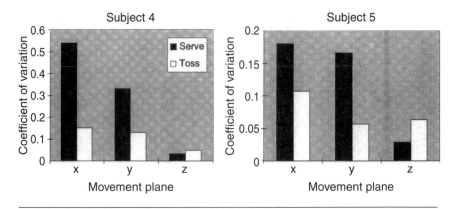

FIGURE 4.4   Three-dimensional variance in ball placement for both conditions for two servers.

planes for part practice was significantly less than variability in the x and y planes for the whole action. It almost appears that when their focus was taken away from making contact between hand and ball, the servers became unnecessarily concerned about spatial consistency in other directions. As a result, variability in the crucial vertical (z) plane was compromised.

In summary, the principles by which a skill might be decomposed for part practice should be established on a sound understanding of the coordination dynamics and key perception–action relationships underlying the skill. With this foundational knowledge, the practitioner may better evaluate the potential effects of separating parts of a skill for isolated practice. It follows that measurements of the effects of separation on known patterns of variability associated with the key relationships can be used as sensitive indexes of transferability. In this way, the likelihood of successfully transferring gains made during practice can be objectively assessed in terms of reconfiguring the parts. For example, if the change effected by task decomposition is too great, then the characteristic variability profile should be disrupted. In this case, the degree of interference determines the extent of the transfer, with significant changes possibly representing a fundamental shift to a coordination that is somewhat unrelated to that to be acquired. In other words, the constraints resulting from partitioning the task are so removed from the original task constraints that the goals of each movement are essentially different and improvements in the whole cannot be predicted (Goodman & Kelso, 1980). On the other hand, if the characteristic stability is preserved, it may be assumed that the constraints on movement are sufficiently similar and so transfer of improvements in the parts is likely.

Given the findings reported here, the prediction that separation of the toss and strike phases of the serving action would lead to positive transfer to the criterion (whole) skill seems to be unlikely. In fact, it would be reasonable to suggest that servers should spend practice time executing the whole action rather than practicing its parts in isolation. For the successful transfer of part-practice regimes, the manipulation of task constraints should preserve the key relationships that describe coordination. Of course, this implication depends on a basic but nontrivial premise that practitioners know these relationships.

Conclusion

Recent ecological approaches to movement have encouraged those interested in sport behavior to examine the coordination and acquisition of skills in an alternative way. The underpinning philosophy and theoretical framework of these approaches include performer, task, and environmental features and have made understanding the key relationships among these elements the pivotal issue. The ensuing methodologies have necessarily focused on detailed analyses of patterns in movement and have consequently brought variability in performance to the forefront. As we have demonstrated, the key variables that describe coordination are specific to the constraints involved and display minimum variation, often despite considerable fluctuations in other variables (Beek & Van Santvoord, 1992). Moreover, they exhibit characteristics of both the movement and perceptual systems of the performer and are governed by a relative organization in that they are not affected by absolute values (see Wallace, 1996). This description of coordinated behaviour has the built-in advantage of accommodating variability across a great range of individual (anatomical) differences.

In addressing problems of movement, coaches and teachers are encouraged to seek solutions that do not reside totally within the individual but that capture the essence of the coordination among performer, task, and environment. Furthermore, the ecological approach invites a review of how sport practitioners treat variability in movement in the context of skill acquisition. A study of serving has demonstrated a clear case for reducing variance in certain influential parameters while showing that fluctuations in other parameters are noncritical and perhaps even complementary. In fact, one interpretation suggests that practices designed to generally reduce variability in movement might ultimately prove to be detrimental to learning. The potential to shed new light on contemporary principles of practice has also been demonstrated in the area of part practice. Again, the need for coaching to be informed by a thorough understanding of the variables influencing coordination has been confirmed. Armed with this knowledge, practitioners are better able to choose an appropriate separation of skills with positive transfer in mind. What is more, practices that separate parts of a skill in the absence of such information are ill-advised and should proceed with caution. The agenda for science and pedagogical practice is clear. An ecological approach should be utilized to uncover the underlying dynamics of the many skills involved in sports. Using the ecological approach would provide the opportunity to re-evaluate the acquisition of other skills and aspects of practice such as instruction, observational learning, and feedback provision.

Chapter 5

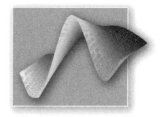

Variability in Motor Output and Olympic Performers

Les G. Carlton, PhD, John W. Chow, PhD, and Jaeho Shim, PhD

Editors' Overview

This chapter examines variability in sport-related tasks attempting to maximize accuracy and minimize variability of outcome. Of particular interest is the relationship between speed and accuracy in the projectile activities that are a component of many sport tasks. While the associations between speed and accuracy are well-known for manual aiming to spatial targets, data from projection tasks are limited. However, these data suggest that the relationship may be fundamentally different in projection. Models of throwing are discussed, and it is clear that variability in movement is maintained within tolerance limits by simultaneously varying key parameters such as the release angle and velocity of the projectile. The infinite number of release angles and velocities that can be combined to achieve the distance required by the throw signals the compensatory role of variability among the important parameters. Research on underhand throwing is reviewed by showing that an equifinal path specifies the movement trajectory for a required throwing height and distance to a target irrespective of the timing of projectile release. Taking the issue of speed-accuracy trade-offs to the context of elite sport performance, data on tennis serving at the 1996 Olympic Games are examined. Data on the variability of motor performance in Olympic athletes have rarely been analyzed, and the task constraints of competitive tennis are ideal for studying the speed-accuracy trade-off in ball games because players systematically adjust the speed of first and second serves. It is argued that these data need to be understood in relation to the variability of the motor patterns used for first and second serves, particularly in light of the use of the racket face to alter the anterior–posterior velocity of the stroke.

The authors thank the International Olympic Committee (IOC) and the Atlanta Committee for the Olympic Games (ACOG) for their permission to collect data during the Olympic Games. Data collection was coordinated by Dr. Ben Johnson of the Georgia State University. We also thank Steve Barrentine, Jake Johnson, and Jeff Johnson for their assistance in data collection. We thank Mary Carlton for her helpful comments on an earlier draft of this chapter.

"Haste makes waste" is an old adage handed down from generation to generation. It suggests that when we try to complete a task quickly, we make mistakes. The same assumption sits behind the concept of speed-accuracy trade-offs in motor tasks. Increasing the speed of performing a task leads to poorer accuracy. Speed-accuracy trade-offs have been observed for a wide range of motor, perceptual, and cognitive tasks. For example, Pew (1969) demonstrated that trade-offs are not specific to task and that performers can control the level of speed or accuracy they wish to maintain. Fitts' law (1954), a description of speed-accuracy trade-offs for aimed movements of the limb, has been found to hold for numerous motor tasks ranging from movements made under a microscope (Langolf, Chaffin & Foulke, 1976) to movements used to position computer mice (Card, English, & Burr, 1978). Speed-accuracy trade-offs are not limited to motor tasks. Regan (1998), for example, observed a shift in the speed and accuracy of news reporting. The demand for online news has led to greater emphasis on speed and as a result, the accuracy of news reporting has deteriorated.

Speed and accuracy are essential elements of most sport activities. In some sports the outcome of a competition depends entirely on the accuracy of performance. Examples include Olympic events such as shooting, curling, and archery. In other sports, a task requiring accuracy is an essential element of outcome, such as shooting in basketball. At the other end of the spectrum, speed dominates the outcome of certain sports. For example, the average speed in competitive running and swimming or the distance a javelin is thrown determines success in those events. In most tasks, however, successful performance demands a combination of speed and accuracy. In baseball pitching accuracy is essential. The pitcher must throw the ball over the plate at the correct height. However, accuracy has little benefit if the velocity of the ball is low. The most outstanding pitchers are able to throw the ball at high velocities without sacrificing accuracy. Similar requirements are characteristic of throwing activities in other sports such as handball, water polo, and cricket.

Many sports require performers to project an object toward a goal or target by striking the object with an implement or a part of the body. Activities such as serving in tennis, kicking in soccer, and shooting in hockey require both speed and accuracy. An accurate tennis serve struck at a low velocity gives the advantage to the receiver. However, not all striking activities benefit by greater speed. In golf, except for the drive and approach shots to the green on longer holes, outcome is a function of accuracy. In fact, it is the variability of performance that determines the outcomes of golf competitions. In a golf tournament, players complete 72 holes and over 250 individual strokes. The successful performer exhibits little variance between the desired and actual paths of the ball. The greater the variance, the farther the ball lands from its intended location and the greater the number of strokes needed to complete the 72 holes. Just as the statistical variance of a set of scores is greatly influenced by an outlier, that is, a score outside the normal distribution of scores, a player's golf score can be greatly influenced by one particularly bad shot or by a round with high variability. A good example is Tiger Wood's performance in the third round of the 2002 British Open golf tournament. Poor weather made controlling the flight of the ball difficult, and many of his shots varied from their intended paths. This variability led to a score of 81 and to the first time in his professional career that he shot a score of 80 or more in a round. His scores for the other three rounds were 70, 68, and 65.

Is there a trade-off between speed and accuracy in sport tasks, and how might such a trade-off be influenced by practice and the constraints of the task? Even though these questions are of great practical importance, there is surprisingly little research on trade-offs for sport tasks. We might ask this question: What do highly skilled performers do when accuracy is critical but speed is of relatively little importance? A number of years ago the public broadcast network in the United States (PBS) televised the singles finals for a number of summer clay court tennis tournaments in cities such as Louisville and Indianapolis. The primary broadcaster was Bud Collins, and as part of the telecast, players in the tournament were given a standard skills test. The test required players to hit ground strokes from balls fed to them at slow speeds, and each player's score was determined by how accurately the player hit the ball to various locations on the court. Shots that landed near the corner of the court or near the baseline received the greatest number of points and balls that landed shorter in the court (near the net) received fewer points. Given that a player's score was determined solely on accuracy, at what speed did the player hit the ball? In general, the player's strategy was to hit the ball very slowly. This strategy suggests that the players believed that there is a trade-off between speed and accuracy and that they could maximize accuracy by hitting the ball with a slow swing. The players used this strategy despite the fact that they had hundreds of thousands, if not millions, of practice trials of hitting the ball at much faster speeds.

The focus of this chapter is the link between speed and accuracy and hence variability in sport tasks. The relationship between speed and accuracy in arm movements and the relationship between variability and accuracy are briefly reviewed. Constraints of speed and accuracy in sport tasks involving projectiles are examined along with existing models and empirical research. Finally, a study on the speed and accuracy of tennis serves from the 1996 summer Olympic Games in Atlanta is presented. This study is unique in that it examines some of the top performers in the world under competitive conditions.

Variability in the Motor Domain

The consistency with which individuals can perform motor tasks has been of empirical and theoretical interest since the early days of research in motor skills, and it is generally regarded as a hallmark of skilled performance (Guthrie, 1935). Fullerton and Cattell's (1892) study of variability in force production and Woodworth's (1899) examination of the fundamental aspects of accuracy in movement provided the foundation for research conducted a century later (see Elliott, Helsen, & Chua, 2001 for a review). Perhaps the best-known description of motor functioning is Fitts' law (Fitts, 1954). Fitts described a nonlinear relationship between the speed and accuracy of aimed movements of the arm. Subsequent research showed that Fitts' description generalized to a variety of tasks, environments, and organisms.

Accuracy and variability are integrally related. Perhaps the easiest way to see this connection is to examine the speed-accuracy relation of aimed hand movements described by Schmidt, Zelaznik, Hawkins, Frank, and Quinn (1979). Schmidt et al. described a linear relationship between the average velocity of movements and the variability of the hand's landing locations (W_e). Rather than fixing target accuracy and measuring the time required to complete movements as Fitts had done, Schmidt et al. fixed the time of the movement and measured the variability of landing locations and so described the relation between the speed of movement (average velocity) and the variability of movement (variability of end points). A direct relationship between speed and variability using the Schmidt et al. paradigm has been documented in a number of experiments (e.g., Wright & Meyer, 1983; Zelaznik, Mone, McCabe, & Thaman, 1988; Zelaznik, Shapiro, & McClosky, 1981).

The link between accuracy and variability was also made in the Fitts' paradigm. Welford (1968) noted that the variability in landing location and target accuracy are directly related, assuming that there are no significant tendencies to overshoot or undershoot the target distance. The mean spatial error plus 2 standard deviations should encompass 95% of the response end points. In Fitts' paradigm an accuracy rate of 95% is assumed, resulting in a direct relation between accuracy in Fitts' paradigm and variability. A similar argument can be made for the relation between the measurements of absolute error and variable error typically used with performance in motor tasks requiring accuracy. Absolute error measures overall accuracy and variable error reflects the standard deviation of performance. If there is no tendency to overshoot or undershoot the goal target (small constant error), absolute error and variable error are proportional.

The point is that the speed-accuracy trade-off can just as well be described as the speed-variability trade-off.[1] The theoretical ideas underlying Fitts' original work, information theory (Shannon & Weaver, 1949), were based on concepts of noise and variability in communication channels. Fitts (1954) argued that the capability of a movement effector to transfer information is fixed. If movement speed is increased, the result must be greater noise, or variability in the movement. Thus Fitts, on theoretical grounds, might have argued for a speed-variability description rather than a speed-accuracy account.

Not all aspects of movement become more variable with increased speed. In rapid-timing tasks, which require moving through a fixed distance in a specified time, variability in timing decreases with increased movement speed. When

---

[1]It should be noted that increases in speed result in increases in variability rather than decreases as the term "trade-off" implies.

the movement time is fixed, increasing the distance of movement, and hence increasing the speed of movement, substantially reduces variability in timing. This fact could be of considerable importance to sport tasks where timing is critical. While the typical instruction would be to reduce speed to increase accuracy, the opposite strategy might be better! Consider the task of striking a baseball with a bat or a ball in table tennis. Slowing down the swing results in greater error in timing and may lead to poorer performance. We say *may* because performance in these tasks requires both temporal and spatial accuracy. Faster movements result in a greater change in spatial position per unit time. Decreasing the variability of timing may or may not result in decreased spatial variability with faster movements (Newell, Carlton, & Kim, 1994). A complete account of the relation between speed and variability in limb movements requires a coherent space-time function (Hancock & Newell, 1985). Evidence suggests that this function is driven by the nonlinear scaling of the force-time properties of the impulse for the movement (Kim, Carlton, Liu, & Newell, 1999).

Speed and Accuracy in Projectile Tasks

In ancient times hunters relied on their ability to throw with speed and accuracy for their survival. While most of us do not have to throw for our dinner, throwing and other tasks involving projecting a ball or object are an integral part of many sports. In many of these tasks accuracy is important, and accuracy is achieved by controlling the direction or speed of the movement, or both. Even among sports requiring the accurate projection of an object, each sport has its own unique requirements. In some sports balls are thrown and in others they are kicked. In others, objects are hit with an implement such as a racket, stick, or bat. Does each of these tasks have the same relation between speed and accuracy, and are the speed-accuracy relations seen in sport tasks consistent with those documented in the literature on motor behavior?

Throwing tasks that demand spatial accuracy have been separated into two categories (Whiting & Cockerill, 1972). In one category the target is vertical with respect to gravity. Tasks such as dart throwing and baseball pitching are examples of this classification. In these tasks the relation between speed and accuracy might be examined by having performers attempt to hit the same target while throwing at different speeds. In the second category the target is horizontal and includes tasks such as pitching horseshoes where the amount of effort is critical to the accuracy of the task. In this group of tasks the projection distance must be controlled, and a speed-accuracy relation might be observed with changes in the distance of the throw. As distance increases, the speed of the released object must be increased, and increased variability in velocity will result in greater variability in distance. In either classification accuracy depends on the speed of the throw and the angle of release. The suggestion, however, is that the accuracy of throws at vertical targets might not be influenced by increases in throwing speeds (Dupuy, Mottet, & Ripoll, 2000).

Models of Throwing Accuracy

Most of the research on variability and tasks involving projectiles has focused on throwing. This appears to be due to the prevalence of throwing in games and sports and to the fact that throwing is viewed developmentally as a fundamental motor skill (Keogh & Sugden, 1985). Unlike in aimed movements of the hand, on-line control cannot be used to guide the projectile to the target. Models of throwing accuracy, therefore, have focused on the mechanical requirements for successful throws and on how performers exploit the laws of physics. As might be expected, models focus on the angle and velocity of release, the heights of release and target, and how these parameters might be manipulated to maximize throwing precision. Current models are also similar in that the throwing action being modeled involves only a few degrees of freedom and that variability is minimized by compensation among release parameters. Two models will be reviewed: one that accounts for variability in hitting horizontal targets and one that focuses on hitting vertical targets.

Throwing Accurately to Horizontal Targets

Dupuy et al. (2000) generated a model of underarm throwing based on a popular French game, *petanque*. The game is similar to pitching horseshoes in the United States. In both sports, an object is projected with an underarm throw to a spatial target placed at ground level. The motion is produced at the shoulder joint and the distance of the throw is critical for success. The speed, angle, and height of release all contribute to the distance of the throw. When the height and angle of release are fixed, distance increases exponentially with increases in the speed of release. When the height and velocity of release are fixed, distance increases as the angle of release increases to approximately 45° and then decreases at larger angles. When release angle and velocity are fixed, distance increases systematically with increases in the height of release. Of the three parameters, the speed of release has the greatest effect on throwing distance (Hay, 1993).

There are an infinite number of combinations of release velocities and angles that lead to the same distance. When the target and the point of release are at the same height, an angle of 45° produces a given distance with the lowest velocity. Unfortunately, when the height of the release and target are not the same, the optimum angle, that is, the angle that produces the greatest distance for a given speed, is not readily obtained. The optimum angle depends on the difference in height between the point of release and the target and on the release velocity (Hay, 1993). An angle of release that is greater or smaller than the optimum can still hit the target, but the velocity at release must be higher. The question becomes, what is the combination of velocity and angle that minimizes variability in throwing distance?

Dupuy et al. (2000) noted that small variations in the speed of release resulted in significant changes in distance. However, because the optimum angle corresponds to the maximum peak of a parabolic function relating the angle of release and the distance of the throw, small variations in angles near the optimum have little effect on distance. To determine the effect of variation in angle on distance, Dupuy et al. numerically differentiated the equation of projectile range with respect to angle (figure 5.1). This process yielded a graphical representation of the relationships among the speed and angle of release and the variation in distance. Two factors are clearly evident from figure 5.1. First, there is a valley for angles of release approaching 45° for releases at high speeds and 35° for releases at low speeds. In this area, small variations in speed and angle have a very small effect on the distance thrown. Second, variations in release angle have a small effect on distance at low velocities (also see Hay, 1993).

To determine if throwers used velocities and release angles consistent with their model, Dupuy et al. (2000) had participants throw baseballs underhanded to targets located 4, 5, 6, 7, and 8 m away. The results showed that the mean speed and angle of release increased with distance. Variability in the distance thrown increased with distance, but interestingly distance had no systematic effect on variability in either speed or angle. The angle and velocity combinations that participants spontaneously chose were in accordance with the

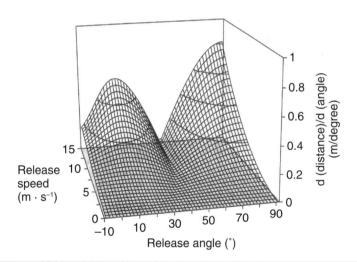

FIGURE 5.1   A plot representing the numerical differentiation of distance with respect to angle as a function of the speed and angle of release. A valley running from near 45° for fast speeds to near 35° for slow speeds represents an area where variability in speed or angle has its least influence on distance.

Reprinted, by permission, from M.A. Dupuy et al., 2000, "The regulation of release parameters in underarm precision throwing," *Journal of Sports Sciences* 18(6): 377. Http://www.tandf.co.uk/journals.

predictions of the model. Participants chose the slowest speed that covered the required distance. The angle of release for the speed chosen was the angle that minimized variability in distance.

Throwing Accurately to Vertical Targets

Like throwing to a horizontal target fixed at a distance (throwing for distance), throwing to a vertical target can be accomplished by an infinite number of speeds and angles of projection. Mueller and coworkers (Mueller & Loosch, 1999; Mueller, Reiser, & Daugs, 1998) have developed a simple model of throwing variability based on tasks such as dart throwing. The task is to use an overarm throw to project an object (e.g., dart) to a vertically oriented target (e.g., dartboard). The arm motion is restricted to the rotation at the elbow, and the recorded outcome is limited to the vertical plane, that is, to whether the projectile (dart) lands high or low on the target (dartboard). As in the model of Dupuy et al. (2000), the speed and angle of release are parameters.

There are two major differences between these two models. First, while Dupuy et al. (2000) focuses on variability in a single velocity parameter (velocity of release), the Mueller model treats velocity as a continuous variable that changes with time. As the angle of the elbow changes, the velocity of the hand also changes. Second, changes in the time of release are seen as having a greater influence on outcome in the Mueller model. This is partly due to the assumption that changes in the angle of release affect both the velocity of release and the trajectory of the object.

How accurate are humans at timing release in rapid throws? Calvin (1983) calculated that the timing precision needed to project objects accurately over long distances was extremely great. Assuming a target height of 10 cm and an elbow-to-hand radius of 40 cm and also that the release occurred within a window of 10° before the top of the throwing arc, Calvin calculated that throws of 7 m have a release window of 1 ms and that throws of 14 m have a window of only 0.1 ms! Empirical examinations, however, have reported much greater variability in release timing. Hore, Watts, Martin, and Miller (1995) found a 10 ms variation in hand opening in a throwing task, and Becker, Kunesch, and Freund (1990) reported that for the release times they studied, standard deviations were 4 to 6 ms. Given these significant timing errors, Hore, Watts, and Tweed (1996) examined whether variability in throw height for fast overhand throws was a function of variability, or "errors," in the velocity of joint rotations, the timing of joint rotations, or the timing of ball release. They found a strong relation between the height of impact on the target and the onset of finger extension, which suggests an important role for the angle of release.

The Mueller model attempts to account for the ability to throw accurately even with significant variability in the angle of release. The basic model parameters are shown in figure 5.2. The object to be thrown is accelerated along a circular path caused by elbow rotation. The angle-velocity profile of the elbow joint is produced in such a way that variations in release angle are compensated by velocity changes. Mueller and Loosch (1999) termed this model the "equifinal path." The model specifies that for a given throwing height and distance, there is an angle-velocity profile of the elbow joint that leads to consistent vertical accuracy. The equifinal path, then, is the spatial-temporal pattern of movement that leads to angle-velocity combinations that result in a target hit, no matter when the object is released.

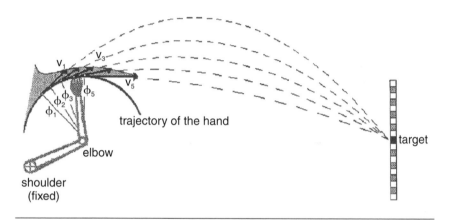

FIGURE 5.2   The equifinal model. Rotations occur about the elbow joint, and dart release can occur at any angle from φ_1 to φ_5. The location of an equifinal landing can be obtained by producing a pattern of hand velocity that yields tangential velocity vectors $(v_1\text{-}v_5)$ matching the upper boundary of the shaded area.

Reprinted, by permission, from M. Mueller and E. Loosch, 1999, "Functional variability and an equifinal path of movement during targeted throwing," *Journal of Human Movement Studies* 36(3): 114.

Do throwers produce a joint angle-velocity profile that matches the pattern specified by the equifinal model? Mueller and coworkers (Mueller & Loosch, 1999; Mueller et al., 1998) compared the angle-velocity profiles used by throwers with the profile specified by the model, using a virtual dart task for both overhand and underarm throwing. Throwers moved a lever attached to their forearms as if throwing a dart. A contact switch between the throwers' index fingers and the lever was used to define the time of release. The contact point of the virtual dart on the virtual target was computed and displayed to the thrower. These experiments showed that over the course of nearly 3,000 attempts, throwers altered their throwing patterns to closely match the equifinal path during the range of release times normally used by the thrower.

Speed-Variability Trade-Offs in Sport Tasks

Research on sport tasks has sought to determine whether the speed-accuracy trade-offs that occur for aimed movements and a variety of other tasks also occur for sport tasks. Experiments are usually loosely formulated around speed-accuracy relations (e.g., Fitts, 1954; Schmidt et al. 1979; Zelaznik et al., 1988) and existing descriptions of variability in force production (e.g., Carlton, Kim, Liu, & Newell, 1993; Schmidt & Sherwood; 1982; Schmidt et al., 1979) or movement kinematics (e.g., Newell, Carlton, Carlton, & Halbert, 1980; Newell, Hoshizaki, Carlton, & Halbert, 1979; Sherwood & Schmidt, 1980). Unfortunately, there is not always a straightforward prediction from existing descriptions of speed-accuracy trade-offs to sport tasks involving object projection. Fitts' law, for example, specifies the time to complete aimed movements, using movement amplitude and the size of the target. The performer has direct control over hitting the target because the movement can be controlled on-line using visual feedback. All performers need to do is slow the movement until they do not miss or only miss on 5% of the attempts. In tasks involving projectiles, performers do not have control of the object after its release, and they cannot simply slow down the movement to ensure accuracy. If they slow down too much, the object will not reach the target! This difference in control suggests that the speed-accuracy relations for projectiles and aimed movements are fundamentally different.

Numerous studies have documented the increase in variability of force production that occurs with increased force requirements in dynamic force production (see Carlton & Newell, 1993 for a review). In order to produce faster movement, the force impulse must be increased, and doing so increases impulse variability. This increase in impulse variability results in an increase in speed variability but does not directly specify an increase in the variability of the outcome. The form of the output variability depends on the specific constraints of the task. For example, Whiting and Cockerill (1972) suggested that throwing tasks like darts and pitching in baseball might not show changes in accuracy with variations in throwing speed (Dupuy et al., 2000). What about tasks in which objects are struck with a racket, stick, or club, such as in tennis, ice hockey, and golf? The specific constraints for each task make the speed-variability function difficult to predict from existing theoretical models. In some tasks, such as making a shot in hockey, accuracy is specified almost totally by the direction of the shot. In other tasks, variability in speed is important for accuracy.

The following review of empirical studies is broken into two sections based on task constraints. The first section reviews studies examining speed and variability in throwing. The specific tasks used in these studies include ball and dart throwing. The second section includes studies on striking activities such as tennis and hockey. The review is focused on sport tasks, but non-sport tasks are also mentioned.

Speed and Variability in Throwing

A common experimental method is used in most studies of speed and accuracy in throwing. Throwing speed is typically varied over a fixed target distance. Perhaps the most systematic study of speed-accuracy trade-offs in throwing was conducted by Gross and Gill (1982). In two experiments, dart throwers were asked to adjust their focus toward either speed or accuracy. Five levels of speed and accuracy weighting were used, and throws were performed under both competitive and noncompetitive conditions. The weighting instructions were very effective in producing variations in throwing speed. The time of flight varied between 400 ms for the speed focus and 725 ms for the accuracy focus. In general, speed increased linearly over the five conditions of varying speed-accuracy emphasis. Radial error, as measured from the target center, increased systematically with increasing velocity. A 75% increase in velocity resulted in a 67% increase in radial error.

These results are consistent with a recent experiment by Etnyre (1998). Again the task was dart throwing, but only two levels of speed were used: a normal speed and a maximal speed. Advanced, intermediate, and novice dart players varied more at the condition of maximal speed. The actual velocities of the throws were not measured, but variability in landing location increased by over 80% when darts were thrown at maximum speed. As expected, more experienced throwers were less variable, but there was no statistical interaction between skill level and throwing speed.

Studies on overhand and underarm throwing provide mixed results. Banuelos (1976) found speed-accuracy trade-offs consistent with the findings from dart throwing, while others have observed greater accuracy at intermediate speeds (Indermill & Husak, 1984) or that accuracy is not influenced by speed (Engelhorn, 1997). Indermill and Husak (1984) had participants throw tennis balls to a vertical target 40 ft (12.2 m) away. Throws were made at 50, 75, and 100% of the thrower's maximum velocity, and accuracy was measured from the center of the target. Throwing at an intermediate speed improved accuracy by 30% over the slower and maximum speeds. Using a training design, Engelhorn (1997) had 10- and 11-year-old girls practice fast-pitch softball throwing over 6 wk. One group of girls focused on accuracy and the other group focused on speed. At the end of 6 wk, the group focusing on speed threw 20% faster than the group focusing on accuracy, but both groups were equally accurate at hitting the target. When the throwers then switched emphases, the accuracy group was able to match the speed of the speed group, but its accuracy deteriorated. That is, there appeared to be a trade-off of accuracy for speed. When throwers from the speed group were told to focus on accuracy, they threw at the same speed as when they practiced, but their accuracy decreased! Unfortunately, a speed-accuracy trade-off cannot be assessed for this group because speed did not change with the switch to an emphasis on accuracy.

Speed and Variability in Striking

A few studies have examined speed-accuracy relations in striking activities. The tennis serve has been the most popular task, but other striking tasks have also been used, including a hockey shot and a task resembling a stroke in four-wall handball. The experimental procedures in these studies were similar to those used for throwing tasks. Speed was directly varied by specifying target speeds and providing feedback after trials or indirectly varied by instructing the performer to focus on speed or accuracy.

The tennis serve appears to be an ideal task for studying the relation between speed and accuracy. Players routinely adjust the speed of the ball on first and second serves. First serves have greater speed, but players are successful in hitting the ball into the proper service area about 40 to 70% of the time. Second serves have a greater focus on accuracy because a second missed serve results in a double fault and a point for the opponent. Second serves have a slower ball velocity and a much higher probability of landing in the proper court, typically greater than 90%. Of course players cannot reduce the speed of the serve too much, or their opponent will have an easy return and will usually win the point. A player with a very fast first serve may win as many as 80% of the points when the first serve is in but only 40% of the points played on the second serve.

Cauraugh, Gabert, and White (1990) directly varied serving speed in a study of skilled male and female tennis players. Maximum speeds ranged from 74 to 115 mi·h^{-1} (121-189 km·h^{-1}), and players were required to hit the ball at speeds of 50, 60, 70, 80, and 90% of their maximum speed. Players attempted to hit a point target at the intersection of the service line (the line running across the back end of the service court) and the center service line (the line that runs down the middle of the court and separates the two service areas). In contrast to the findings from studies on throwing tasks, there were no differences in the variability of ball landings or the variability of serve speeds. Unfortunately, data were only analyzed for the conditions of 70, 80, and 90%. By limiting the range of speeds, Cauraugh et al. ensured that players hit the ball with patterns of movement similar to those used during practice. The downside of this strategy is that the limited range of speeds makes it difficult to obtain a speed-variability function for this task. Consistent with the finding that the speed and accuracy of tennis serves are not related, Johnson (1957) found no correlation between serve speed and accuracy for skilled women players. In this study, speed was not experimentally varied and participants always hit first serves, and it appears that these correlations were possibly computed across subjects.

A lack of a speed-accuracy trade-off was also observed in two studies that trained participants under speed or accuracy instructions. In one, Southard (1989) studied an arm swing used to hit a stationary ball to a target, and in the other, Belkin and Eliot (1997) studied a hockey shot. Southard found that practice under speed instructions resulted in greater speed, with accuracy equal to participants trained under accuracy instructions. Belkin and Eliot obtained similar findings. Both the speed and accuracy groups completed a posttest with equal stress on speed and accuracy. Speed instructions increased speed but had no effect on accuracy.

The only evidence suggesting that increased speed may lead to poorer accuracy in striking tasks comes from a study by Atkinson and Speirs (1998) examining the effects of time of day on the performance of tennis serves. A significant negative correlation between speed and accuracy was found for first but not second serves. While there were no differences in accuracy between first and second serves early in the morning, first serves hit in the afternoon were less accurate than second serves. Racket velocity was greater for first serves at all times of day, but it was only measured in the anterior–posterior plane.

Summary

In throwing tasks, spatial accuracy is influenced by projection speed. The exact relation between speed and accuracy is not clear. In some studies increases in speed resulted in systematic decreases in accuracy (Etnyre, 1998; Gross & Gill, 1982), and in others accuracy was greatest at intermediate speeds (Indermill & Husak, 1984). Whether these differences are due to differences in task (both Etnyre and Gross & Gill used a dart throw and Indermill & Husak used a ball throw) or some other factor is not known. In contrast to the influence of speed on accuracy in throwing, speed does not typically affect spatial accuracy in studies on striking. It also appears that training participants for speed does not result in a loss of accuracy, at least not when participants perform under instructions for both speed and accuracy.

There are a number of limitations in previous studies of speed and accuracy in sport tasks. Most of the studies reviewed did not specifically measure variability, and only a few directly manipulated speed over a wide range. Statistical correlations between speed and accuracy calculated either between subjects or within subjects with emphasis on a single speed provide limited enlightenment on this issue. Differences in the tasks, the dimension in which accuracy or variability is measured, and the skill levels of the participants make general conclusions about the effect of speed on accuracy impossible.

Olympic Project

The findings from Cauraugh et al. (1990) indicated that increasing the speed of serves up to 90% of the player's maximum has no detrimental effect on accuracy. Why then do skilled tennis players hit the ball slower on second serves? We were interested in examining the speed-variability relation for world-class athletes, particularly tennis performers, and the techniques that players use to generate both fast and accurate serves. The competitive environment is ideal for such an investigation because performers systematically change the speed of the serve as the demands for accuracy change. Among elite performers, ball speeds for first serves are typically 25% faster than for second serves. While studying elite performers in a natural competitive environment has the advantage of providing information about the strategies used for coping with increased requirements for accuracy, the link to typical speed-accuracy laboratory manipulations is not perfect. In laboratory tasks performers are generally asked to produce the same basic action but at varying speeds. Variation in accuracy is assumed to be a function of change in speed rather than change in strategy. Changes in speed and accuracy for first and second serves may also relate to variations in the action pattern (Chow et al., 2003).

We were interested in observing performers during competition for two additional reasons. First, the possibility of several world-class men and women tennis players coming to our laboratory for testing seemed remote. Second, competitive conditions allow for an examination of how players actually perform, including how they adjust the speed and accuracy of their serves. Fortunately the International Olympic Committee (IOC) allows research projects to be conducted during the Olympic games if the research has applications for performance enhancement or injury reduction. The primary focus of the IOC Olympic Research Program is biomechanics, although any area of sport science is considered, and scientists from all over the world are eligible to apply. The program is administered through the IOC Subcommission on Biomechanics and Physiology, and it provides scientists access to Olympic venues and facilities for collecting data. However, investigators are not allowed direct access to the athletes.

We started our project by developing a model of the serve and the factors responsible for the location of ball landing (figure 5.3). Based on principles of projectile motion, the displacement of the ball from the time it leaves the player's racket to the time it lands on the court surface is determined by the location of the ball when it impacts the racket, the postimpact velocity (speed and direction) of the ball, gravitational forces, and fluid dynamics related to air resistance and ball spin (Magnus effect). The location of the ball at impact and the postimpact velocity of the ball are, for the most part, under the direct control of the server.

Ball Location at Impact

In general, players attempt to maximize the height of the ball as it impacts the racket. A greater height at impact allows the ball to clear the net and land in the court at a high velocity. When hit from a greater height, the ball can land shorter in the court and closer to the net, and this increases the range of locations for vertical landing in the service court. Short players, even if they were capable of hitting the serve at 140 mi·h⁻¹ (230 km·h⁻¹), would not be able to get the ball over the net and down to the ground because a) when the ball contacts the racket there is not a direct line of sight from it to the service line

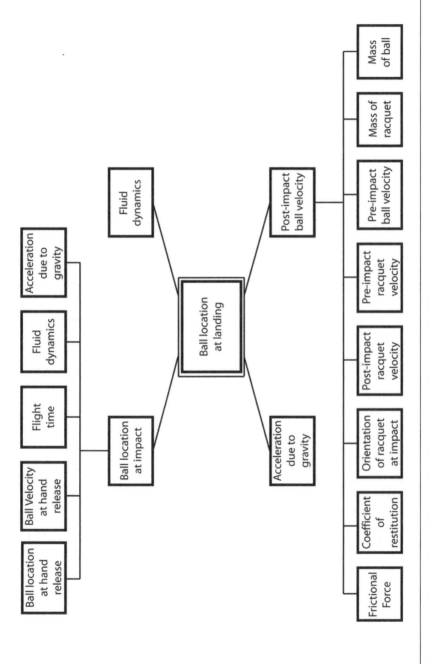

FIGURE 5.3   The mechanical factors that determine the location of ball landing in the tennis serve.

(the line of sight would go through the net), and b) due to the high speed there is insufficient time for gravity to drop the ball onto the court.

Postimpact Ball Velocity

In general, players attempt to hit the ball with high speed and to locate its landing toward one of the two corners of the service court. The postimpact velocity (direction and speed) of the ball is influenced by a variety of factors (figure 5.3). The server has direct control of the orientation of the racket at impact and of the pre- and postimpact velocities of the racket. The velocity of the racket includes anterior–posterior, vertical, and lateral components. First serves have greater anterior–posterior velocity while second serves are believed to have reduced anterior–posterior velocity but greater vertical and lateral velocities (Groppel, 1984). The server has some control over the preimpact velocity of the ball, but this factor seems to minimally affect the landing location of the ball.

It appears from observation that most intermediate tennis players achieve a higher success rate for second serves by slowing down their swing. A slower speed reduces force output and leads to reduced variability in the force produced. The direct effect is lower variability in the speed produced and potentially lower variability in the distance the ball is hit—a speed-accuracy trade-off. It is generally believed that highly skilled performers do not slow their swing between first and second serves (e.g., Groppel, 1984), but there are little data from competitive conditions to determine what players actually do during a tennis match. One of the goals of the Olympic project was to examine how elite performers adjust the velocities of the ball and racket and how these changes in velocity influence variability during competition.

Data Collection

The data were collected at the stadium court of the Stone Mountain Tennis Center in Atlanta, Georgia, during the 1996 Summer Olympic Games. The playing surface was hard court. The most popular matches were often scheduled on this court and as a result data were gathered on many of the top players and some of the best servers in the world. Data were gathered on 14 players: 7 males and 7 females. Five of the female and 3 of the male players had a current world ranking of 14 or higher. Top players competing on the stadium court included Monica Seles, Conchita Martinez, Lindsay Davenport, Arantxa Sanchez Vicario, Gabriela Sabatini, Andre Agassi, Goran Ivanisevic, Thomas Enquist, and MaliVai Washington.

The landing location of the serve, the speed of the ball, and the three-dimensional kinematics of the serving motion were recorded. Landing locations were recorded by an experienced line judge on a court-scaled form, and speed was recorded from a radar gun operated by the court staff and displayed at courtside. Landing locations were verified using a SVHS camera placed at one end of the court along the center service line at a height of 10 m. The actual size of the service box was used for spatial reference, and landing locations were digitized for subsequent analysis. Two high-speed (200 Hz) video cameras, one located next to the SVHS camera and one 23 m to the right, were used to record serves hit from the right, or deuce, side of one end of the court. The preimpact velocity of the racket was determined from high-speed video recordings by using standard techniques for 3-D motion analysis. The number of serves completed for analysis of landing location and the number recorded for kinematic analysis varied by match. The minimum number of serves completed by each player in a two-set match is 24. Half of these serves are to the right (deuce) court and half are to the left (ad) court. Because kinematic patterns were recorded from only one end of the court on the deuce side, the potential number of serves for analyses was reduced by 75%. Lighting conditions, intermittent rain, and other technical problems associated with field-based research significantly reduced the number of serves where information on the preimpact velocity of the racket was available.

Location of Ball Landing

The mean and standard deviation of ball landing location were computed. Both the depth of serve (anterior-posterior location) and serve direction (lateral location) were analyzed. Radial error, the absolute deviation between each serve's landing location and the server's point of aim, was also analyzed. Unfortunately, the players did not tell us where they were aiming before each serve. However, the observed distribution of the landing locations suggests that players aimed for one of two court locations. The point of aim varied for each player and also depended on the side of the court the performer was serving and whether the serve was a first or second serve. Consistent with this description, the locations of ball landing for the top-seeded men's (figure 5.4) and women's (figure 5.5) players were distributed into two sectors representing the two corners of the service box. While it is possible that players varied their aim within these two sectors, two factors suggest that they did not, or if they did, the change they made was very small. First, the landing distributions themselves suggest that the players did not have precise enough control to vary their point of aim on each trial. For example, first serves hit to the left of the deuce court (as viewed by the server) were wide and long by as much as 1 m. Even if the server was aiming directly for the singles sideline (the line marking the outside edge of the service box), the distribution of the lateral landing locations would vary by 2 m, assuming a normal distribution of locations to the left and right of the point of aim. A 2 m deviation in lateral landing location encompasses most of the measured landing locations in each sector. Second, previous research examining the accuracy of first serves for skilled players (Johnson, 1957) found the range of landing locations to be as much as 12 ft (3.66 m) in lateral direction and 18 ft (5.5 m) in depth or anterior–posterior location. The distributions in the present data were well within this range.

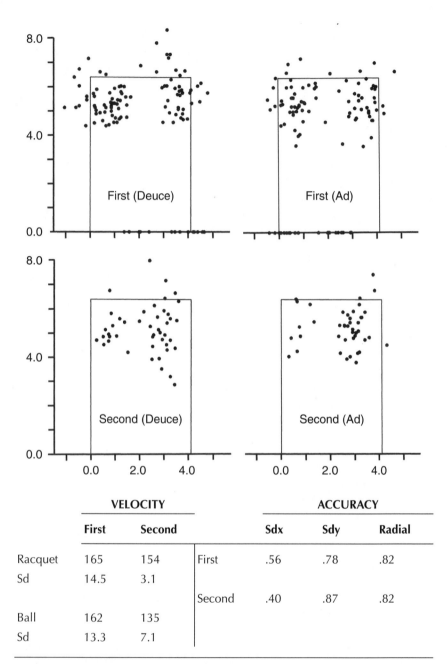

	VELOCITY			ACCURACY		
	First	**Second**		**Sdx**	**Sdy**	**Radial**
Racquet	165	154	First	.56	.78	.82
Sd	14.5	3.1				
			Second	.40	.87	.82
Ball	162	135				
Sd	13.3	7.1				

FIGURE 5.4   Locations of ball landing for the number one seeded men's competitor at the 1996 Olympic Games. The 0.0, 0.0 coordinate marks the intersection of the net and the border of the left service box (as viewed by the server). The units are in meters. The means and variabilities of selected velocity and accuracy measures are presented in the lower portion of the figure.

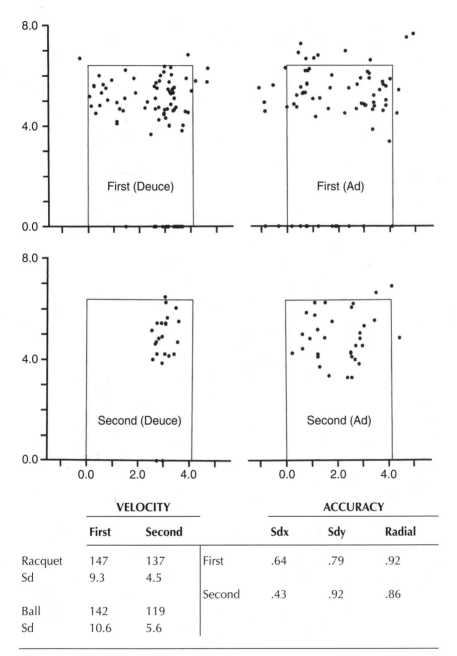

FIGURE 5.5   Locations of ball landing for the number one seeded women's competitor at the 1996 Olympic Games. The 0.0, 0.0 coordinate marks the intersection of the net and the border of the left service box (as viewed by the server). The units are in meters. The means and variabilities of selected velocity and accuracy measures are presented in the lower portion of the figure.

An examination of landing locations in figures 5.4 and 5.5 suggests that the width of the landing distribution was greater for first serves but that the distributions of serve lengths were similar between first and second serves. The data from all 14 servers are summarized in table 5.1. The average landing location in each sector, or the assumed point of aim, varied systematically for first and second serves. Mean landing areas for second serves were consistently more toward the middle of the court than areas of first serves. The mean landing

TABLE 5.1   Mean Spatial Landing Locations and Spatial Variability for First and Second Serves

	FIRST SERVES				SECOND SERVES			
	DEUCE		AD		DEUCE		AD	
	Left	Right	Left	Right	Left	Right	Left	Right
Males								
X (m)	0.69	3.54	0.73	3.62	1.05	3.11	1.14	2.98
SD	0.61	0.48	0.53	0.54	0.47	0.31	0.39	0.39
Y (m)	5.71	5.86	5.81	5.85	5.02	4.94	5.03	4.85
SD	0.77	0.86	0.84	0.79	0.90	0.67	0.61	0.61
RE (m)	0.85	0.82	0.85	0.79	0.85	0.62	0.66	0.62
Females								
X (m)	0.66	3.08	0.84	3.37	1.19	2.91	1.28	3.07
SD	0.65	0.61	0.54	0.64	0.38	0.41	0.48	0.53
Y (m)	5.41	5.59	5.64	5.66	5.17	5.01	4.88	5.03
SD	0.84	0.80	0.90	0.93	0.89	0.89	0.62	0.84
RE(m)	0.94	0.87	0.77	0.96	0.66	0.83	0.49	0.83

	FIRST SERVES COMBINED					SECOND SERVES COMBINED				
	Left	Right	Left	Right	Mean	Left	Right	Left	Right	Mean
X (m)	0.67	3.31	0.79	3.50		1.12	3.01	1.21	3.02	
SD	0.63	0.54	0.53	0.59	0.57	0.43	0.36	0.43	0.46	0.42
Y (m)	5.56	5.72	5.72	5.75	5.68	5.09	4.98	4.96	4.95	4.97
SD	0.80	0.83	0.87	0.86	0.85	0.90	0.79	0.61	0.72	0.81
RE (m)	0.90	0.84	0.81	0.87	0.87	0.75	0.74	0.57	0.72	0.73

Note: All locations are referenced from the intersection of the net and the center service line (middle of the court). The service line (back edge of the service box) is 6.4 m from the net, and the outside edge of the service box is 4.12 m from the center service line. X = lateral location, Y = anterior-posterior location, RE = radial error.

location of serves hit to the right in the add court (to a right-handed opponent's backhand), for example, was located 0.6 m from the sideline for first serves and 1.1 m from the sideline for second serves. The serve landed short of the service line by an average of 0.72 m for first serves and 1.43 m for second serves.

The variability of lateral landing locations was consistently smaller for second serves. This trend was observed in 13 of the 14 players. On average, second serves were 29% less variable in the direction of the serve. However, there were no meaningful differences in the variability of depth (anterior–posterior landing location) between first and second serves. Of the 14 players, 8 were more variable in depth on the first serve and 6 were more variable on the second serve. The reduced variability in direction on second serves decreased the radial error for second serves by 16%. On average, women players tended to vary slightly more in both direction and depth than men players, and landing locations were slightly closer to the lines for men players. Radial errors were 11% greater for women players. One limitation of using the tennis serve is that a percentage of the serves hit the net and so those landing locations were not recorded. The effect these unrecorded locations on the distribution of landing locations is not clear. More first serves hit the net than second serves, and this difference might artificially reduce the variability in landing location for first serves.

Ball and Racket Speeds

The speeds of the ball and racket as functions of type of serve, landing sector, and gender are presented in table 5.2. As expected, the speed of the ball on first serves (161 km·h⁻¹) was significantly greater than that on second serves (128 km·h⁻¹), and men served faster than women on both first (22% faster) and second (15% faster) serves. Even though there were large differences in the speed of the ball between first and second serves, the speed of the racket was very similar. As expected, the speed of the racket was greater for men than women for both first (23% faster) and second (20% faster) serves. The data on racket speed should be regarded with some caution because data were only available for 9 servers and for only a few trials for each player.

The increased speed of the ball for first serves was associated with increased variability. For both first and second serves the standard deviation (SD) of ball velocity was approximately 5% of the mean speed of the serve. This figure is quite low considering that players appear to change speed as part of their strategies. Players sometimes hit first serves with kinematic patterns and ball speeds consistent with second serves. Like in the speed of the ball, variability in the speed of the racket was greater for first serves, and variability scores for men and women were nearly identical. The limited number of trials available for analysis makes interpreting these scores tenuous. More data were available for the top-seeded players because they played more matches on the stadium court. The data for these players are included in figures 5.4 and 5.5. Consistent

TABLE 5.2   Mean Speeds and Speed Variability of the Ball and Racket (km·h⁻¹) for First and Second Serves

	FIRST SERVES				SECOND SERVES			
	DEUCE		AD		DEUCE		AD	
	Left	Right	Left	Right	Left	Right	Left	Right
Males								
Ball	173	185	182	171	136	145	142	129
SD	8	8	8	10	8	7	5	7
Racket	200	163	182	166	160	154	157	156
SD	20	25	22	22	5	20	16	17
Females								
Ball	140	148	150	139	127	119	120	113
SD	7	9	8	9	5	8	9	6
Racket	139	133	136	135	130	132	131	131
SD	6	13	9	10	6	4	4	4

	FIRST SERVES COMBINED					SECOND SERVES COMBINED				
	Left	Right	Left	Right	Mean	Left	Right	Left	Right	Mean
Ball	156	166	166	155	161	132	132	131	121	128
SD	7	8	8	9	8	7	7	6	6	6
Racket	159	143	151	146	146	142	141	140	140	140
SD	12	18	15	15	15	5	10	9	9	9

with the overall results for all subjects, the speed of the racket was slightly slower on second serves and variability was smaller, mirroring the variability changes in the speed of the ball.

Olympic Project and Speed-Accuracy Trade-Offs

In some respects, the data from the Olympic competitors are startling. While it is assumed that second serves in tennis are significantly more accurate and less variable than first serves, the data suggest that this is not the case for the depth of serve. The depth was equally variable for both serves. This is significant because variability in depth (anterior–posterior landing location) appears to be much more important for serve success. Only 2% of the second serves analyzed in this study were missed because they landed too wide, and variability in depth was five times more likely to cause a second serve to be missed. The first serves that were missed followed the same pattern, with 70% of them due to variability in depth.

Then why are players so accurate in hitting second serves, hitting over 90% into the proper service area, when they are able to get in only about 60% of their first serves? The answer appears to relate to changes in the patterns of movement for the two serves and to a change in the point of aim. In comparison to first serves, second serves are hit with greater vertical and lateral racket velocity and less anterior-posterior velocity (Chow et al., 2003). This puts greater topspin on the ball, and the ball is hit at a higher projection angle with respect to the horizontal. Thus, in the second serve the ball is hit higher, with more topspin, and with less forward velocity. The greater projection angle allows the ball to clear the net and the reduced speed and greater topspin allow the ball to fall into the court at a shorter distance from the net. This can clearly be seen in the mean landing positions of first and second serves; second serves landed 0.78 m closer to the net. The servers' variation in movement pattern between first and second serves results in similar distributions of landing depths for first and second serves, only the distribution for second serves is closer to the net. It appears that players are adept at manipulating factors related to the location of ball landing (see figure 5.3) and do so to maximize the probability of winning a point.

Similar variability in depth between first and second serves might not be surprising given that the speed of the swing is similar between serves. While the forward velocity was lower for second serves, possibly leading to less variability, the vertical and horizontal velocities were higher. The increased velocities in these dimensions might lead to greater variability and counteract the advantage gained by reduced variability in the forward dimension.

In second serves, the speed of ball was 25% slower than in first serves, and radial errors were smaller for second serves mostly due to reduced variability in ball direction. Directional variability for tasks involving projectiles has not been studied extensively. In studying a throwing task, Banuelos (1976) found that throwers had greater directional accuracy when given instructions to be accurate rather than fast and accurate. Directional variability has received little theoretical attention. Models of variability in throwing, for example, have focused on variability in distance (Dupuy et al., 2000) or height (Mueller et al., 1998). This is probably because variability tends to be greater in the distance or height dimension, such as with throwing tasks and aimed movements of the hand to targets (e.g., Mueller & Loosch, 1999). This pattern is also true for tennis serves (e.g., Johnson, 1957; present data). Studies for variability of force production have focused on the magnitude of force produced and its variability (for an exception, see Schmidt & Sherwood, 1982). A recent study of variability in force direction conducted in our laboratory and with a task involving two-joint leg extension (Vandermeulen Luyt, 2002) found that variability in force direction was independent of the amount of force produced.

Even in this study, variability was measured in the vertical plane, or in height, rather than in the lateral dimension.

The Olympic Games, like other international competitions, test the skill of highly practiced performers. Those with greater skill are able to perform tasks with greater speed and accuracy than players who are less skilled. Previous studies of tennis serving (e.g., Johnson, 1957) have found that players with the highest serve velocities did not tend to be more variable. Similarly, in studies involving training under instructions for speed or for both speed and accuracy, typically subjects following instructions for speed increase speed while maintaining accuracy (Belkin & Eliot, 1997; Engelhorn, 1997; Southard, 1989). In the Olympic project, players in the men's competition hit serves with greater speed and less variability than the serves of their women counterparts. The question that these examples raise is whether or not such findings are true examples of deviations from speed-accuracy trade-offs. Our opinion is that they are not and that they instead reflect differences in skill as it is typically defined (e.g., Guthrie, 1935). Our observation is that even in aimed movements of the hand, there are some individuals that are both faster and more accurate than others, but these individuals still conform to speed-accuracy trade-offs.

Very little is known about the effect of long-term practice on variability in movement. Moderate practice leads to reduced but persistent variability (Norrie, 1967), but the amount of practice used in experimental studies is trivial compared to that completed by skilled sport performers. Skilled performers in Olympic tennis, for example, have completed hundreds of thousands of serves and have perfected swings that meet the accuracy demands of the task while giving the ball incredibly high speed. Could these performers be less variable if they slowed their swings? It is unlikely that we will answer this question by monitoring performance under competitive conditions. The cost of reducing speed—a more effective return by the opponent—is too great for players to employ this strategy. More research with elite performers, under both performance and experimental conditions, is necessary to unravel the link between practice and speed-accuracy trade-offs.

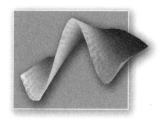

Chapter 6

Genetic and Environmental Constraints on Variability in Sport Performance

Joseph Baker, PhD and Keith Davids, PhD

Editors' Overview

Why do some athletes benefit more than others from training and practice? A frequent observation of interindividual variation in response to training and practice raises important theoretical and practical questions about the nature of genetic and environmental constraints on skill acquisition and performance. This problem is a manifestation of the long-standing debate of nature versus nurture, which argues the precise proportion of performance variation in a population accounted for by genetic characteristics or environmental influences. The relationship between genetic and environmental constraints on responses to practice and training is complex, requiring a careful interpretation of the data in the extant literature and a comprehensive theoretical model to explain research findings. In this chapter, the theories of practice emphasizing the role of environmental constraints in explaining variability in expertise are evaluated, and the evidence favoring the role of genetic constraints in variability of interindividual responsiveness to training and practice is examined. The biological determinism underlying some recent interpretations of the roles of genetic diversity and environmental context on variation in human motor performance is rejected for an interactive model that is captured well by dynamic systems theory. The challenges for future research on the interacting constraints of genetics and environment are (1) to locate the primary and secondary influences on performance and (2) to understand the dimensions of their interactions in order to improve practical intervention programs such as those dedicated to talent identification and development.

What governs an athlete's response to training and practice? Are elite performance institutes justified in putting large amounts of funding into genetic testing of athletes to micro-manage personalized training programs? (Dennis, 2005). The frequent observation of interindividual variations in responsiveness to training and practice raises important theoretical and practical questions like these on the genetic and environmental constraints on skill acquisition and performance. How these constraints shape variations in performance is of increasing interest in psychology, physical education, movement science, biology, and sports medicine, and in this chapter we examine current theory and data on environmental and genetic influences on expertise and performance. This issue is manifested in the long-standing debate of nature versus nurture, which seeks to identify the precise proportion in which genetic characteristics and environmental influences contribute to variation in performance. Much has been written about this particular dualism, and resolving the debate has proved difficult (for excellent analyses see Lewontin, 2000 and Johnston & Edwards, 2002).

The relationship between genetic and environmental constraints on responses to practice and training is a complex issue that requires careful interpretation of the data in extant literature and a comprehensive theoretical model to explain research findings. We begin this chapter by evaluating theories of practice that emphasize environmental constraints in explaining variability in achieving expertise. We then examine the evidence that favors the role of genetic constraints on performance variability. We conclude by outlining the theory of dynamic systems as a powerful explanatory framework for interpreting the interactional influences of genetic diversity and environmental context on variation in human motor performance.

Nurture Perspective of Expertise Development: Deliberate Practice

One of the most radical perspectives regarding the role of practice in performance variation is the framework of deliberate practice presented by Ericsson and colleagues (Ericsson, Krampe, & Tesch-Römer, 1993). They proposed that individual differences in performance in any domain can be accounted for by the amount and type of practice previously performed. Likewise, they suggested that genetics play a minimal role in determining individual achievement and that this role can be circumvented by optimal amounts of quality practice. While many presumptions of this theory remain to be proven, deliberate practice is largely based on two previously observed guidelines: the 10-year rule (Simon & Chase, 1973) and the power law of practice (A. Newell & Rosenbloom, 1981).

The 10-Year Rule

In their classic study of chess expertise, Simon and Chase (1973; Chase & Simon, 1973) made the first suggestion that interindividual variation in performance can be explained by quantity and quality of training. This hypothesis was based on findings indicating that differences between expert (grand master) and lower (master and novice) levels of skill were attributable to the ability to organize information into more meaningful chunks rather than to a superior memory. Since then, researchers examining experts and novices have found no reliable differences in static, physical capacities such as visual acuity, reaction time, or memory (hardware) but have found consistent differences in domain-specific strategies for information processing (software) (for a review see Starkes, Helsen, & Jack, 2001). In a recent overview of the last 30 years of research on expertise in sport, Singer and Janelle (1999) summarized the characteristics that distinguish the expert:

1. Experts have greater task-specific knowledge (McPherson, 1993; McPherson & French, 1991).
2. Experts interpret greater meaning from available information (Abernethy, 1987; 1990; 1991).
3. Experts store and access information more effectively (McPherson, 1993).
4. Experts are better at detecting and recognizing structured patterns of play (Allard & Starkes 1980; Chase & Simon, 1973).
5. Experts are better at using situational probability data (Abernethy & Russell 1984; 1987).
6. Experts make decisions that are more rapid and appropriate (A.M. Williams, 2000).

In sport, research examining interindividual variation in cognitive abilities has been somewhat limited to sports and physical activities with dynamic task constraints demanding a high level of decision making. However, existing evidence suggests that in fields where the distinguishing characteristics between experts and nonexperts are domain-specific abilities in information processing, these differences result from training rather than innate ability. An interesting question is the role of other genetic constraints, such as differences in power or endurance, which we examine later in this chapter.

The 10-year rule stipulates that a 10-year commitment to high levels of training is the minimum requirement to become an expert. This 'rule' has been retrospectively applied to the study of expert careers, with some success in domains such as music (Ericsson, Krampe, & Tesch-Römer, 1993; Hayes, 1981; Sosniak, 1985), mathematics (Gustin, 1985), swimming (Kalinowski, 1985), distance running (Wallingford, 1975), and tennis (Monsaas, 1985).

The perspective of deliberate practice (Ericsson et al., 1993) extends the work of Simon and Chase (1973) by suggesting that it is not simply any training that differentiates individual performance, but engagement in deliberate practice. By definition, deliberate practice is not intrinsically motivating, it requires effort and attention, and it does not lead to immediate social or financial rewards. Further, involvement in deliberate practice depends on the learner accessing effective resources (facilities, coaches, financial support), providing the necessary physical and mental intensity for progressively adapting to appropriate training loads and possessing the ability to maintain involvement without intrinsic forms of motivation such as enjoyment. In the framework of deliberate practice, future experts perform training that develops required skills under continuously evolving conditions in which stress and recovery are optimally balanced to maximize training adaptations and minimize training plateaus.

Power Law of Practice

Research examining the accumulated effects of prolonged practice and the rate of learning has suggested that performance increases monotonically according to a power function. This finding, known as the power law of practice (or the log–log linear learning law) (A. Newell & Rosenbloom, 1981), has been demonstrated in numerous domains. According to the power law of practice, learning occurs rapidly at the start of practice, but this rate of learning decreases over time as practice continues (see figure 6.1).

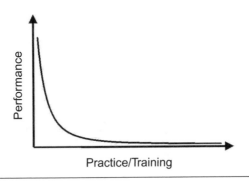

FIGURE 6.1 Example of the power law of practice for performance on a response time task.

Central to the notion of deliberate practice is the *monotonic benefits assumption.* Ericsson et al. (1993) proposed that, contrary to the power law of practice, a monotonic relationship exists between the number of hours of deliberate practice performed and the performance level achieved. Their original research with musicians indicated that the difference between expert and nonexpert pianists and violinists was the amount of time spent practicing while alone (i.e., deliberate practice). The best musicians had spent at least 10,000 h practicing alone while their less successful counterparts had spent no more than 7,000 h.

Ericsson et al. further argued that it is not simply the accumulation of hours of deliberate practice that leads to superior performance. The accumulation of such hours must coincide with crucial biological and cognitive development. Early specialization is an important element predisposing future success. Figure 6.2 illustrates the relationship of chronological age, time spent in deliberate practice, and performance. Performers beginning deliberate practice at later ages (performers b and c), even with the same commitment to training, are unable to match the quantity of training accumulated by performers starting

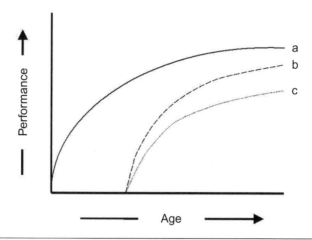

FIGURE 6.2   Relationship of chronological age, performance, and hours of deliberate practice.

From K.A. Ericsson, R.T. Krampe, and C. Tesch-Römer, 1993, "The role of deliberate practice in the acquisition of expert performance," *Psychological Review* 100 (3): 363-406. Copyright © 1993 by the American Psychological Association. Reprinted with permission..

earlier (performer a). The assumption that future experts must specialize early becomes increasingly important in sports where peak performances typically occur at younger ages (e.g., diving, gymnastics, and figure skating for women), although the necessity for early specialization in sports where peak performance occurs later (e.g., basketball, field hockey) has recently been questioned (Baker, 2003; Baker, Cote, & Abernethy, 2003a).

Deliberate Practice in Sport

Although the theory of deliberate practice was developed through research with musicians, Ericsson and colleagues have indicated that it should also apply to expertise in sport (Ericsson et al., 1993; Ericsson, 1996). To date, researchers examining the theory of deliberate practice in sports have investigated figure skating (Starkes, Deakin, Allard, Hodges, & Hayes, 1996), karate (Hodge & Deakin, 1998), wrestling (Hodges & Starkes, 1996), soccer (Helsen, Starkes, & Hodges, 1998), middle distance running (Young & Salmela, 2002), field hockey (Baker et al., 2003a; Helsen et al., 1998), triathlon (Baker, Deakin & Cote, 2005; Hodges, Kerr, Starkes, Weir, & Nananidou, 2004), basketball (Baker et al., 2003a), and netball (Baker et al., 2003a). These studies have encountered some problems with applying the original framework of deliberate practice to the sport domain. For example, Starkes and colleagues (Helsen et al., 1998; Hodges & Starkes, 1996) found that athletes tended to rate relevant practice activities as very enjoyable and intrinsically motivating, contrasting with a key component of the definition of deliberate practice. Further, there is concern regarding which forms of athletic training constitute deliberate practice. In the original work of Ericsson et al. (1993), only practicing while alone met the requirements for deliberate practice. In studies of deliberate practice in sport, there are few, if any, training activities that meet the original criteria set in the definition by Ericsson et al. (1993). Helsen et al. (1998) suggested that the specifications for deliberate practice in sport should be extended to include all relevant forms of training. This is particularly important in team sports where both individual and team practices increase skill and improve performance.

The relationship between hours spent in practice and attainment is typically consistent with the tenets of deliberate practice. Expert athletes accumulated more hours of training than nonexperts (Helsen et al., 1998; Starkes et al., 1996; Hodge & Deakin, 1998). Not only do experts spend more time in practice, but they also devote more time to the specific activities deemed as being the most relevant to developing the essential component skills for expert performance. For example, Baker, Côté, and Abernethy (2003b) found that expert athletes from basketball, netball, and field hockey accumulated significantly more hours in video training, competition, organized team practices, and one-on-one coaching than nonexpert athletes.

Deliberate Practice and Interindividual Variation in Performance

The essence of the perspective of deliberate practice seems to be "all individuals are created equal." In a review of studies on skill acquisition and learning, Ericsson (1996) concluded that, with few exceptions, the level of performance was determined by the amount of time spent performing a "well defined task with an appropriate difficulty level for the particular individual, informative feedback, and opportunities for repetition and corrections of errors" (p. 20-21). Continually modifying the task difficulty allows future experts to perpetuate adaptations to greater training stress. Informative feedback and opportunity for repetition allow the performer to master skills more easily and to progress more quickly.

Data from the Ericsson et al. (1993) study of expert musicians support the relationship between hours of deliberate practice and level of performance. Specifically, the study found that expert musicians spend in excess of 25 h/wk in deliberate practice (training alone) whereas less successful musicians spend considerably less time in deliberate practice (amateurs spend <2 h/wk). These notable differences in weekly hours accumulate to enormous divisions after years of training. Similar relationships have been found in chess (Charness, Krampe, & Myr, 1996). Prior research on the training histories of athletes and the characteristics that distinguish individual athletes provides evidence for the powerful role of appropriate training in building the expert sport performer.

Influence of Other Activities

Recently, researchers have provided evidence that challenges one of the basic tenets of the theory of deliberate practice, specifically, that early specialization is necessary for the development of expertise. Baker et al. (2003a) studied experts from field hockey, basketball, and netball and found that these players performed a wide range of sports during early stages of development. As the athletes developed, their broad involvement in sports gradually decreased until they specialized in their main sport (figure 6.3). Moreover, Baker et al. (2003a) reported a negative correlation between the number of other sports played and the number of sport-specific training hours performers required before making their respective national teams. These findings suggest that participation in indirectly related activities may augment the physical and cognitive skills necessary for an athlete's primary sport. For example, many of the athletes participated in various forms of football (including rugby, Aussie rules, and touch football), a sport that also requires dynamic, time-constrained decision making as well as physical elements such as cardiovascular fitness and coordination.

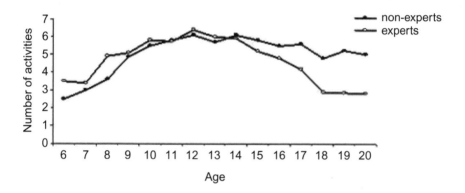

FIGURE 6.3   The number of sporting activities performed each year by experts and nonexperts from basketball, netball, and field hockey.

From P.A. Kolers, 1975 "Memorial consequences of automatized encoding," *Journal of Experimental Psychology: Human Learning and Memory* 1: 689-701. Copyright © 1975 by the American Psychological Association. Reprinted with permission.

Research by Côté (1999; Côté & Hay, 2002) has indicated that playlike activities (termed *deliberate play*) during the early stages of training benefit expertise development in many sports. Deliberate play represents the antithesis of deliberate practice in that it is made up of activities designed for enjoyment that require active and pleasurable participation. In early development, activities that are inherently enjoyable and motivating may be necessary to provide an impetus to continue training when more diligent, effortful practice is required. Without this pleasurable involvement, athletes may drop out of sport (Petlichkoff, 1993).

The above relationships are not unexpected. During early stages of development, improvement comes rapidly and easily because there is so much room for it. During this time, it is likely that any form of relevant participation provides improvement, regardless of whether this participation is direct involvement through sport-specific training or indirect involvement through sports that share basic characteristics. However, as performance improves, enhancement becomes increasingly difficult until focused training on specific areas of weakness becomes the only means of advancement. At this point, deliberate practice becomes the most effective form of training (see Baker, 2003 for a more thorough review).

Challenges of Deliberate Practice

Despite the evidence favoring environmental effects on responses to practice and training, the issues in the nature/nurture area are enormously complex. In her thought-provoking paper on the theory of deliberate practice in sport, Starkes (2000) raised some important questions regarding the relationship between expertise and responsiveness to training and practice. Starkes' examination of the data on the elusive element of athletic success attempted to contrast two theories purporting to explain athletic achievement: the sport commitment model of Scanlan and colleagues (Scanlan, Carpenter, Schmidt, Simons & Keeler, 1993) and the theory of deliberate practice (Ericsson et al., 1993). Despite the arguments proposed by these researchers, both theories end with the feeling of "the chicken or the egg." For example, the sport commitment model provides few indications of whether the commitment required of performers of international caliber is developed or is predominantly inherited. There seems a hopeless correlation among the innate factors influencing the propensity to enjoy sport and the willingness to invest time and effort into countless hours of practice and the influence of positive learning experiences (which the coach can do much to foster).

Deliberate Practice and Intraindividual Variability in Performance

K.M. Newell and McDonald (1991) have argued that practice is a necessary but not sufficient condition for developing motor expertise. Traditional approaches to practice have tended to overemphasize the amount of required time to be spent in practice to the detriment of understanding how the quality of specific practice activities affects expertise. For example, earlier in this chapter we noted how the theory of deliberate practice is grounded in the power law of learning. Despite the fact that the power law has been called "the ubiquitous law of learning" (A. Newell & Rosenbloom, 1981, p. 2), there has been recent criticism of this view, particularly as it relates to intraindividual variability in performance.

K.M. Newell, Liu, and Mayer-Kress (2001) have pointed out that performance can change in persistent and transitory ways as a function of learning and development and that previous research has emphasized identifying persistent changes rather than transitory changes. A number of variables can be used to assess intraindividual change in performance over time, but task outcome has been the main variable used in studying learning curves. The power law of learning has been the generally accepted law of learning primarily because data from two of the best-known studies on learning, one by Crossman (1959) and one by Snoddy (1926), fit the power law well. The power law of learning has had some passionate advocates, including Logan (1988), for example, who advocated that any theory providing data that do not fit the power law should be immediately rejected.

But, as K.M. Newell et al. (2001) have indicated, careful analysis of the data from Crossman (1959) (late in practice) and Snoddy (1926) (early in practice) shows occasional significant departures from the power law. The notion that there may be many functions of change over time supports a broad vision of the factors that can influence change. K.M. Newell and colleagues (2001) criticized two main methodological practices: (a) blocking trials and (b) averaging scores over participants in studies of intraindividual change as a function of learning and development. Trial blocks and averaging scores over individuals ignore the fact that laws of learning should reflect both transitory and persistent changes, whereas the power law treats transitory effects as random behavior, possibly masking the persistent trends in intraindividual variations. Traditionally, this behavior has been viewed as the result of noise or effects such as the warm-up decrement (the result of early trials within a session that bring the performer back up to the stable performance point reached in earlier practice). K.M. Newell et al. (2001) admit that it is not clear to what extent averaging practices has affected the data on learning, but future research clearly needs to consider how ubiquitous the power law of learning actually is. Another point is that most experiments on motor learning have been conducted with a span of a few hours at most. Using a short duration for measuring learning and coming up with learning curves naturally limits the range of curves that can be exhibited by learners. Hence there is an inherent methodological bias that predisposes outcomes toward the curve of the power law. That is, in real life several functions of change can emerge in learning curves from multiple timescales of motor learning.

In contrast, the timescale of transitory change during learning is much shorter than that of the persistent changes. But these variations should not be dismissed as random or as the result of noise (K.M. Newell et al., 2001). Changes in the outcome of action over time are the product of many interacting subsystems, each with its own timescale that is continuously evolving over real time. Contrary to the power law edict that larger absolute gains in performance occur early in learning before tailing off, the greatest absolute changes in learning may occur any time during practice, particularly if the performer is learning a new pattern of coordination. The longer a performer has been practicing, the more likely there will be sudden discontinuous jumps in learning due to developmental changes occurring over the life span. Exponential learning curves are most likely to be found in the learning of simple motor tasks such as the linear positioning and timing tasks of laboratories. This is because new patterns of coordination do not need to be learned and qualitatively new patterns do not need to be picked up.

To summarize, this criticism of the traditional literature is reflected by the assumption of monotonic benefits proposed by Ericsson and colleagues (1993). The theory of deliberate practice places a narrow emphasis on the main constraints of time and effort spent practicing, regardless of how much innate ability the performer brings to a learning situation or of the nature of the activities that take place during practice (Ericsson, 1996; Ericsson & Charness, 1994; Ericsson & Lehmann, 1996; Ericsson et al., 1993). Starkes (2000) argued that this emphasis on a limited number of constraints leads to "a very environmentalist theory", and the implication is that the constraints on skill acquisition may range far wider than implied by the theory of deliberate practice (Davids, 2000). Sternberg (1996) has highlighted the fact that the current version of the theory of deliberate practice ignores the issue of genetic constraints; is difficult to disconfirm because its operational definitions are weak; has confounded talent, motivation, and level of practice; and has no strong experimental work involving control groups.

It is clear that acquiring expertise in sport takes time, although the time and amount of deliberate practice should not be viewed as the only constraints on skill acquisition. The overarching theoretical question is: In what mechanisms does interindividual variability in performance manifest itself? For example, the issues of hereditary influences, such as baseline differences in motivation, should not be ignored merely because the work in this area is ongoing and currently inconclusive. A perspective led by constraints proposes that there are many route maps to a high level of performance. All in all, these arguments suggest that a major focus of research should be on understanding the differences among top athletes rather than on overemphasizing perceived commonalities, such as time and amount of practice, that influence the acquisition of expert skill in movement (Davids, 2000).

Perhaps the most critical challenge facing proponents of the theory of deliberate practice concerns the role of genes in constraining responsiveness to prolonged training and practice. Regarding possible innate qualities that may predispose an individual to successful performance in a domain, Ericsson and colleagues have conceded only one quality—height—as being beyond circumvention through deliberate practice. Further, Ericsson et al. (1993) provided evidence that several characteristics thought to be innate were in fact trainable. For example, while the ability to distinguish and name the 64 notes in music, referred to as perfect pitch, is difficult for adults to acquire, it is relatively easy for children to attain (Takeuchi & Hulse, 1993). This finding lends support to the assumption of Ericsson et al. that proper training at appropriate times of development is crucial to expert performance. Moreover, Ericsson et al. (1993) suggested that physiological parameters could also be modified through deliberate practice. Research indicating that endurance athletes develop a cardiovascular adaptation known as athletic heart syndrome (George, Wolfe, & Burggraf, 1991) that reverts to near normal when training has stopped may denote the influence of training rather than genetic predisposition.

In the remainder of this chapter we examine the evidence for genetic constraints on performance variability. Numerous genes that contribute to variability in performance are being identified in the literature on molecular biology and exercise and sport physiology (for reviews see Davids, Glazier, Araújo, & Bartlett, 2003; Frederiksen & Christensen, 2003). Although certain general traits have been linked to heritability (e.g., intelligence) (T.J. Bouchard, 1997), it is widely accepted that the refinement of these traits into domain-specific abilities (e.g., pattern recognition, strategic thinking) occurs through exposure to optimal preparation in specific environments. There is little evidence to support the idea that there is a single gene predisposing an athlete to superior performance in a specific domain (e.g., a gene for hand-eye coordination or a genetic predisposition to play ball games), and the application of this idea has begun to occur in support services for elite sports performance (Dennis, 2005).

Genetic Constraints on Physical Performance

The search for the genetic basis of many human capacities such as physical performance has engendered strong arguments in the literature, with some molecular biologists calling it the "biological counterpart" to the holy grail (Kevles & Hood, 1992) and some sport scientists asserting that genetics are responsible for up to half of the variation in physical performance among individuals within a population (Hopkins, 2001). Interpretation of the extant literature is complex because the research on genes and physical performance expands almost weekly and there is considerable rhetoric among the genuine conclusions that can be drawn. It can be concluded that there is a great deal of equivocality in the existing research on the genetic basis of physical performance (Davids et al., 2003).

Nevertheless, it is possible to interpret existing data on interindividual variability in health and performance based on the interaction of genetic and environmental constraints. For example, adiposity is considered a constraint on performance in some sports and physical activities, and although increasing adiposity (within limits) may not harm performance in certain sports such as Sumo wrestling or rugby union and league, performance in endurance activities may suffer considerably from unfavorable levels of adiposity. The interactive role of genes and environment is emphasized by the growing consensus in the study of human obesity that the contribution of genetic factors is exacerbated by different environmental constraints including caloric availability (e.g., Barsh, Farooqi, & Rahilly, 2000). Genetic propensity toward adiposity has less of a constraining influence on individuals in environments where caloric availability is lower, whereas these same individuals would be at greater risk of obesity in calorie-rich environments. Environments can be categorized as high or low risk, depending on the prevalence of other significant cultural constraints including the availability of training facilities, work patterns imposed on traditional mealtimes, and the fall in popularity of physically active pastimes leading to a greater emphasis on static activities such as playing computer games and watching TV. Thus, the interaction of genes and environment on the phenotypic expression of behavior can be best understood by considering individual risk rather than by considering them as defective behavior (i.e., as in the medical model). This is an important point when considering the effects of spending time practicing in sport. Given interindividual genetic differences, variations in physical performance are more likely to assert themselves under intensive practice regimes.

In fact, during the past decade there has been increasing research on the role of genetics in defining the level of athletic performance attainable by individuals. As we note in the following sections, research has focused on genetic and environmental contributions to physical (typically endurance) performance (e.g., Rankinen et al., 2000), although there have been isolated attempts to evaluate relative contributions to the acquisition of motor skill (e.g., Fox, Hershberger, & Bouchard, 1996).

Genetic Contribution to Motor Skill Performance

L.R. Williams and Gross (1980) studied the performance of 22 monozygotic (MZ) and 41 dizygotic (DZ) twins on a stabilometer balance task over 6 d to examine the genetic contribution to learning and performance. The prediction was that interindividual variation in performance and learning would be less in the MZ group as compared to the DZ group. This prediction was supported by data indicating a greater intrapair resemblance in the MZ group only when the learning profiles of the twins were compared over time. Intraclass correlations were used to estimate the proportion of the total phenotypic variance in performance and learning that was accounted for by heritability. Heritability effects were reported to be low during the earliest stages of learning, but they became increasingly powerful as practice continued. Furthermore, the proportion of variance in performance accounted for by systematic variation of the environment due to the manipulation of constraints by coaches and teachers, was highest during the early stage. Although heritability is made up of genetic and environmental components, these findings imply that there is potential for influencing performance and learning by manipulating task constraints during practice.

Other work has been more ambitious in its aims. A study of performance in pursuit rotor tracking by Fox and colleagues (1996) examined the performance and learning of MZ ($n = 64$ pairs) and DZ ($n = 32$ pairs) twins reared apart. Performance outcome was scored by the time spent on target over 75 trials and was expressed as a proportion of the perfect score, 20 s. Fox et al. (1996) observed that the performance of the groups was very similar, with both substantially improving over the five trial blocks of the first day. Patterns of variability for both groups were also similar. Over practice, some participants improved more than others, which led to increases in variability within groups by the third day of the practice regime. However, statistical analysis did not reveal significant differences between the variances of the MZ and DZ twins over trials. The authors noted that there was greater variability in correlations with task performance in the DZ group over trials, although this effect may have been partly due to the smaller number of DZ pairs studied. The slope of the regression line for the DZ intraclass correlations for the last 2 d was close to zero, implying that the contribution of environmental factors decreased as practice continued. Despite the large intergroup differences in the number of participants, the authors concluded that the consistently larger intraclass correlations for performance in the MZ group as compared to DZ group pointed to a significant genetic component of performance (see figure 6.4).

The authors proposed that a model combining genetic and environmental effects best fits the data. The influence of heritability (reflecting both genetic and environmental factors) was high from the first trial block (proportion of contribution to performance variance = 0.66) to the last trial block (proportion = 0.69). The fact that the influence of heritability was high for the first of the initial 5 trial blocks (0.66, 0.53, 0.52, 0.55, and 0.52, respectively) might be taken as evidence that individuals rely on innate capacities for the first few practice trials of a novel task. Conclusions by the authors of a clear distinction between MZ and DZ for dependent variables such as percent time on target, rate of improvement of performance over trial block, and improvement after a time of rest were based on genetic influence. More work is needed, however, since the authors seem to confuse performance with skill acquisition. Although "skill acquisition" is the phrase used in the title of the paper, only 75 trials were examined and it could be argued that performances of both groups were measured.

The issue of the potential confounding effects of unequal sample sizes in the study by Fox et al. (1996) is nontrivial. In complete contrast to the findings obtained by Fox et al. (1996), other work examining differences in the performance of pursuit tracking between equal numbers of pairs ($n = 35$) of MZ and DZ twins proposed that the strength of the genetic constraints on performance systematically diminished throughout the course of practice, fitting a monotonic trend over trials (Marisi, 1977). Joseph (2001) has outlined a number of other methodological concerns with studies on twins. Classical methodology in research with twins compares the correlation or concordance rates for measurements from same-sex DZT (dizygotic, reared together) and MZT (monozygotic, reared together) twins. Identical (MZ) twins share 100% of the same genes while fraternal (DZ) twins share only 50% on average. Greater similarity in MZT twins is taken as evidence of the powerful influence of genetic constraints. The assumption is that both types of twins share the same environment, although it has been argued that data are confounded by MZT participants having a greater environmental similarity than DZT participants (Joseph, 2001).

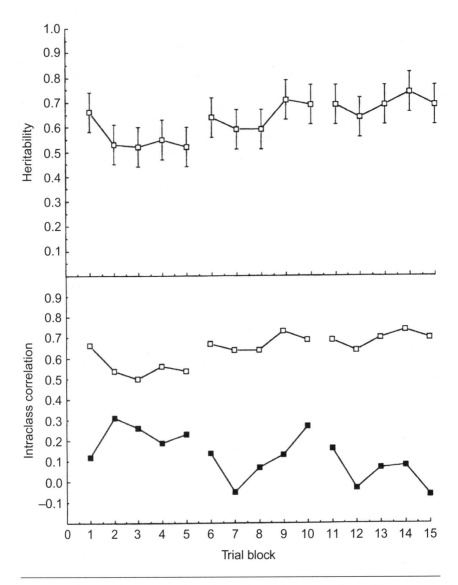

FIGURE 6.4 Data from Fox et al. (1996) on the performance of pursuit rotor tracking in monozygotic (*n* = 64 pairs) and dizygotic (*n* = 32 pairs) twins reared apart.
The top graph purports to show a high influence of heritability on skill practice in
the first few practice trial blocks and the maintained influence of heritability over
trials. The bottom graph shows the differences between monozygotic (open squares)
and dizygotic (filled squares) twins in the magnitudes of intraclass correlations for
performance, indicating that there is a significant genetic component of performance.

Reprinted by permission from Nature, P.W. Hershberger, S.L. Bouchard, and T.J. Jr., 1996, "Genetic and environmental
contributions to the acquisition of a motor skill," *Nature 384:* 356-358. Macmillan Publishers Ltd.

Another favorite methodology is to study MZ (monozygotic, reared apart) twins separated at birth and raised under different socioeconomic and cultural constraints. Such a comparison is believed to provide an ideal analysis of the effects of nature and nurture. Genetic inferences from studies on separated twins are based on the assumption that the shared environments of the twins were not systematically more similar than those of unrelated and randomly paired individuals, the so-called *unequal environment assumption*. According to Joseph (2001), the problem is that comparisons of separated twins reared in distinct environments are almost impossible to achieve in reality. He argued that there are many difficulties in obtaining pure samples that fit the stringent criteria needed for this type of test of genetic and environmental constraints. Twin studies adopting this methodology can be contaminated in many different ways including:

- The twins are separated only after being raised together a long time (years).
- They are raised by members of the same family.
- Their placement families are correlated for many factors to ensure equitable living conditions.
- In contrast to the assumption of minimal contact, the twins remain aware of each other and maintain contact.
- They are brought to the attention of researchers because they are perceived to be very similar and worthy of further study.
- Data on both twins are collected by the same researchers rather than by independent observers, which leaves the data open to bias and expectation.

Often an important error in twin studies is the assumption of different socioeconomic and cultural backgrounds, which is difficult to achieve because of historical constraints. That is, two people born on the same day and brought up at the same time and in the same culture, possibly sharing similar class and ethnic values, may be expected to show a great deal of similarities because of the so-called cohort effect (a constraint on group affiliations). One important way in which cohort effects can be ruled out as an explanation for the data of studies on twins is using closely matched pairs of biologically unrelated strangers as controls to the MZ participants. One difficulty in interpreting the data from studies on twins is that information about participant recruitment is often not reported and there is a lack of case histories to help independent judgments of the data.

These significant problems have led to the conclusion that there has not been a clear demonstration that MZ twins are reared in uncorrelated environments to support the unequal environment assumption. According to Joseph (2001), "significant MZ personality and behavioural correlations can be explained plausibly on the basis of the various environmental similarities shared by separated identical twins and by inflated figures resulting from bias and error in the various studies" (p. 24).

Genetic Contribution to Variability in Physical Performance

Not all research on genetic constraints has adopted the twin studies approach. The significant interindividual variations observed in response to training of the cardiovascular system has led many investigators to question the extent to which genetic diversity may be responsible for the data (e.g., Feitosa et al., 2002). In the past few years, the role of the ACE[1] gene has received considerable attention in the literature on exercise physiology, molecular biology, and sports medicine. In the next section, we evaluate the evidence for its role as a genetic constraint on variation in physical endurance.

The ACE Gene

The ACE gene is one of a number associated by research with interindividual variability in performance in physical endurance (Alvarez et al., 2000; Montgomery et al., 1999; Montgomery & Payne, 2004; Myerson et al., 1999; Nazarov et al., 2001; Taylor, Mamotte, Fallon, & van Bockxmeer., 1999; A. G. Williams et al., 2000; A.G. Williams et al., 2004; Woods, Humphries, & Montgomery, 2000; Woods et al., 2001; Woods et al., 2002). In muscle, the angiotensin I-converting enzyme degrades vasodilators (i.e., bradykinin and tachykinin) and stimulates production of the vasoconstrictor angiotensin II during physical performance (Sonna et al., 2001). To date, three variants of the human angiotensin I-converting enzyme (ACE) gene have been found. The presence or absence of a fragment containing 287 base pairs characterizes the I (insertion) or D (deletion) allele, respectively, leading to 3 variants (II, ID, and DD).

Increasing ACE activity is linked with the D allele, affecting the degradation of bradykinin and the synthesis of angiotensin II. DD participants show increased conversion of angiotensin I to angiotensin II, the latter having a vasoconstriction effect. However, angiotensin II seems to stimulate endogenous factors for the growth of muscle cells, contributing to a hypertrophic response useful for power development. Degradation of bradykinin results in lower substrate metabolism and less efficient vasodilation. Therefore, lower ACE activity may be associated with an increased half-life of bradykinin that alters substrate metabolism. Increased angiotensin II is associated with the DD genotype and may facilitate muscle bulk for power sport performance. It is estimated that

---

[1] ACE stands for angiotensin-converting enzyme.

25% of the population have the II genotype, 50% the ID genotype, and 25% the DD genotype (Jones, Montgomery, & Woods, 2002).

One approach to research on the ACE gene has been to examine whether a particular genotype occurs more frequently in specific populations as compared to controls. If a polymorphism is found to prevail more in a specific population as compared to matched controls, then either the polymorphism or its locus on the chromosome may be responsible for different frequencies of appearance. Alternatively, the polymorphism may be in linkage disequilibrium, that is, closely associated with a different locus on the chromosome that is actually responsible.

For example, the earliest work with army recruits found that the type II polymorphism of the gene is associated with lower ACE activity in muscle and an increased response to physical training (Montgomery et al., 1998). Recruits with the ACE genotype II differed by as much as 1,100% in response to repetitive upper-arm exercises when compared to peers with the DD genotype. Individuals with a heterogeneous genotype (DI) were associated with levels of performance between those of both homozygous genotypes. In sport, a higher prevalence of the II genotype has been found in elite endurance athletes including mountaineers able to climb to 7000 m without the aid of oxygen, Olympic endurance runners, and elite rowers (Gayagay et al., 1998; Montgomery et al., 1998; Myerson et al., 1999).

Interpreting the data from studies on the genetic constraints in physical performance and in the acquisition of motor skill is rather complex and there is enormous potential for confusion amidst the rhetoric. Initially, the data favoring a strong genetic constraint on physical performance seemed compelling. While most researchers studying genetic variations in human performance agree with Hopkins' (2001) opinion that athletes are born and made, a clear interpretation of the data on the ACE gene is needed to understand how athletic performance emerges under interacting constraints.

A good example of the appropriateness of this conclusion in the face of rhetoric that human physical performance is *strongly* influenced by genetic factors (e.g., Myerson et al., 1999) was provided in a study by C. Bouchard and colleagues. They attempted to establish the proportion of influence attributable to genetic and environmental constraints on familial resemblance for maximal oxygen uptake ($\dot{V}O_2max$) during exercise on a cycle ergometer in sedentary individuals (C. Bouchard et al., 1998). For this purpose, the exercise performance of fathers, mothers, sons, and daughters was measured in 86 nuclear families. Maximum heritability including genetic and nongenetic causes for physical performance accounted for 51% of the total adjusted phenotype variance. Several models of interacting constraints were tested, and results showed that there was 2.6 to 2.9 times more variance between families than within families.

Unfortunately, the approach taken in this study meant that genetic and familial environmental influences could not be "fully quantified separately," although "inferences about their respective contributions to the phenotype variance could be made by inspection of the pattern of familial correlations" (p. 255). As is well known, however, correlations do not imply causation. The emphasis on the constraints imposed by the shared familial environment is also important. While this explanation for heritability of maximal oxygen uptake may be valid, it does not preclude the influence of *wider* environmental constraints such as sociocultural changes in society, including effects of media images, changing fashions in society, government education programs, and peer pressure.

Despite the fact that the maximal heritabilities reported in this study were inflated by familial, nongenetic contributions, the effects of the maternal transmission of mitochondrial DNA to the fertilized zygote were seen as optimally allied to the father's environmental contribution. The authors argued that the data "revealed" that "maternal influence, perhaps by mitochondrial inheritance, accounts for as much as 30% of the familial transmission" (p. 257). The authors' conclusion was that "based on the present results, we estimate that 'mitochondrial' heritability is in the range of 30-35%" (p. 257). This highly speculative interpretation of the data is based on correlational statistics, a limited range of environmental constraints considered as affecting model construction, and no evidence from DNA analysis.

This study exemplifies the complexities involved in understanding genetic and environmental constraints on physical performance. In order to enhance understanding of the literature on genetic constraints on behavior, it is worth reiterating what is already known in this area of work. As most geneticists studying physical performance understand, genes work in combination to influence biological function. This understanding refutes the idea of successful athletes being differentiated by the presence of a single gene (for a similar argument in developmental theory see Johnston & Edwards, 2002). It has also become clear that genes are not biologically determinate, since even the most ardent geneticists agree that the transmission of genetic information between generations is less than perfect (e.g., Jones, 1999). DNA is simply a copy of information that is read by cellular machinery in the production of proteins that create the individual part by part. However, somewhere along the line the view of DNA as an information bearer has been replaced with the fallacy of DNA as a plan or master molecule (Lewontin, 2000).

Genes and Variability in Movement Systems

Therefore, the presence of genetic material should not be viewed as a blueprint for success in sport. As Johnston and Edwards (2002) have pointed out, it is "a very long step from polypeptide sequences to behaviour—a step . . . that covers much incompletely understood territory" (p. 26). An attempt to see genes as building plans is one of the great artificialities in human conceptualizations of nature (van Geert, 1994), but it has become a central dogma of how people think about the process of evolution (Oyama, 2000). Genes simply contain the information to synthesize proteins with properties that lead to clustering. Lewontin (2000) criticized "biological determinism," the rejection by the medical model view of polymorphism and the implicit notion of variability as deviation from a perfect ideal. Genetic diversity is the norm and biological systems are not determined by DNA. There is no single, standard DNA sequence that we all share, and estimates are that we differ in DNA sequencing by 0.1% (about 3 million nucleotides), including sequences inherited from parents. It takes more than DNA to produce a living organism, and those other components cannot be computed from DNA sequences. According to Lewontin (2000), "a living organism at any moment of its life is the unique consequence of a developmental history that results from the interaction of and determination by internal and external forces" (p. 147).

A major argument against the conceptualization of genetics as a blueprint is found in evidence that identical twins are not actually identical. A study of phenotypically identical twins showed that their fingerprints differ and that the shape of their brains can differ by as much as 40% (Yates, 1993). Heritability of a trait is constrained by genetic and environmental factors to some extent, and research in behavioral genetics is concerned with explanations of hereditary influences at the level of populations, not individuals.

Nonetheless, the evidence linking the ACE gene and physical performance continues to accumulate. Although some work on endurance performance in elite athletes has failed to support the more functional role of the I allele of the ACE gene (e.g., Taylor et al., 1999), this study was made up of 120 performers chosen from sports with task constraints emphasizing a high level of aerobic fitness (including 26 hockey players, 25 cyclists, 21 skiers, 15 track and field athletes, 13 swimmers, 7 rowers, and 5 gymnasts). An alternative explanation for the data is that such a mixed group of athletes may not have had the requisite levels of phenotypic homogeneity to lead to valid estimates of the genetic basis of performance. Moreover, it has become clear that carriers of the D allele have an advantage in training and performance when task constraints emphasize power over a shorter duration (Myerson et al., 1999; Nazarov et al., 2001). In fact, the D allele has been related to increased gains in quadriceps strength following 9 wk of isometric training (Folland et al., 2000). It is possible that the D allele may confer some performance and training benefits in task constraints requiring power (perhaps through its effect on greater angiotensin II and muscle hypertrophy), and similarly the I allele may have an effect under task constraints requiring endurance. The implication is that variability at the level of individual genes provides functionality and adaptability in movement systems that need to perform a variety of activities in a complex environment. This suggestion also emphasizes that in experiments on variants of the ACE gene and sport performance, a clear understanding of differences in task constraints is needed to ensure that homogenous cohorts of athletes are carefully examined in order to avoid the loss of genetic association.

Finally, research on the ACE gene is progressing rapidly, and there are some indications that its role in constraining physical performance may be somewhat different than originally perceived. For example, there has been some doubt cast on the relationship between the I allele and responsiveness to endurance training that was originally proposed in some studies (e.g., Gayagay et al., 1998; Hagberg et al., 1998; Montgomery et al., 1998). The locus of the ACE gene has been identified as chromosome 17q23, and genomic scanning for candidate genes for baseline $\dot{V}O_2$max performance or responsiveness to training failed to confirm evidence of linkage (C. Bouchard et al., 2000). These findings on a sedentary population were supported by a frequency analysis that failed to find a relationship between the accumulations of alleles I and II and endurance performance in 192 elite athletes (skiers, runners, and cyclists) and 189 controls (Rankinen et al., 2000). Interestingly, the highest frequencies reported for both the elite athletes and controls were for the ID genotype (0.46 and 0.47, respectively). Nevertheless, future research needs to ascertain (a) whether or not the effect of the I allele of the ACE gene on endurance performance is mediated via peripheral muscle effects and changes in efficiency, and (b) whether or not the effect of the D allele on performance in power tasks is mediated via increased angiotensin II acting as a local hypertrophic factor in muscle.

To summarize, the main difficulty with current research on the ACE gene is that investigators seem to have conducted research on samples with mixed phenotypes leading to equivocality of findings. Sometimes, the label given to specific populations has not been accurate (e.g., elite versus subelite athletes) (Jones, Montgomery & Woods, 2002). The strongest associations between II and DD polymorphisms and endurance and power performance, respectively, have been found in homogenous cohorts of elite athletes of specific sport disciplines. The conclusion by Jones, Montgomery & Woods (2002) is that "the ACE I/D polymorphism should not be considered a 'gene for human performance,' but a marker for modulation such that one would expect an excess of the I allele in the truly elite endurance athlete, with a concordant excess of the D allele represented in the more power-oriented events. Therefore, the study of mixed cohorts is unlikely to prove fruitful" (p. 187).

One problem with this explanation for equivocality by Jones, Montgomery & Woods (2002) is that it is *post hoc*. That is, there is a question mark over the predictive power of using the ACE gene polymorphism to explain performance in endurance and power sports. It seems that the linkage is clear only with pure samples of elite athletes, and where no effects are found it might be possible to argue that the samples were not pure. The lack of clarity in the literature was confirmed by Jones, Montgomery & Woods (2002), who stated that "the ACE genotype has never been associated with endurance performance in the untrained state. Any effect appears to require a period of gene-environment interaction. A high level of aerobic fitness is an essential, but not sole, requirement for elite endurance" (p. 188). A final point is that there is a high level of individual variation in the data on the ACE gene and endurance and power performance. Jones, Montgomery & Woods (2002) argued that "there will always be elite endurance athletes who are of the ACE DD genotype, and many champions in anaerobic sports of the II genotype. Whatever the data may conclude, elite athletes are still made and not born, though perhaps some may be made elite in one discipline more easily than others" (p. 189).

Concluding Remarks: A Case for Dynamic Systems Theory

We have evaluated the strengths and weaknesses of theoretical ideas and empirical research for theories of learning and performance that posit major effects for environmental and genetic constraints. It was concluded that neither approach, each emphasizing the unitary role of one category of constraints, provided enough explanatory power to account for data on variability in performance, suggesting it may be premature to include genetic testing as part of athletic screening programs (e.g., Dennis, 2005). It was noted that the implicit basis of the perspective of deliberate practice is the adage "all individuals are created equal." The analysis of the literature on genetic constraints on variability in performance does not support this conclusion, but this analysis should not be taken to imply that performance is biologically determined. Rather, the effects of interacting constraints on health and performance have been noted, since despite variations in genetic structure, the maximal heritability of particular traits includes strong environmental components.

A theoretical perspective based on dynamic systems, in which interacting constraints explain variability in behavior, may provide an adequate overarching framework for interpreting data (Davids et al., 2003; Davids, et al., 2004). Genetic diversity may be responsible for a small part of the differences in training or performance response in individuals and performance benefits may be observed only when there is a favorable interaction with important environmental constraints. The effects of the available environment on phenotypic expression were noted in research on causes of obesity in human health. The implication of these findings and of data from studies on endurance performance is that elite athletes of a less favorable genotypic disposition can succeed with the appropriate training environment. However, it can be concluded that performers with a more favorable genotype who appropriately interact with their training environments are more likely to receive a greater response to training. The current data on genetic constraints in the acquisition of motor skills are unclear due to various methodological weaknesses and conflicting findings, and more work is needed to identify genetic mechanisms underlying variations in performance. Moreover, the emphasis on constraints placed by dynamical systems theory implies new ways of looking at the whole nature versus nurture argument. This theoretical perspective provides an overarching framework that encompasses an extensive variety of organismic and environmental constraints on human behavior.

Part III

Issues in Measurement

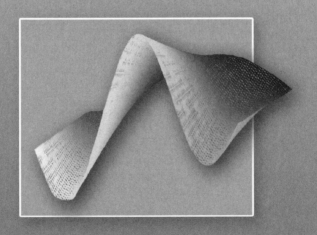

Chapter 7

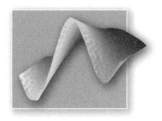

Coordination Profiling of Movement Systems

Chris Button, PhD, Keith Davids, PhD, and Wolfgang Schöllhorn, PhD

Editors' Overview

Advances in methodologies for motion analysis have provided opportunities for fine-grained analyses to reveal tendencies of movement coordination in individuals. The resultant shift in focus toward analyses centered on individuals is beginning to reveal the nature of specific adaptations to interacting organismic, task, and environmental constraints. An exciting development is the plotting of individual kinematic characteristics of movement coordination over several trials. This chapter presents one method for analyzing inter- and intraindividual characteristics of performance based on the implementation of an algorithm that recognizes patterns. One implication from this chapter is that there needs to be a greater emphasis on individualized approaches in science, such as case studies and single-subject designs in motor learning and control. Moreover, reference to optimization processes in the literature on biomechanics and motor control should be associated with individual movement outcomes and not with an idealized, hypothetical optimal pattern of movement that always achieves the same outcome (e.g., throwing a javelin to a maximum distance). This reemphasis in performance analysis naturally leads to practical approaches such as differential learning and an approach led by constraints, which use variability as a mechanism for forcing individual performers to adapt their movements to interacting constraints during practice. It is argued that these findings suggest that coordination profiling may be needed for interpreting the variability and stability demonstrated by each athlete as she attempts to construct functional, goal-directed motor patterns during each performance.

The human motor system is blessed with more degrees of freedom than it actually needs for achieving most everyday tasks. The different ways in which individuals exploit apparently redundant degrees of freedom can be observed from detailed analyses of patterns in movement that show subtle variations in trajectory from one performance to the next, regardless of the person's skill level (e.g., Button, McLeod, Sanders, & Coleman, 2003; Müller & Sternad, 2004; Berthier, Rosenstein & Barto, 2005). It has been proposed that a level of functional variability exists within the motor system to help it adapt and consistently achieve its overall goals (a control feature called "piece-wise determinism" by Riley and Turvey, 2002). As we demonstrate in this chapter, variability in movement is particularly important in many sport skills in which the adaptability of complex motor patterns is necessary within dynamic performance environments.

The revelation of this important feature of motor behavior has recently shifted the attention of the research spotlight away from examining the behavioral tendencies of groups of individuals and toward the analysis of individual performance. As we demonstrate in this chapter, the analysis and interpretation of variability in movement has rapidly become one of the main priorities for scientists of movement seeking to understand the control processes underpinning motor behavior (Newell & Corcos, 1993; Newell, Deutsch, & Morrison, 2000; Riley & Turvey, 2002; Müller & Sternad, 2004; Berthier et al., 2005). The enhanced focus on variability in movement at an individual level has resulted from changes in theoretical influences in the literature on motor control and from advances in data collection and analysis techniques. To illustrate our arguments for an individual-centered approach to variability, we provide examples from a variety of motor tasks such as prehension, catching, discus, and javelin throwing.

Theoretical Evolution of Variability in Movement

Variability in motor performance has been considered from a variety of theoretical perspectives (e.g., Newell & Corcos, 1993). Traditionally, cognitive science views higher levels of variability as a problem for movement systems during task performance (Newell & Slifkin, 1998). This is because the main focus of models from cognitive science on motor behavior has been on system *control* by movement representations such as motor programs stored in the memory. Due to the influence of engineering and computer sciences on the development of motor control theory in the 1950s and 1960s, variability in output was viewed as a form of system noise (Williams, Davids, & Williams, 1999).

In cognitive science, the approach of information processing views the performer as a sort of human communications channel in which the relationship between input signals and system output is linear and deterministic.[1] Therefore variability in signal processing and programming is seen as a problem of

---

[1] More recently, Todorov and Jordan (2002) have argued for a more valuable role of variability within a computational theory of coordination that they term *optimal feedback control*. These authors suggest that the traditional separation in computational approaches of trajectory planning and execution has led to the misconception that optimal control necessarily predicts stereotypical movements. Within the model of optimal feedback control it is proposed that variability is permitted within redundant (task-irrelevant) dimensions as a product of feedback being used to correct deviations that interfere with task goals.

system control (Newell & Slifkin, 1998; Slifkin & Newell, 1999). In control system theory, the ratio of the strength of the control signal to the noise in the system determines the amount of variability present in system behavior and subsequently the quality of control. In this view of the human performer, noise can be eliminated or minimized through practice and task experience. For this reason, the *magnitude* of the variability in performance has been viewed as an important feature for assessing the quality of system control (Schmidt, 1985). As we shall see in subsequent sections of this chapter, these theoretical approaches have typically neglected the important *structural* role that variability might play during goal-directed movement.

Additionally, developments in postmodern scientific approaches such as dynamical systems and chaos theory have led to alternative views concerning variability in movement (Kelso, 1995; Latash, Scholtz, & Schöner, 2002). In these newer theoretical approaches, the emphasis has shifted away from the concept of motor programs controlling the system in a hierarchical fashion to concepts such as self-organization under constraint (Thelen, 1995). For example, it has been suggested that the microscopic variance in the components of a movement system facilitates self-organizing behavior of the whole system at a macroscopic level (Davids, Button, & Bennett, in press). Furthermore, variability plays an important functional role in exploring boundaries of stability and generating valuable information to encourage adaptability and transfer within motor learning (Zanone & Kelso, 1992; Berthier et al., 2005). These ideas indicate that the emergent behavior of a dynamic system does not evolve because of a cleverly constructed plan or pure chance, but because of the pressures of key constraints that shape and guide its evolution. Successful movement behaviors, those that allow a performer to achieve her task goals, can emerge from varied movement production and selection during practice. Selection in skill acquisition results from feedback on goal achievement, the observation of which led Turvey and Fitzpatrick (1993) to refer to practice as a process of "chaos + feedback."

Another recent theoretical concept that particularly relates to this chapter is the role played by the performer's *intrinsic dynamics* in shaping patterns of coordination. Kelso (1991) defines intrinsic dynamics as the order pattern dynamics that reflect the internal coordination tendencies of an individual motor system. Thelen (1995) highlighted the importance of organismic constraints by referring to intrinsic dynamics as "the preferred states of the system given its current architecture and previous history of activity" (p. 76). The intrinsic dynamics of each individual are unique and shaped by many constraints including genetic factors, learning experiences, and environmental influences. The manner in which a performer moves to satisfy these constraints is determined by the way he matches his intrinsic dynamics with the specific dynamics of the task to be performed (Corbetta & Veriejken, 1999). By knowing the intrinsic dynamics, one can specify which element within the movement repertoire actually changes due to environmental, learned, or intentional influences (Zanone and Kelso, 1992).

In summary, the traditional conception of variability in movement as system noise has been replaced by a more positive view of variability as a functional factor in the underpinning organization of the system. Furthermore, due to the potentially unique matching of intrinsic dynamics with task dynamics, each person may exploit system variability in a slightly different way. In the next section, we describe how technological advances and new analytical tools have allowed us to develop our awareness of this new view of variability in movement.

Data Collection and Statistical Analysis

The last 30 years have seen comprehensive changes in the way patterns of human movement are analyzed and interpreted. Such developments have been fueled by the introduction of cine filming, high-speed digital photography, 3-D analysis, and more recently computer modeling and simulation (Allard, Stokes, & Blanchi, 1995). Such techniques allow researchers to look at patterns of coordination with greater depth and sensitivity than was previously possible (for an excellent early example involving catching a ball, see Alderson, Sully, & Sully, 1974). The development of sophisticated measuring devices has also facilitated research examining complex tasks that require multiple degrees of freedom rather than simplistic, laboratory-based tasks (e.g., linear positioning, reaction time, and pursuit rotor), which characterized much of the earlier research in motor control (Williams, Davids, & Williams, 1999).

Advances in techniques for *data collection* have meant that alternative methods for *data analysis* have also been required. For example, the statistical analysis of outcome or error data from research in motor control has traditionally been carried out with pooled group data. This type of analysis was presumably conducted in an effort to establish laws of action that are generalizable to a wider population. Indeed, the type of analysis demanded by inferential statistics forms a cornerstone of traditional science. However, as patterns in movement are being analyzed in more depth, researchers are identifying subtle individualities, or signature patterns of movement, in even very simple tasks (Beek, Rikkert, & van Wieringen, 1996; Port, Lee, Dassonville, & Georgopoulos, 1997; Button, Bennett, & Davids, 1998). From a perspective based on dynamic systems, it has been argued that pooled group data has limited value, prompting Kelso (1995) to point out that:

> because each person possesses his or her own "signature," it makes little sense to average performance over individuals. One might as well average apples and oranges. This does not mean that putative laws and principles of learning cannot be generalized across individuals; laws wouldn't qualify as such if it were not possible to do so. It only means that the way the law is instantiated is specific to the individual. (p. 147)

The argument that we propose is that individual analyses of kinematics are preferable to the traditional pooling of group data if one is interested in unraveling the complex processes governing motor control.

Variability can be defined in statistical terms as the variance of data dispersed about the mean, and it is usually quantified by the size of the standard deviation (Riley & Turvey, 2002). While the standard deviation is beneficial if one is interested in the *level* of variability in performance on a specific task at a discrete point in time, it is of little use if one is interested in changes in the variability of selected measurements of coordination in movement over time by participants in a group, such as during development or as a result of learning (Newell & Slifkin, 1998; Riley & Turvey, 2002). Statistics such as the standard deviation, the coefficient of variation, and the range assume that there is little association among discrete measurements taken at different times during performance. Traditional analyses of motor behavior at discrete time intervals assume that each point of measurement is independent of the others. For example, in biomechanical analyses of movement there has been a typical focus on measuring variables such as relative timing and the magnitudes of discrete kinematic and kinetic variables (Slifkin & Newell, 1999). A good example of the emphasis on discrete measurements of kinematic variables is the report that elite javelin throwers achieve higher peak speeds of distal segments of the arm than novice throwers and that 50% of peak speed is generated in the last 50 ms before release (for an overview of statistical procedures in biomechanics and motor control, see Mullineaux, Bartlett, & Bennett, 2001).

However, performance analysis of complex motor tasks such as the javelin throw as a continuous time series is predicated over *selected portions* of the movement and not isolated points from the throw (over the whole javelin throw or during the final 50 ms of the movement). The analysis of time series allows key kinematic variables to be plotted against each other as the pattern of movement unfolds. Values of a particular variable can be compared earlier and later in the movement. In this way, one can examine the *structure* of variability in movement rather than simply the *magnitude* of variability in a given performance. In a similar vein, phase plots have allowed researchers to demonstrate how variability within patterns of movement such as gait (Clark, 1995; Heiderscheit, Hamill, & van Emmerik, 1999) can help satisfy task constraints. Phase plots display the velocity characteristics of a moving body against its position as a function of time, and by overlaying trials one can gain a clear picture of how these derivatives relate (see figure 7.1). The data in figure 7.1 demonstrate how phase plots can distinguish different coordination tendencies in a basketball free throw, such as increased consistency at ball release for expert players. Time-continuous variables are further discussed in the Applications to Throwing sections with examples from discus and javelin throwing.

In this section we have discussed how technological advances and new analytical methods have helped us gain a more detailed appreciation of variability in movement. In the next two sections we describe specific techniques (coordination profiling and cluster analyses) that can be employed to carry out this level of analysis (e.g., Button, Bennett, & Davids, 1998; Button, 2002; Schöllhorn, 1998, 2000).

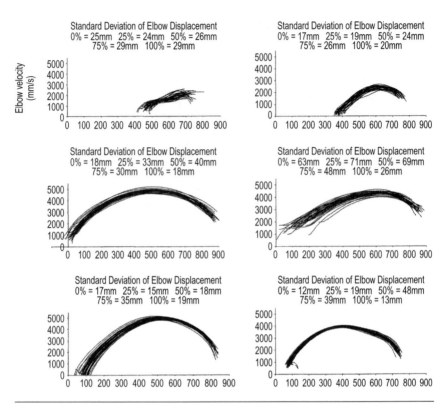

FIGURE 7.1   Phase-plane plots of linear displacement against velocity for the elbow during the basketball free throw (adapted from Button et al., 2003). The graphs represent participants across a range of expertise, from novices (graphs 1 and 2) to national team players (5 and 6). Within each graph the data from 30 experimental trials are overlaid. The intertrial standard deviation of elbow displacement was calculated at 0%, 25%, 50%, 75%, and 100% of normalized movement time.

Reprinted with permission from *Research Quarterly for Exercise and Sport*, Vol. 74, pp. 257-269, Copyright 2002 by the American Alliance for Health, Physical Education, Recreation and Dance, 1900 Association Drive, Reston, VA 20191.

Coordination Profiling

Coordination profiling requires that a small number of participants performs multiple trials of a motor task in an experimental design that uses repeated measures.[2] The kinematics of each trial are then analyzed with conventional statistical tools (e.g., analysis of variance, simple main effects) and are presented separately for each individual. Where they are of potential interest, commonalities or differences among individuals are highlighted within the analysis.

---

[2] The assumptions of homogeneity and sphericity that are checked before applying conventional statistics on group data should also be confirmed with multiple trials (Thomas & Nelson, 2001). Furthermore, given that only a few trials may be possible in order to maintain participant motivation or because of limited resources, calculating effect size within coordination profiling is also recommended.

Using this approach, the experimenter is limited to making generalizations about an individual's behavior rather than the behavior of a wider population. The following experiments demonstrate the value of examining coordination in this way.

Applications in Prehension

Button, Bennett, and Davids (1998) were interested in examining the coordination in discrete and rhythmic reach and grasp movements. In the rhythmic condition, 6 participants grasped plastic dowels in time to a metronomic beat, whereas for the discrete condition the participants had to complete each grasp within a predetermined time. Based on previous work (Wallace et al., 1994), the relative time of the final closure of the hand within the reach (T_{rfc}) was chosen to characterize the coordination of grasp and transport components of the task. The movements of the index finger, thumb, and wrist were recorded in three dimensions with an on-line motion analysis system with a sampling frequency of 100 Hz. The analysis of T_{rfc} was performed at two levels, one using the conventional within-group approach and one using coordination profiling.

Interestingly, no differences in T_{rfc} between the rhythmic and discrete conditions were found with the conventional pooled group analysis. However, there was a large amount of within-participant variability in the coordination data. When the data on each individual were analyzed separately, some alternative findings became obvious (see table 7.1). Two participants (3 and 6) tended to grasp early in the discrete condition as compared to the rhythmic condition, 2 (4 and 5) tended to grasp late in the discrete condition, and 2 (1 and 2) showed no significant difference between conditions! This interindividual variability masked any overall effects when the T_{rfc} data were pooled across participants. In fact, the high levels of individual variability in task performance were interpreted as a result of the competition between specific and nonspecific control parameters (e.g., the participants' intentionality and the auditory beat specifying movement time). In other words, it is likely that some individuals prioritized properly grasping the plastic dowels whereas others prioritized coupling their action with the metronome. Guiard (1997) also found differences in patterns

TABLE 7.1 Mean Relative Phasing of Final Hand Closure Within Overall Movement Time (T_{rfc}) for a Prehension Task

	Participant					
Condition	1 (–)	2 (–)	3 (**)	4 (*)	5 (*)	6 (*)
Rhythmic	147	115	254	122	124	150
Discrete	125	114	181	172	143	86

Individual data are presented within discrete and rhythmic conditions. Where * denotes a significant main effect for condition, p < 0.05; ** corresponds to p < 0.01 and – is a nonsignificant effect, p > 0.05.

of coordination (and individual variability) while directly comparing discrete and cyclical tapping movements. As in the study of Button et al. (1998), the contention is that participants' patterns of movement differed in the rhythmic conditions because of differential abilities (due to intrinsic coordination tendencies) to combine rhythmic movement with other task constraints. The important point for this chapter is that if the individual analyses had not been conducted, it is unlikely that this important finding would have emerged.

Applications in Catching

Button (2002) set out to determine the role of auditory information in the coordination of an interceptive action (one-handed catching). A machine serving tennis balls, which emitted a clicking noise before releasing each ball, was used to project tennis balls to skilled catchers. In a nonauditory condition, participants carried out 20 trials wearing earplugs and headphones emitting white noise. Patterns of movement were also collected from a control condition in which auditory information was available. As in the previous example, the Elite motion analysis system was used to record profiles of movement.

There were no differences between conditions for the outcome variable in the study, that is, the number of balls caught. However, coordination profiling of the kinematics revealed both intertrial and interindividual variability. Initiation time generally increased in the nonauditory condition (7 out of 8 participants), which was coupled with alterations in either the maximal opening or closing velocity of the hand or the maximal velocity of the wrist. Furthermore, these attunements were idiosyncratic in that each individual found a different solution to the experimental manipulation. High levels of standard deviation in these variables also indicated that each participant's grasping pattern varied considerably from trial to trial. It was suggested that this variability is functional, as it allowed the performers to adapt to small variations in ball flight, time of movement initiation, and limb positioning. More generally, it seems that the intention to catch the ball allowed skilled catchers to flexibly rearrange their patterns of movement to adjust to major and minor variations of the task. For example, one strategy that was employed in a number of trials was altering the location of contact between ball and hand.

A 3-D space plot (see figure 7.2) shows how one skilled catcher adapted to the lack of auditory information by catching the ball in front of the body, whereas a cushioned catch, closer to the body, was typical in the auditory trials. Other kinematic adaptations included increasing the wrist velocity and the velocity of opening the hand in response to the experimental manipulation. The data showing such high levels of on-line variability are difficult to reconcile with the idea that catching movements may be preprogrammed. As constraints on performance change, perhaps through the unforeseen occlusion of information that is typically available, skilled performers are able to immediately reassemble a perception–action coupling by substituting other available sources of information to achieve the same task goals. That is, through experience they

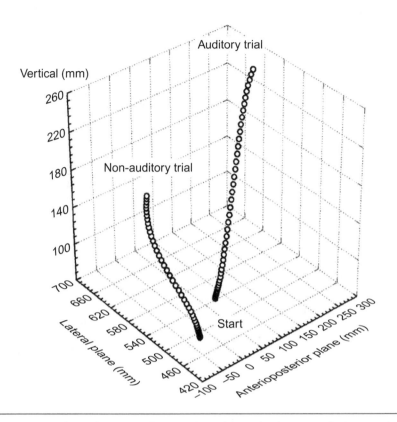

FIGURE 7.2   Three-dimensional space plots of wrist displacement during sample trials taken from participant 8. The location of contact with the ball is represented relative to the start position of the hand.

Reprinted, by permission, from C. Button, 2002, Auditory information and the coordination of one-handed catching. In *Interceptive actions in sport: Information and movement* (London, United Kingdom: Routhledge), 191.

might become better attuned to multiple information sources that can be used to guide the timing and coordination of the arm and hand in catching (see also Van der Kamp, Vereijken, & Savelsbergh, 1996).

Cluster Analyses and Time-Continuous Variables of Intra- and Interindividual Athletic Performance

In this section, we describe an alternative type of individual analysis that has proven particularly useful in understanding the performance data of elite athletes. First, it is necessary to explain the concept of studying similarity in analysis of movement. Consider the case of moving two fingers cyclically with an increasing frequency, shifting from an out-of-phase to an in-phase pattern (Haken, Kelso, & Bunz, 1985). Both patterns can be considered as a system consisting of different interactions of its elements (two fingers). Two advantages accompany this choice. First, the interaction of the two cyclic elements can be described by one variable (the angle between each finger), and second, the time-course data of a single cycle can be compressed into a time-discrete variable, the relative phase. This kind of data reduction corresponds to assigning time-continuous (process) data to time-discrete (product) parameters, and here it is possible because of the monotony and cyclicity of the movement. If the two fingers performed two totally different and noncyclic movements, other variables of description would need to be chosen. For a corresponding transfer of that approach to noncyclic or ballistic movements, the relative phase of two sinusoidal time courses can be considered as a coarse measurement for the *similarity* of the shape of the curves within a certain time interval. Taking similarity as a measurement for the interaction of two moving limbs has the advantage of serving a more general application (Rosen, 1983). However, the investigator has to choose among different measurements of similarity, and therefore the subsequent mathematical modeling becomes more complex. Considering similarity as a measurement for closeness, complementary measurements for dissimilarity or for distance satisfy the same intention (Everitt, Landau, & Leese, 2000) and are taken in the following approach correspondingly. Furthermore, similarity takes over the role as a more generalized order parameter (Schöllhorn, 1998) and opens a door to a principle of Gestalt psychology that has been stated for visual perception and recognition (Metzger, 1975). According to this principle, humans tend to cluster visually perceived objects by their (holistic) gestalt similarity.

Transferring or extending the process-oriented approach for data analysis to ballistic movements offers an alternative for analyzing intra- and interindividual variability or fluctuations, with alternative practical consequences for motor learning. Besides this, a time-course approach provides an auspicious alternative for assessing the effects of training or therapy that could hardly be diagnosed by a traditional time-discrete approach. In this discussion, time discrete is associated with a stroboscopic investigation of a continuous process by selecting the intensities of striking variable characteristics at certain instants. Alternatively, the time-continuous approach takes the complete time course of a variable or a movement.

A central problem for comparing complex ballistic movements is unifying the several single variable time courses into which the movement was previously decomposed for a more complete description. Different statistical procedures have been suggested in movement science. Data reduction by classifying variables by their time-course characteristics is obtained by linear transformation algorithms such as Karhunen-Loeve transformation (Haken, 1996), principal component analysis (Mah, Hulliger, Lee, & O'Callaghan, 1994; Olree & Vaughan, 1995; Schöllhorn, 1993), and orthogonal reference functions (Schöllhorn, 1995). More recently, Bauer and Schöllhorn (1997) suggested a nonlinear transformation procedure based on self-organizing maps (SOM) for data compression. Self-organizing maps (SOMs) are artificial neural networks that are adapted in an unsupervised learning process to project data points from some input space to a position in a usually low dimensional output space (Kohonen, 1995; Ritter, Martinetz, & Schulten, 1992). A SOM is given in terms of weight vectors, which map a data point to a neuron located in the output space of the map. While the mapping rule of winner takes all that applies to the SOM is identical to that of a regular vector quantizer, the SOM has the additional characteristic of neighborhood preservation. Two applications of comparisons on similarity in patterns of quantitative movement by nonlinear classifying neural nets are reported in the following sections.

Applications to Throwing (Discus)

Two discus throwers were filmed in selected competitions and training sessions during 1 y, resulting in data for 45 trials of a decathlete and 8 trials of a specialist. The positions and angular velocities of all body and limb joints were extracted during the final delivery phase, which starts (for a right-handed thrower) when the left foot touches down and ends when the hand releases the discus. This movement results in sequences of 51 time-normalized, 34-dimensional feature vectors $v_i(t)$ per trial i. The data were further processed by normalizing the individual dimensions to a mean of 0 and a variance of 1. SOMs were trained to project the individual feature vectors to an $N = 11 \times 11$ neuron output space. Learning parameters were $\sigma_{init} = 4.0$, reduced to $\sigma_{final} = 0.2$ during training, $\varepsilon = 0.9 \rightarrow 0.01$, 2×10^5 learning steps.

The sequence $v_i(t)$ of the feature vectors that constitute the original pattern of movement is transformed by the SOM into a sequence of excited neurons $r_i(t)$ (figure 7.3). Instead of considering a distance or similarity between sequences $v_i(t)$ and $v_j(t)$ directly in the 34-dimensional input space, we now could operate in the two-dimensional output space, with all the redundant, noisy dimensions suppressed. This resulted in a distance matrix:

$$d(i,j) = \sqrt{\sum_{t=1}^{51}(r_i(t) - r_j(t))^2} \tag{7.1}$$

The distances of all trials to a reference trial (number 5 of the specialist throws) as an exemplary cut through the distance matrix is shown in figure 7.4. The left-hand figure displays the distances of all eight trials of the specialist to the reference trial (number 5) in chronological order. All eight trials were exclusively throws in different competitions. Five trials were recorded before and three trials recorded after a specific training (Mendoza & Schöllhorn, 1990) during which the athletes were supported with objective feedback about their foot positions, the twisting angle between their hip and shoulder axes, and the twisting angle between their shoulder and arm axes. Because the first five

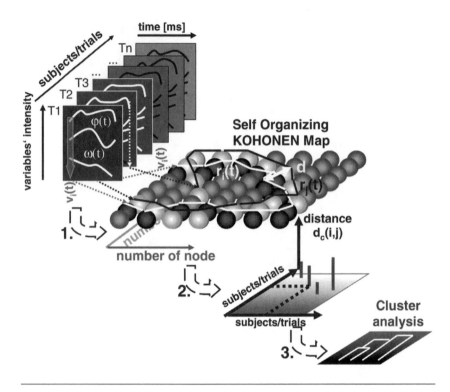

FIGURE 7.3   Schema of time-continuous data processing by a self-organizing Kohonen map and cluster analysis.

trials can be separated from the last three disjunctively, the learning or training process may be considered as successful. In the right-hand plot of figure 7.4, the distances of all the trials of the decathlete, relative to the reference trial, are displayed chronologically. The trials were filmed during different training sessions (T1-T5), in which the athlete received the same feedback training as the specialist, and during different competitions (C). The trials clearly fell into several clusters of similar distances to the reference trial. Assigning the clusters to specific units of training and competition leads to the interpretation that in each training session the decathlete has day-dependent strategies. The decreasing distance in training session T4 reflects a higher similarity between the decathlete's throwing pattern and the specialist's (reference) throwing pattern. Due to the increasing distance in training session T5 and the following competitions, a successful learning process cannot be assumed. Nevertheless, although both participants were high-performance athletes, executing hundreds of throws each week, they displayed continuous fluctuations in their throwing patterns within training and competition, which therefore verifies the low probability of repeating the same movement. In order to evaluate this clustering phenomenon in a more quantitative fashion, a clustering algorithm to the distance matrix $d(i,j)$ (equation 7.1) was applied. The cluster algorithm (average linkage, included in the SPSS package) yields a clustering hierarchy of similarities among trials (figure 7.5). At first glance, a clear separation in the trials of both athletes is recognizable. In more detail, the specialist's trials are clustered into five trials (S1-S5) before and three trials after (S6-S8) the feedback training. In the decathlete's trials, a clustering by training sessions (T2-T5) is primarily visible. Single trials of the training sessions are mixed up with the competition throws (C1-C4). The strategies that decathletes apply in different training sessions need further research.

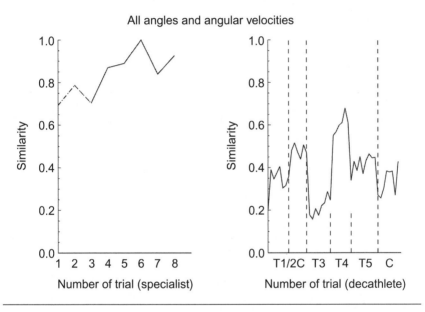

FIGURE 7.4   Distance $d(i,k)$ of projected trajectory $r_i(t)$ from the reference trajectory (trial 5 of the specialist). The dotted lines separate groups of throws that were performed during one training or competition.

Finally, in the cluster hierarchy, five groups of at least five trials were determined that are most similar among each other in the rescaled cluster distance delivered by the average linkage algorithm. Dividing the mean distance within one cluster by the mean distance between it and the other clusters revealed a ratio of 3.29 ± 0.62, which means that the different clusters have on average more than three times as much distance between them than within them (for further details see Bauer & Schöllhorn, 1997).

As the recognition of the two athletes, as well as the clustering into training sessions, were found only by implication of all variable time courses, the

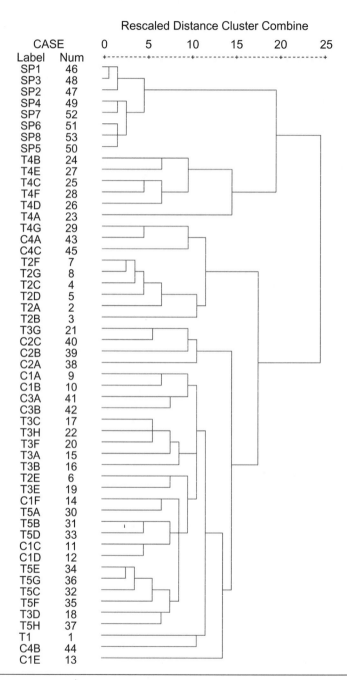

FIGURE 7.5 Clustering dendrogram of discus throws resulting from the average linkage algorithm. The horizontal lines indicate at what level of the rescaled distance the RESP movements are grouped into one cluster. The dendrogram was calculated for the average distance matrix obtained with the two-dimensional SOMs.

applied approach seems to identify phenomena which correspond to the gestalt or topology of a movement (Bernstein, 1967). Thereby the identified clusters can be considered as groups of different qualitative patterns of movement. Accordingly, the separation seen in the specialist's throws displays learning on a more qualitative level. Similar results could not be achieved by either single variables or time-discrete parameters.

Applications to Throwing (Javelin)

Our final application of individual analysis addresses the problem of individuality and generality in sport techniques in further detail and especially addresses the relationship of an ideal throwing technique as a general prototype and individual styles in javelin throwing. The ideal throwing technique is associated with the best human solution for the problem of throwing a javelin as far as possible, and therefore it is assumed that this technique is applied by world-class javelin throwers. Most often, an ideal technique serves as a general prototype (Brisson & Alain, 1996) that has to be imitated several thousand times in order to reach the world-class level. Whereas the previous study distinguished several discus throws of 2 athletes, in the present study 51 trials of 8 male and 19 female javelin throwers were analyzed (Schöllhorn & Bauer, 1998). The male throwers were finalists of the 1987 World Championship in Rome, and the female group consisted of 10 world-class heptathletes and 19 javelin specialists at the national and international levels. From 2 female specialists, 10 and 6 throwing trials were filmed, respectively, in different competitions during a time span of at least 3 y. The final throwing phase, from touchdown of the right foot (right-handed thrower) to when the hand releases the javelin, was described by the same main joint angles and angular velocities used in our previous example. The data were analyzed in the same manner as the previous study, with the exception of revealing the best results by a 3-D output space with $5 \times 5 \times 5$ neurons for the SOM.

A distance matrix is shown in figure 7.6. The higher the vertical bars, the more dissimilar are the throwing patterns. Due to the symmetry of the distance data, only one half of the matrix is displayed. This distance landscape provides a qualitative impression of the data structure. Three characteristics attract attention: The trials with numbers higher than 44 (in the background) show higher distances in comparison to the others, and two groups (trials 1-10 and 38-43) of throws display lower distances. Assigning the trial numbers to the throwers identifies the male group of throwing patterns (higher distances) and the groups of throwing patterns of the 2 female athletes with multiple throwing trials.

A coarse verification of this grouping is given by the cluster analysis (figure 7.7). The 10 (suffix $P*$) and 6 (suffix $T*$) trials of the 2 female specialists are clearly clustered into separate groups (shaded). These two clusters correspond to the recognition of a person by her time course of movement on the basis of 200 ms video recording. Statistically, the probability of accidentally revealing

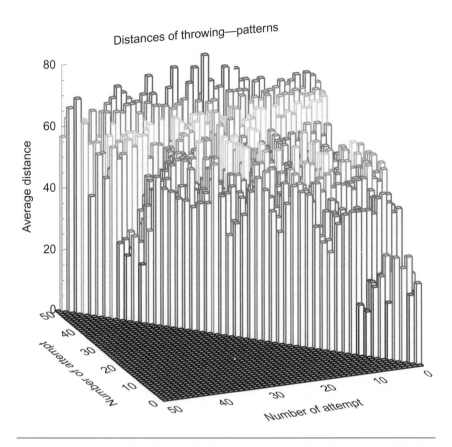

FIGURE 7.6   Distance landscape of all 51 patterns of javelin throwing, with three areas of interest highlighted (shaded).

these clusters of individuals is far below typical significance levels, and it emphasizes the power of this approach. From an epistemological point of view, in this case the individuality in patterns of movement is proven and not guessed at by an indirect derivation from finding no common structure in an investigated collective. Although both athletes' throws had the same range of distances (55-68 m), the throws were not in the same cluster but were separated into extra clusters. This separation identifies individual throwing styles independent of the athletes' performances. Most intriguingly, the throwing styles of both athletes could be identified although the athletes tried to improve their throwing patterns by training over 3 y. Most probably, the achieved improvement in performance was associated with conditional parameters rather than coordination.

The men's (4th letter, M) cluster could be identified only according to tendency. Only 4 out of 8 throws by men were grouped in a cluster separate from

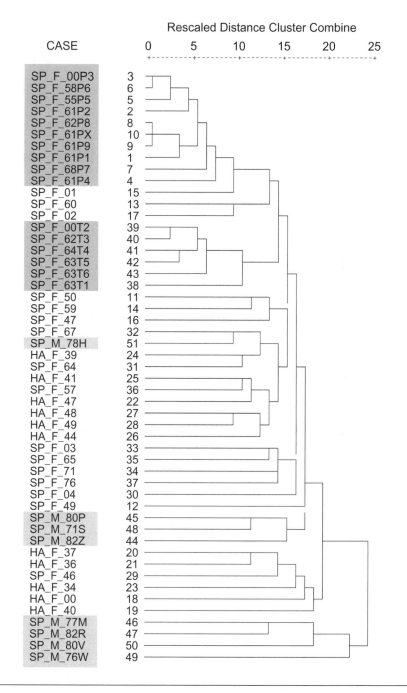

FIGURE 7.7   Clustering dendrogram resulting from javelin throws, as computed by the average linkage algorithm.

the female cluster of throws. Three trials of other men's throws were clustered separately but within the large female cluster. The throwing patterns most similar to those in the male cluster are displayed by a group of heptathletes (HA). Whether the athletes themselves cause these patterns of movement or the patterns are influenced by an external teacher or coach, the relative distances have to be taken into account. The finding that the mean distances within the male clusters are larger than the mean distances within the female cluster provides evidence for national influences. Keeping in mind that all the male throwers were finalists of the world championship and came from different countries, whereas all the female throwers originated in one nation, it seems that throwing patterns in javelin are strongly influenced by a nation's philosophy about the ideal throwing technique. Because no relationship between the thrown distances and the throwing patterns could be diagnosed by the cluster analysis of any set of variables for either men or women, strong evidence is given for the existence of not one but several best solutions. Additionally, being able to identify individual throwing styles by analyzing a duration of just 200 ms leads us to rethink the idea of the ideal throwing technique and its pure imitation in learning strategies. We question whether the athlete learns a coach's conception of a movement technique or acquires a technique that is optimized to his boundary conditions. To solve such problems, the movement and sport sciences need more emphasis on single case studies (Yin, 1988). Practical consequences, which cope with the problem of the low probability of repeating the same movement and the problem of individual patterns of movement related to prototypes, are suggested by the differential learning approach (Schöllhorn, 2000). Thereby the athletes are confronted with many different exercises in order to induce a self-organizing and self-optimizing process as well as to prepare them for the adaptational process that is needed in any repetition.

General Discussion and Implications

Due to the detailed analyses conducted at the individual level that were used in the experiments we described in this chapter, we have been able to uncover interesting individual differences across participants in a range of different tasks. From fine, static motor tasks like prehension to dynamic, explosive tasks like javelin throwing, an enhanced emphasis on variability has highlighted important implications for motor control and learning. For example, coordination profiling indicated that each performer can exploit intra- and interindividual differences in a unique way to achieve task goals despite any minor spatial and temporal variations or experimental perturbations. The presented time-course approach involving self-organizing neural nets (see Applications to Throwing sections) provides a sensitive tool for analyzing individual performance characteristics and their variabilities as well as for recognizing individual patterns of movement and processes of motor learning. If the individual data were pooled across all participants, these subtle differences would only be represented by large standard deviations, which are often underemphasized by researchers or neglected.

In the applications we described, experienced performers were often employed as participants. However, interindividual variability is perhaps more apparent among very inexperienced performers. For example, Ulrich, Ulrich, Angulo-Kinzler, and Chapman (1997) noted that infants already show preferred phasing patterns when producing spontaneous kicking movements. For novices learning a new task, it is possible that the behavioral requirements of the novel task closely match their preexisting intrinsic dynamics, leading to a relatively successful performance straight away. Such matching may explain precocial behavior in sport demonstrated by some athletes who can perform incredibly well from an early age. The problem for the learner arises when there is a conflict in what he brings into the situation and what is eventually required from him. So the reason why novices sometimes produce successful patterns of movement very early in learning is linked to the fit between the intrinsic dynamics of the movement system and the task demands. Where there is a good fit between the two, positive transfer occurs. Where the task dynamics and intrinsic dynamics clash, negative transfer results.

Practitioners such as coaches or physical educators can use the concepts described in this chapter to enhance learning. The traditional emphasis on reducing error during the practice of a skill by encouraging consistency in motor patterns should be revised to acknowledge the valuable role of variability in moment-to-moment control as well as in long-term learning. A struggling learner can be viewed as a system that is temporarily trapped in a stable attractor state that does not correspond well with a behavioral solution satisfying task demands. As Corbetta and Veriejken (1999) suggest to practitioners, a strategy of perturbing the movement system may be necessary to help the learner let go of previous movement experiences. Techniques such as altering task constraints like rules, space, equipment, and number of opponents are useful ways to induce variability in movement and encourage exploration for alternative solutions. Altering task constraints question the traditional concepts of repetition and breaking down skills during practice to minimize variability in movement. Note that the learner may need additional encouragement and reassurance at this important stage, as performance could fluctuate as a consequence of the motor reorganization.

In this chapter, we have argued for and demonstrated the value of employing individualized analyses in research on movement in order to gain a clearer picture of how performers exploit variability. As more and more studies employ methods such as coordination profiling and cluster analysis, researchers are becoming increasingly convinced that a linear, causal relationship between the commands of the CNS and motor output cannot exist. For example, Latash (1996) suggested that the brain "does not care" exactly how the degrees of freedom in the system interact to produce goal-directed activity. Instead, varied movement trajectories emerge from the interplay among the specific task, environmental, and organismic constraints unique to each situation. This is particularly apparent within sport, where such factors change frequently and unexpectedly. As we have demonstrated, expert performers are increasingly recognized as having an ability to continually adapt their techniques as perceptual demands change. The mechanisms by which humans progress to this level of control as a function of learning or relearning provide a fruitful focus for future research.

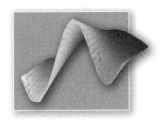

Chapter 8

Clinical Relevance of Variability in Coordination

Joseph Hamill, PhD, Jeffrey M. Haddad, MS,
Bryan C. Heiderscheit, PhD,
Richard E. A. Van Emmerik, PhD, and Li Li, PhD

Editors' Overview

This chapter shows that there are a number of potential reasons why variability is important during gait. A significant factor seems to be variation in the point of force application, which prevents repetitive strain injuries. Moreover, comparisons of gait in runners with and without patellofemoral pain reveal why lower levels of variability may be problematic. One of the practical implications from these findings is that integrating motor control theory and clinical biomechanics could identify the potential onset of injury due to the apparent inverse relationship between variability in coordination and the degree of pathology in runners. Indeed, increasing variability in coordination may be a sign of successful rehabilitation after injury. An important point in this chapter is that an interpretation of variability based on dynamic systems does not signify that all observed variability is beneficial but rather that all variability is not detrimental to performance. As long as basic postural requirements for stability are met, healthy movement systems can use variability in a functional way to explore task constraints. This chapter demonstrates the clinical relevance of variability by describing research on using an artificial constraint (a taping procedure) to help runners find more variability in coordination of the lower limb in order to reduce patellofemoral pain. These data exemplify how biomechanical analyses can be allied to the theory of motor control in assessing the relative merits and deficiencies of increasing or decreasing variability in key joint and limb couplings in the human motor system.

As discussed in chapter 3, the notion of variability has changed dramatically over the last decades. Due to research stemming from a perspective of dynamic systems, variability, once thought to be noise and detrimental to normal function, is now believed to be an essential element in normal, healthy functioning. This is not to imply that all variability is good. Rather, the perspective of dynamic systems has challenged the notion that all variability is bad. The actual role of variability in movement is currently a significant question being addressed in the movement sciences.

The Russian physiologist Nicolai Bernstein was one of the first individuals to measure and document variability in normal biological movement. Bernstein, in studying the repeatable movement of hammering, found that despite invariance in the end point of the hammer, large variability was present in its trajectory (Bernstein, 1967). He suggested, therefore, that variable trajectories could lead to the same motor solution (figure 8.1). Bernstein speculated that variability in movement emerged from the multiple degrees of freedom (DOF) inherent in biological systems and that coordination required these DOFs to be organized into functional units specific for a given context. He considered this tenet the primary problem in motor control. Bernstein's insights complement what is today considered the perspective of dynamic systems on motor control. According to this perspective, given the vast number of DOFs and the context specificity of movement, traditional models of motor programming for control cannot explain coordination. Essentially, a 1:1 mapping cannot exist between the motor commands and the associated motor outputs. Rather, coordinated movements and behaviors require units of action to be assembled into temporary linkages of controllable units (now termed coordinative structures), which are functional over specific purposes (Turvey, 1990). Coordinative structures are organized at all levels of the nervous system, and they emerge from constraints imposed on the DOFs of the system through an interaction of the individual, task, and environmental dynamics (Newell, 1986; Turvey 1990). This type of control essentially devolves responsibility from higher cognitive structures, places greater responsibility on the lower levels of the nervous system, and ultimately reduces the inherent DOFs into manageable units (Turvey, 1990).

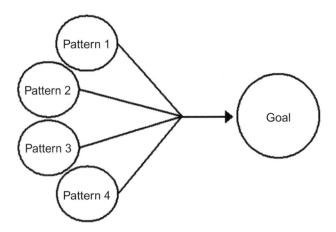

FIGURE 8.1   Multiple patterns of movement are available to achieve the same goal.

Bernstein's views came under scrutiny in the then Soviet Union, where Pavlovian ideas dominated at that time. Pavlovian doctrine regarded the motor system as being mainly reflexive in nature. Turvey (1990) states, "Reflexes, for example, were not elements of coordinated actions for Bernstein but, rather, elementary coordinated actions and, therefore, part of the problem of coordination rather than contributors to its solution" (p. 938).

It is now believed that the multiple DOFs, while providing an interesting challenge to control theorists, are responsible for the tremendous plasticity observed in the motor system. This motor adaptability can be seen in performers first learning a motor skill. The unskilled performer essentially becomes rigid and invariant, thus freezing many DOFs. In contrast, a skilled performer exploits and utilizes many DOFs, making her performance more graceful and adaptable (Vereijken et al., 1992). Thus, biological adaptability in movement emerges from the redundancy in the system, specifically from the coordination of multiple DOFs. This redundancy provides a variable family of motor solutions to a particular task (see figure 8.1).

In this chapter we discuss both traditional and more modern views of variability in movement, including what is currently regarded to be the clinical relevance of variability in two of the most important functions of the human motor system: gait and posture.

Variability in Traditional and Dynamic Systems Views

Traditionally, variability in the motor system was believed to be synonymous with pathology. This way of thinking emerged along two different lines. First, the locomotor and postural systems of patients with various motor pathologies qualitatively appeared highly variable. Second, according to principles of basic physics, variability was synonymous with instability. For example, to avoid falls, the center of mass (COM) must be kept within the base of support. Variability in the motor system that would cause the COM to translate closer to the limit of the base of support would be viewed as an instability. This belief, when applied to human systems, predicts that increasing the variability of the COM increases the incidence of falls.

As mentioned at the beginning of this chapter, recent theoretical and empirical constructs emerging from the dynamic systems perspective on movement control have challenged the notion that all variability is pathological. In many biological systems, variability is now considered the healthy norm in certain processes where highly stable systems may indicate pathology or disease. For example, a highly stable (repeatable) interbeat interval (the time in between heartbeats) indicates cardiac disease, and a certain degree of variability in the interbeat interval is considered the healthy norm (Glass & Mackey, 1988).

The role of variability in movement is not as clearly developed as its role in the heartbeat literature. Empirical research has focused primarily on measuring variability during posture and gait. Recently, the literature on posture and gait has suggested a potential benefit of variability under many different paradigms. This is not to say that variability is always beneficial, but rather that variability is not always detrimental. In the literature on postural control, the benefit of variability is seen as having a mostly sensorimotor nature. In the literature on gait, the sensorimotor function of variability is also considered important. However, there may also be certain anatomical benefits associated with variable patterns of gait. Specifically, variability may be necessary to prevent excessive wear and tear on the joint structures (Hamill, Van Emmerik, Heiderscheit, & Li, 1999).

Dynamic Systems Concept of Variability in Movement

Traditionally, a variable COM was thought to reflect a degenerative system of postural control in which variability increased the risk of a fall (Woollacott, Shumway-Cook, & Nashner, 1986). Clinicians expended great effort in not only diagnosing variable motor patterns but also improving postural stability by reducing center of pressure (COP) and COM excursions. These clinical beliefs emerged from studies examining the role of the sensory systems on balance control. These studies found that the visual (Lee and Lishman, 1975), vestibular, and somatosensory systems (Berthoz, 2000) highly impact postural dynamics. Further, a decrement in these perceptual systems (either experimentally or pathologically induced) increased variability in the COM during upright stance. These basic findings have been documented repeatedly and led to the notion that variability is pathological.

Although a high degree of variability can indeed be detrimental to upright stance, some variability may enhance the perceptual and motor factors involved in maintaining upright stance, and thus variability is functional. One basic question, however, emerges from the previous discussions: Given that variability typically correlates with pathology, how does the dynamic systems perspective demonstrate that variability can be functional? In the remainder of this section, we discuss the answer to this question.

Variability in Postural Control

Ecological psychology has developed along a pseudoparallel course to that of the dynamic systems perspective. Like the dynamic systems approach, the ecological approach stresses the importance of the dynamic interaction of the organism with the environment. Perception emerges from this dynamic interaction (Gibson, 1979). From the ecological perspective, perception cannot be studied devoid of the motor system and its link to the environment. Rather, movement is an active component in perception. The literature on postural control has often been written from this perspective and has thus stressed the importance of the interaction between the sensory and motor systems.

In an ecological perspective, the motor and sensory systems are complementary and work in parallel rather than series. It is through this interaction that the theoretical importance of variability may surface. Specifically, the motor system can enhance the information obtained by the sensory systems. Riccio and McDonald (1998) suggested that variability at higher frequencies may provide environmentally relevant information at bandwidths that do not interfere with the conscious detection from our perceptual systems. High-frequency variability may thus be used by the sensory systems. Riccio and McDonald (1998) suggest that the environmentally relevant information is then concatenated by the perceptual and motor systems in order to reduce it to a temporal scale over which meaningful information can be extracted or compensatory adjustments be made. The exact method that the perceptual systems use to concatenate this information is unknown. Riccio and McDonald (1998) suggest that simple summary statistics may be calculated over different frequency ranges. This allows the information to be transformed to a temporal scale, which is usable by a somewhat slower motor-effector system. This type of variability may provide information regarding the texture of the environment and is essentially exploratory. The information can be used by the person to control actions within the given environmental and internal constraints and to anticipate possible perturbations.

In this theoretical framework, variability can be healthy and exploratory. In some pathological situations, however, COP excursions are less variable and rigid. This rigidity suggests that the basic postural demands must be met before the system utilizes variability in an exploratory manner. This trade-off helps resolve the question posed earlier. Essentially, no conflict exists between the dynamic systems perception of variability and the traditional findings. Rather, there is a trade-off between variability and stability. As long as the basic requirements for the postural stability of the movement are met, the system may exhibit some variability as an exploratory tool. Thus in some conditions where the individual is not able to satisfy the basic postural requirements, variability may indeed be pathological. However, in other conditions variability may be an exploratory tool rather than a symptom of pathology and therefore functional. If variability can be functional, the etiology of variability in specific diseases should be examined, and ultimately the clinical treatments of various pathologies may need to be reassessed.

Recent empirical evidence supports this theoretical framework from the perspective of variability. Van Wegen, Van Emmerik & Riccio (2002) found that young subjects exhibit greater center of pressure excursion than healthy older subjects in quiet standing (figure 8.2). When asked to lean forward, the younger subjects were able to lean further relative to the boundaries of their base of support. In the leaning conditions, not only did the older subjects not lean as far, but their postural variability at the maximal lean condition was greater. Thus, variability was greater in the older subjects in the leaning condition but lesser in the quiet stance condition. Although these results seem counterintuitive, a simple yet interesting explanation can be derived from the data. In the leaning condition, the COP was displaced relative to the line of gravity, imposing a torque on the body and increasing the postural demands.

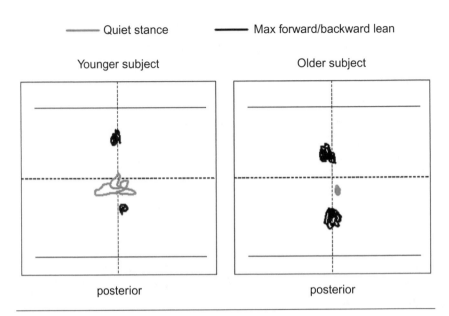

FIGURE 8.2   Examples of patterns in the center of pressure representing quiet stance and maximum forward and backward leans for young and old subjects.

Reprinted, by permission, from R. Van Emmerik and E.E.H. Van Wegen, 2002, "On functional aspects of variability in postural control," *Exercise in Sport Science Reviews* 30: 117-193.

The young subjects were essentially able to stabilize their bodies in response to this new postural demand and to lean forward relative to their base of support (thus successfully completing the task). Older subjects were not able to lean as far and their movements were more variable, indicating that they were not able to stabilize their bodies to successfully accomplish the new postural task. Thus, in the leaning condition, the variability observed among older subjects was actually destabilizing and not beneficial. In the quiet stance condition, the older subjects experienced a greater postural demand as compared to their younger counterparts. They could not beneficially utilize variability and thus stabilized their COPs in order to successfully complete the task. Again, it appears that the human body is able to use variability as an exploratory means only if the basic elements of the task are met (see also Van Emmerik & van Wegen, 2002).

We previously discussed how postural variability (delivered to the system by the motor apparatus) can enhance the information given to the sensory systems. Stochastic variability within the systems or artificially delivered to the cutaneous receptors may also aid postural control. Stochastic resonance has been demonstrated to have functional importance in various physiological systems, including human muscle spindles (Cordo, Inglis, Verschueren, Collins, Merfeld, Rosenblum, Buckley, & Moss, 1996). Through this mechanism, stochastic noise applied to the sensory systems helps amplify weak signals to a level where they can be perceived. Without the applied noise, the sensory signal remains outside of the detectable range. Priplata, Niemi, Salen, Harry, Lipsitz, & Collins (2002) found that this phenomenon of stochastic resonance also aids postural control. In this study, elderly subjects stood on a force platform while stochastic noise was delivered to their feet via shoe inserts. The postural stance of the elderly subjects resembled that of their younger counterparts when the shoe insert producing stochastic noise was used. These results indicate the potential use of stochastic resonance to enhance somatosensory function in older adults as well as in individuals experiencing peripheral neuropathies or strokes.

Variability in Gait Studies

Similarly to traditional postural studies, in some of the more common stride characteristics variability has been associated with decreased performance and pathology. One of the more common gait parameters, stride duration, has been used as a differentiating measurement among various groups. In one of Hausdorff's many papers on this topic (Hausdorff, Cudkowicz, Firtion, Wei, & Goldberger, 1998), he measured stride duration throughout a 6 min walk among two groups of healthy subjects: a young group (mean age of 22 y) and an elderly group (age greater than 70 y). Additionally, a third group was included that matched the ages of the healthy elderly group but that had a history of falls. The coefficient of variation was then determined for each subject, based on the standard deviation and the mean of the stride duration during the 6 min walk. When compared between the healthy young and elderly groups, the variability of the stride duration (as reflected in the coefficient of variation) was relatively consistent. However, the elderly group with a history of falls displayed 2 to 3 times the variability in stride duration than either healthy group. This led the authors to conclude that increased variability in stride duration is associated with the risk of falling.

In a similar experiment, Hausdorff and colleagues (1998) again investigated variability in stride duration and locomotion dysfunction. The coefficient of variation of stride duration was calculated among individuals with Parkinson's disease and Huntington's disease while they walked at a self-selected pace for 5 min. When compared to a healthy control, both the group with Parkinson's disease and the group with Huntington's disease displayed significantly increased variability in stride duration. Interestingly, the average stride duration between groups was the same, suggesting variability to be the more differentiating measurement. Variability was thus a measurement with which these various gait pathologies could be examined.

A different approach to assessing stability in gait has been pursued. It is based on nonlinear dynamic stability analyses, in the form of Lyapunov exponents (Rosenstein et al., 1993). Lyapunov exponents measure the degree of convergence of patterns in state space, with the magnitude of the exponent indicating the stability in the system. Stability assessments based on this Lyapunov procedure have recently been applied to human locomotion (Dingwell et al., 2001). These measurements of local stability capture very small ongoing perturbations to locomotion, such as those provided by the stride-to-stride fluctuations that occur during gait. Dingwell et al. (2001) showed that stride-to-stride variability is a poor indicator of local dynamic trunk stability. They also found age-related declines in this dynamic stability. The relation between variability and stability in the trunk, however, needs further examination, especially under more challenging postural conditions.

The work by Hausdorff also found that the variability in gait is not random but fractal. Using detrended fluctuation analysis (DFA), Hausdorff et al. (1996) showed that the stride interval obtained over long durations of overground locomotion contains self-similar fractal structure with long-range correlations. The self-similarity indicates that variability in the stride interval is not attributable to uncorrelated random fluctuations in the form of white noise. The fluctuations in the stride interval exhibited long-range power law correlations, which are signatures of fractal processes. In these fractal patterns, fluctuations at one timescale are statistically similar to fluctuations at another. The fractal nature of fluctuations in the stride interval indicates positive correlations in the duration of subsequent steps at timescales ranging from milliseconds to seconds to hours.

Among older adults and individuals with neurological disease (e.g., Huntington's disease), the fluctuations in the stride interval were observed to be more random (lacking self-similarity) (Hausdorff et al., 1997). These changes in the structure of variability do not necessarily relate to the magnitude of the variability, as no differences in the magnitudes of the variability in the stride interval between young and older individuals were observed. These observations clearly demonstrate the importance of assessing the structure of variability in gait measurements. Hausdorff and colleagues (1996, 1997) concluded from their results that variation in the stride parameters during gait is not random but is structured such that early fluctuations can affect the gait dynamics at a later time. Although these changes in the structure of variability (i.e., more random versus more structured $1/f$-type self-similar noise) identify a loss of complexity with disease (Lipsitz, 2002), the link to stability in gait is at best incomplete.

To suggest that all variability has deleterious effects or that all variability is beneficial would be a significant overstatement. Rather, the beneficial effects depend on the dynamics of the system (i.e., fixed-point or limit-cycle attractors) (Vaillancourt and Newell, 2002). It is more plausible to propose that variability may be classified in either category depending on its observed effect on the movement or task of interest. As previously mentioned, to define the role of variability in movement, variability must be considered in respect to its effect on the task. The uncontrolled manifold hypothesis proposed by Scholz and Schöner (1999) incorporates this concept. Generally, this hypothesis states that in performing a specific task, the involved elements (i.e., joints, muscles) are restricted to a particular range of operation such that the desired task is successfully achieved. Provided the elements stay within the restricted range, they remain uncontrolled. The elements can and will show greater variability, provided that successful task completion is not threatened. This concept can be illustrated in a sit-to-stand task. The horizontal momentum of the COM is an important variable for the successful completion of this task. Configurations of joint angle and joint velocity that alter the COM horizontal momentum threaten successful completion. Therefore, these configurations can be partitioned into those that maintain an invariant COM horizontal momentum and those that do not. Utilizing this approach, Reisman et al. (2002) observed that during repeated trials of the sit-to-stand task, a variety of configurations of joint angle and velocity occurred that maintained the COM horizontal momentum. Fewer configurations were displayed that changed the horizontal momentum. Thus, it appears that variability in joint coordination is inherent to the movement and does not need continuous on-line control unless it jeopardizes the successful completion of the task.

Variability in Gait Pathology

Several studies have concluded that variability in coordination provides the flexibility required to locomote in various environments (Clark and Phillips, 1993; Holt et al., 1995). Recently, this notion of control flexibility has been extended to include patterns of movement resulting from lower-extremity injury. Hamill et al. (1999) used coordination dynamics to suggest that coupling variability can relate to overuse injury. In particular, they explored patellofemoral pain (PFP) during running. The authors used the variability of the continuous relative phase (CRP) of the coupling of contiguous joints or segments that relate to the knee (see chapter 3 for a detailed description of these analyses). Their hypothesis was that the low variability in joint-segment coupling represented the injured condition while high variability indicated the healthy condition. They suggested that the low variability in the injured condition may further stress soft tissue such as cartilage, tendon, and ligament and that this repeated stress may lead to degenerative changes. On the other hand, the high variability of the healthy condition created multiple combinations of coupling actions that would not repeatedly stress the soft tissue. However, these authors could not determine whether the low variability was a result or cause of the knee pain.

Heiderscheit et al. (2002) tested the hypothesis on low variability in coupling in a study on patellofemoral pain. Using the same joint and segment couplings used by Hamill et al. (1999), they examined subjects with unilateral PFP and healthy, matched controls. Rather than using CRP, Heiderscheit et al. used an angle–angle representation of the coupling and a modified vector coding technique (Sparrow et al., 1987). Figure 8.3 presents the results of one coupling, internal and external rotation of the thigh and internal and external rotation of the leg. In this figure, we see that the variability of the control subjects is the same bilaterally. However, the PFP subjects clearly have less variability in the coupling of the involved limb than in the noninvolved limb.

A further hypothesis tested by Heiderscheit (2000) involved relieving the pain in the PFP knee by taping. The variability of the thigh–leg rotation coupling

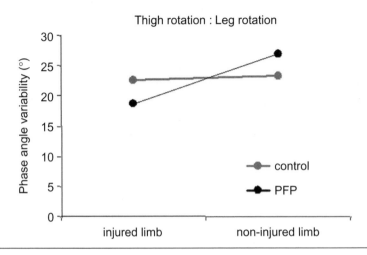

FIGURE 8.3   Mean thigh–leg rotation coupling for unilateral PFP patients versus controls.

Adapted, by permission, from B.C. Heiderscheit, J. Hamill, and R.E.A. Van Emmerik, 2002, "Variability of stride characteristics and joint coordination among individuals with unilateral patellofemoral pain," *Journal of Applied Biomechanics* 18: 119.

is presented in figure 8.4. In both the control subjects and the noninvolved limb of the PFP subjects, there was no significant change in the variability of the coupling after taping. However, with the taping applied to the PFP limb, there was a significant increase in the variability of the coupling. This suggests that the low variability is a product of the pain that the individual suffers while running. In effect, the subject appears to adjust her running mechanics to avoid pain, thus reducing the variability in the coupling.

In a recent set of studies conducted in our laboratory, we investigated the variability in lower-extremity coupling in males and females performing an unanticipated cutting maneuver (Pollard, 2002). The thesis of these studies involved the overwhelming evidence that females have a greater propensity for injuring the anterior cruciate ligament (ACL) than males and that the majority of these injuries occurs during noncontact, cutting activities. We used the same vector coding technique and couplings used in the Heiderscheit et al. (2003) study. Figure 8.5 illustrates the mean variability in the thigh–leg rotation coupling for all subjects across the stance phase of a cutting maneuver. During the 25% to 45% interval of stance, the subjects change the locomotor direction, and it is at this time in the stance phase that the subjects may be at their most vulnerable position regarding the tension on the ACL. Pollard (2002) observed that women have significantly less variability in joint coupling than males do during this interval. The author concluded that the reduced variability and the resulting reduced movement flexibility may place females at greater risk for injury.

As stated previously, it is a gross oversimplification to refer to high variability as completely beneficial. It appears that a certain amount of variability in

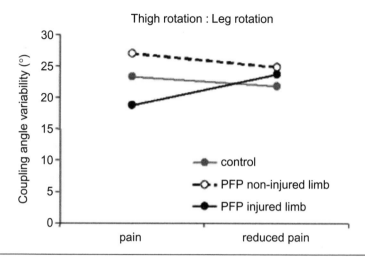

FIGURE 8.4   Mean thigh–leg rotation coupling for unilateral PFP patients versus controls in conditions of tape and no tape.
Adapted from Heiderscheit 2002.

coupling is beneficial but that too much variability may be disadvantageous. Thus, in an optimal performance, consistency and variability must be balanced (Turvey, 1990). Delineation of the appropriate levels of variability and consistency has yet to be performed for posture and locomotion. This delineation might be specific to task and dynamics.

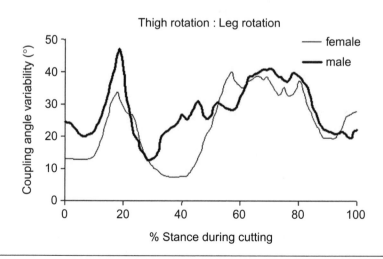

FIGURE 8.5   Mean thigh–leg rotation coupling for males and females during the stance phase of an unanticipated cutting maneuver.
Adapted from Pollard 2002.

Further studies have investigated variability in several populations with pathologies such as Parkinson's disease, cerebral palsy, and tardive dyskinesia. In a study by Van Emmerik et al. (1999), coordination of the pelvis and thorax during locomotion was compared between individuals with Parkinson's disease and age-matched, nonimpaired individuals. Axial coordination (pelvic–thoracic coupling) and stride duration were assessed while subjects ambulated on a treadmill at varying speeds (0.2-1.4 m/s). The nonimpaired individuals displayed distinct increases in the variability of axial coordination at speeds coinciding with changes in the pattern of axial coordination. The individuals with Parkinson's disease, however, displayed a reduced variability in axial coordination at the faster speeds as compared to the nonimpaired individuals. Further, many of the subjects with Parkinson's disease did not demonstrate the pattern change in axial coordination that was apparent in the nonimpaired group. The authors concluded that the reduced variability among the subjects with Parkinson's disease contributed to the axial rigidity by preventing a change in the pattern of axial coordination. Further, the two groups displayed similar variability in stride duration, suggesting that traditional stride parameters are not sensitive enough to detect differences in coordination when the speed of locomotion is controlled.

Reduced variability in the coordination between joints has also been identified in the affected limbs of children with spastic hemiplegic cerebral palsy (Jeng et al., 1996). The observed stereotypical coordination was attributed to the reduced variability resulting from neural and mechanical deficits. While the affected limb displayed a more consistent pattern of movement, the nonaffected limb revealed an increase in variability as compared to nonimpaired children. The authors concluded that the increased variability of the nonaffected limb provided a means of adaptation or compensation for the deficits of the affected limb.

The stereotypical patterns of movement and postural problems observed in individuals with tardive dyskinesia have also been associated with reduced variability in posture and coordination. Tardive dyskinesia is a movement disorder marked by involuntary stereotypical movements that can occur secondarily to prolonged use of neuroleptic medication. Individuals with this disorder display reduced variability in the movement trajectory of the center of foot pressure (Newell et al., 1993).

Clinical Relevance of Variability

As is evident from the examples in the literature on posture and gait, variability in joint coordination may play a functional role in human movement. Variability is a part of the dynamics of movement and as such can be altered by changes in the movement itself. Several techniques have been used to clinically alter variability in movement. Wagenaar and Van Emmerik (1994) incorporated an external auditory rhythm for individuals with Parkinson's disease to move their arms and legs in temporal synchrony and observed a reduction in the characteristic axial rigidity. Using an orthotic device has also been regarded as an environmental change that can affect the overall system dynamics (Kamm et al., 1990). Without containing instructions for a different pattern of movement, the orthosis can disrupt the current pattern and provide an avenue to seek a potentially better one.

Variability can also indicate an impending change in the pattern of movement. In dynamic systems theory, the information regarding variability in movement can be valuable to the clinician in treating movement disorders. In general, the observed dynamics of particular variables are utilized to understand the process of pattern change. Once the process is determined in nonimpaired individuals, it can be applied to individuals with movement dysfunction. Scholz (1990) provided an excellent review of the dynamic systems theory and how it can be incorporated into therapeutic practice.

From a clinical perspective, treating movement dysfunction may be most effective when the system is in transition (i.e., with increased pattern variability). If a consistent, stable pattern is observed, attempts to improve the movement dysfunction may be ineffective (Kamm et al., 1990). From a dynamic systems perspective, variability indicates that the system is in a more flexible state, which allows therapeutic interventions to be more effective. Kamm et al. (1990) discussed providing a safe, yet progressively unstable environment for the patient, thereby allowing the patient to explore the movement boundaries. For example, altering the locomotion speed or surface to make it more challenging may elicit a change in the movement coordination displayed by the patient. This change in the pattern of movement is typically preceded by an increase in its variability.

Conclusions

The traditional notion clearly identifies variability in movement as a characteristic of the unhealthy or pathological state. The dynamic systems perspective has forced us to rethink this notion. In fact, there is ample evidence indicating that variability is inherent to movement and is exploited by the system dynamics. Variability is an integral part of the solution to the problem of performing tasks well (Todorov and Jordan, 2002). Therefore, the notion of abolishing variability in clinical practice needs to be reconsidered with respect to the individual, task, and environment. Rather than be a liability, variability in movement may be a beneficial, adaptive mechanism.

Chapter 9

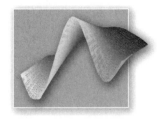

Measuring Coordination and Variability in Coordination

Jonathan S. Wheat, PhD and Paul S. Glazier

Editors' Overview

This chapter reviews tools for measuring movement coordination and its variability and draws attention to the capacity of enhanced technology in motion analysis for providing detailed measurements of the coordination among limb segments and joints of the body. The review is highly relevant for theorists of motor control interested in measuring movement coordination and its variability during complex actions with multiple degrees of freedom such as locomotion. Key differences in methodological assumptions in the literature on biomechanics and motor control are identified, such as in assumptions regarding the definition of phase angle used when describing coordination between two segments. Decisions in measurement protocol, such as whether conventional linear statistics or circular statistical techniques should be used, can greatly influence the level of variability found in coordination. Although the literature is currently focusing a lot of attention on continuous relative phase and vector coding techniques, no single ideal technique exists for measuring coordination and its variability over time. Consequently, researchers need to be aware of the strengths and limitations of existing methods and should state the rationale for using particular methodologies in their research studies to help readers interpret what amount of variability in the data is likely due to measurement errors and discrepancies. Measuring coordination and its variability is an issue that continues to challenge researchers in the movement sciences.

As Glazier, Wheat, Pease, and Bartlett highlighted in chapter 3, traditionally in biomechanics, data from isolated joints (e.g., displacement, velocity, angle, force, and so on) are presented as a function of time, with much research focusing on the relative timing and magnitude of time-discrete kinematic variables. Glazier and colleagues drew attention to studies that have investigated the coordination between joints and body segments. It has recently been suggested that the coordination or coupling relationships between segments may be an important line of investigation owing to the fact that motor behaviors may be distinguished by the coordination between entire limbs and body segments (Tepavac and Field-Fote, 2001). Also, the coordination between adjacent anatomical structures, such as the subtalar and knee joints, has been implicated in the etiology of injuries (e.g., Lafortune, Cavanagh, Sommer, and Kalenak, 1994; McClay and Manal, 1997; Stergiou and Bates, 1997; Nawoczenski, Saltzman, and Cook, 1998; Stergiou, Bates and James, 1999). However, quantifying the coordination between two body segments is problematic. In this chapter we outline, from a biomechanical perspective, various techniques that are commonly used in research on motor control in order to measure coordination and, arguably more importantly, variability in coordination. We also highlight the major benefits and limitations of these methods.

Measuring Coordination and Variability in Coordination

In the late 1960s, Grieve (1968, 1969) proposed that the angular time series of two joints be plotted against each other on what was called a relative motion plot. These plots, also known as angle–angle diagrams, have since been used to distinguish normal and pathological gait (Hershler and Milner, 1980; Miller, 1981; Charteris, 1982), compare symmetrical and asymmetrical gait (Whitall and Caldwell, 1992), identify differences between same-field and opposite-field hitting in baseball players of different expertise (McIntyre and Pfautsch, 1982), and examine changes in coordination during the practice of a soccer kick (Anderson and Sidaway, 1994). However, as Tepavac and Field-Fote (2001) highlighted, angle–angle diagrams are excellent for qualitative purposes but quantifying the data can be problematic. Parenthetically, the problem of how to quantify the coordination between body segments is effectively the same as of how to quantify the data in an angle–angle diagram. Many techniques have emerged to quantitatively evaluate the coordination or coupling between body segments, including discrete relative phase (van Emmerik and Wagenaar, 1996; LaFiandra, Wagenaar, Holt, and Obusek, 2003), continuous relative phase (Hamill, van Emmerik, Heiderscheit, and Li, 1999; Heiderscheit, Hamill, and van Emmerik, 1999; Post, Daffertshofer, and Beek, 2000; van Uden, Bloo, Kooloos, van Kampen, de Witte, and Wagenaar, 2003), vector coding techniques (Whiting and Zernicke, 1982; Sparrow, Donovan, van Emmerik, and Barry, 1987; Tepavac and Field-Fote, 2001; Heiderscheit, Hamill, and van Emmerik, 2002), and other techniques such as cross-correlation (Amblard, Assaiante, Lekhel, and Marchland, 1994) and normalized root mean squared difference (Sidaway, Heise, and Schoenfelder-Zohdi, 1995). In the following sections we review these techniques, focusing mainly on methods of relative phase and vector coding, and we discuss their relative merits and limitations in quantifying coordination and variability in coordination.

Relative Phase

Both discrete relative phase (DRP) and continuous relative phase (CRP) are based on the assumptions that the two oscillating segments under scrutiny are of a one-to-one frequency ratio and they exhibit a sinusoidal time history (Hamill et al., 2000). Clearly, segmental motions in gait and sport do not always meet these assumptions, and problems can arise when using relative phase to quantify the coordination between body segments in such activities. Care should therefore be taken when interpreting relative phase in relation to intersegment coordination, especially if these assumptions are violated. However, alternative techniques are available, such as relative Fourier phase (Lamoth, Beek, and Meijer, 2002; see the section "Continuous Relative Phase"), to transform the data and ensure that they satisfy the assumptions.

Discrete Relative Phase   DRP is a point estimate that illustrates the latency of an event in the motion of a segment with respect to the motion of another segment (Kelso, 1995). When the relative timing of the events between two segments is important, as in investigating the relationship between subtalar inversion-eversion and knee flexion-extension (Lafortune et al., 1994; McClay and Manal, 1997; Stergiou and Bates, 1997; Nawoczenski et al., 1998; Stergiou et al., 1999), DRP may be an important variable. DRP has already been used to measure the phase difference between thoracic and pelvic rotations during treadmill walking (Lamoth et al., 2002), determine the effect of load carriage on trunk coordination (La Fiandra et al., 2003), and examine the transition between walking and running in human locomotion (Diedrich and Warren, 1995). DRP can be calculated using the following equation:

$$\Phi = \frac{t_{\max\varphi 1(j)} - t_{\max\varphi 2(j)}}{t_{\max\varphi 1(j+1)} - t_{\max\varphi 1(j)}} \times 360° \tag{9.1}$$

In this equation, t is time, $max\varphi 1$ is the maximum rotation of segment 1, $max\varphi 2$ is the maximum rotation of segment 2, and φ is the phase difference during the cycle j.

Hamill et al. (2000) suggested that, when considering the example of knee flexion-extension and subtalar inversion-eversion, in which it might be appropriate to study the stance phase in isolation, foot strike could be used as the initial point of the cycle. They also suggested that the length of the stance phase could represent the time of the cycle. Therefore, in this example $max\varphi 1$ is maximum subtalar eversion, $max\varphi 2$ is maximum knee flexion, and the period of time (the denominator) is simply the duration of the stance.

Since DRP is calculated in the range of $0° \leq \varphi \leq 360°$ and there is redundancy in the angles (e.g., $0°$ and $360°$ are equivalent), DRP is a circular variable. Therefore, to avoid phase wrapping (Burgess-Limerick, Abernethy, and Neal, 1991; Lamoth et al., 2002), the average DRP over several cycles and the variability of coordination should be calculated using circular statistics (see Batschelet, 1981 or Mardia, 1971 for an overview).

One advantage of DRP is that it requires no further manipulation of the data other than that which is normally carried out in the calculation of joint angles (Hamill et al., 2000). However, problems may arise if the data do not meet the assumptions of having sinusoidal time histories and a one-to-one frequency ratio. There would certainly be a problem if definite peak values could not be ascertained or respective peak values changed between cycles. In other words, patterns of angular displacement that contain multiple maxima and minima might impede the calculation of DRP if the magnitudes of the peaks changed from cycle to cycle, such that selecting a peak in each cycle that correctly corresponds to peaks in other cycles is difficult. This phenomenon would be most detrimental to calculating variability in coordination, as erroneously high variability may be calculated simply because the magnitudes of the separate peaks change between each cycle. Changes in respective peak values are not a problem in most of the examples from the literature on coordination cited earlier in this section. They might become a problem if DRP is used to analyze other sport techniques or joint motions with more peaks and troughs in the angular displacement time series. Changes in the magnitudes of the peaks from cycle-to-cycle might introduce ambiguity into the definition of the required peak value. Another obvious disadvantage is that DRP provides only one measurement per cycle of movement.

Continuous Relative Phase CRP indicates the phase relation between two oscillating segments at each sampled data point throughout the cycle of movement. Both CRP and variability in CRP have been used to examine running injuries (Hamill et al., 1999; Heiderscheit et al., 1999), the coordination of finger oscillations (Kelso, 1981, 1984), the coordination of thorax and pelvis rotations (van Emmerik and Wagenaar, 1996; Lamoth et al., 2002; LaFiandra et al., 2003), patterns of coordination in walking and running (Li, van den Bogert, Caldwell, van Emmerik and Hamill, 1999), one-legged hopping (van Uden et al., 2003), and intralimb coordination following obstacle clearance (Stergiou, Scholten, Jensen, and Blanke, 2001; Stergiou, Jensen, Bates, Scholten, and Tzetzis, 2001). The CRP between two oscillating segments at any given instant is defined as the difference between the respective phase angles of each segment. Hamill et al. (2000) recently highlighted that before CRP can be calculated, the displacements and velocities of the segments need to be normalized to eliminate the effects of differences in the amplitudes of the range of motion of each segment—this issue is discussed later in this section. Also, the displacement and velocity data should be interpolated to a fixed number of data points so that ensemble averages and variability can be calculated. These displacement and velocity data are then used to construct a phase-plane portrait (normalized angular velocity versus normalized angular displacement) for each segment; a typical phase-plane portrait is illustrated in figure 9.1. Phase-plane portraits graphically represent all possible states of the segment (Clark, 1995), as the behavior of a dynamical system may be captured by a variable and its first derivative with respect to time (Rosen, 1970).

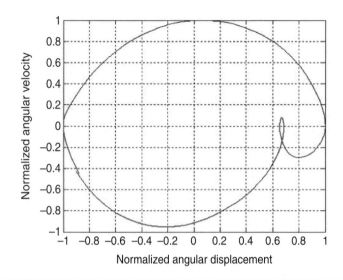

FIGURE 9.1   An example of a phase-plane portrait for hip flexion-extension.

The Cartesian coordinates of each data point on the phase plane are then converted to polar coordinates. The phase angle component is given by the following equation:

$$\varphi(t) = \tan^{-1}\left(\frac{\dot{\theta}(t)}{\theta(t)}\right) \tag{9.2}$$

In this equation, $\dot{\theta}$ is normalized angular velocity, θ is the normalized angular displacement, and φ is the phase angle at time t.

The CRP between the two segments can be calculated as the difference between their phase angles, which is usually achieved by subtracting the phase angle of the distal segment from that of the proximal segment. For example, the CRP between the shank and the foot during running is calculated using the following equation:

$$\Phi(t) = \varphi_{shank}(t) - \varphi_{foot}(t) \tag{9.3}$$

In this equation, φ_{shank} is the phase angle of the shank, φ_{foot} is the phase angle of the foot, and Φ is the CRP at time t.

In calculating the component phase angle, the output of $\tan^{-1}(y/x)$ takes on values between $-90°$ and $+90°$. Therefore, the output data need manipulating to ensure that the component phase angles are calculated within a suitable range. In the literature on studies using CRP, a discrepancy exists in the definition of the range of component phase angle used. In motor control (see Scholz, 1990 for an overview), a range of $0° \leq \varphi \leq 360°$ has typically been used, but the recent application of this technique in biomechanics has brought with it a new range of $0° \leq \varphi \leq 180°$. Hamill et al. (2000) suggested that this new range is necessary because there is redundancy in the angles in the original range ($0°$ and $360°$ mean the same thing). Presumably, this new definition is preferred because it avoids discontinuities in the component phase angles, which can be problematic if conventional linear statistical analyses are used.

Changes in the definitions of the component phase angle, however, affect the values of the computed CRP. Wheat, Bartlett, and Milner (2003) investigated the effect of using different definitions of component phase angles on CRP. In this study, test data were created for two segments using sine and cosine functions. Data from a sine function served as the angular displacement of one segment. Similarly, as cosine is the first derivative of sine, data from a cosine function served as the angular velocity of the same segment. The CRP of the two segments was manipulated by adding a given amount to the angles inputted into the sine and cosine functions for the second segment. Three conditions were tested in which the segments were 180°, 90°, and 45° out of phase. In the 180° out-of-phase conditions, constant CRP values that instantaneously switched between 180° and −180° were apparent for the range of $0° \leq \varphi \leq 360°$, but they were not evident when the phase angles were defined in a range of $0° \leq \varphi \leq 180°$ (figure 9.2). Instead, a gradual shift between 180° and −180° was seen. Similar results were obtained for the 90° and 45° out-of-phase conditions.

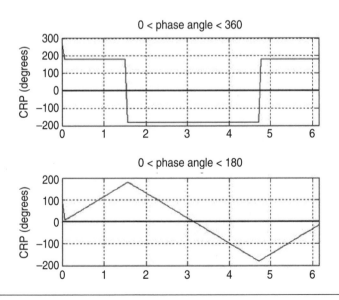

FIGURE 9.2 Continuous relative phase calculated with two different definitions of component phase angle.

It appears that if information about the coordination between segments is required, the range of $0° \leq \varphi \leq 360°$ is most suitable because the range of $0° \leq \varphi \leq 180°$ does not yield correct results. In other words, if Kelso had used the range of $0° \leq \varphi \leq 180°$ in his work monitoring nonlinear phase transitions in finger movement, he would never have been able to record the antiphase ($\pm180°$ out-of-phase) relationship. Recently, other ranges have also been used, including $-180° \leq \varphi \leq 180°$ (e.g., Lamoth et al., 2002), which is effectively the same as $0° \leq \varphi \leq 360°$, and $0° \leq \varphi \leq 90°$ (e.g., Kurz and Stergiou, 2002), which has the same problems as $0° \leq \varphi \leq 180°$. As already suggested, presumably the definition of $0° \leq \varphi \leq 180°$ (and $0° \leq \varphi \leq 90°$) was used to avoid the discontinuities in the component phase angles and, subsequently, in the CRP data during the analysis of most movements. These discontinuities can introduce anomalies that may cause erroneously high variability with conventional linear statistical techniques. However, this problem is easily solved if the recommended circular statistical techniques are used (see Burgess-Limerick et al., 1991; Lamoth et al., 2002). If researchers wish to present CRP data graphically as a function of time but do not want to present data containing discontinuities, they should manipulate CRP data to a suitable range after calculation, as Lamoth et al. (2002) have done. Authors should certainly state their definitions of phase angle so the reader can make an informed and correct interpretation of the results (Wheat et al., 2003).

As mentioned previously, the need to normalize the data in a phase-plane portrait has been identified (e.g., Hamill et al., 2000). Normalization adjusts for amplitude differences in the ranges of motion and centers the phase-plane portraits about the origin (Hamill et al., 2000; Lamoth et al., 2002). Hamill et al. (2000) presented data highlighting the effects of different normalization techniques on CRP and variability in CRP. Differences were seen in both CRP and variability in CRP among the four techniques discussed. The authors suggested that ultimately the choice of a normalization procedure will likely depend on specific aspects of the research question. Conversely, Kurz and Stergiou (2002) suggested that normalization is not required when calculating component phase angles. They investigated the effects of three different conditions of normalization—two normalization techniques and no normalization—on calculating phase angles within two different ranges, which appear to be $0° \leq \varphi \leq 180°$ and $0° \leq \varphi \leq 90°$. They suggested that certain combinations of parameters produced "errors" in the calculated CRP. They proposed that normalizing the data on a phase plane is not required because of the properties of the arctangent used in calculating the component phase angles. They suggested that CRP is not affected by differences in amplitude between segments since the arctangent is based on a ratio (velocity / displacement) and the differences in amplitude are removed during the calculation of phase angle (Kurz and Stergiou, 2002). However, Peters, Haddad, Heiderscheit, van Emmerick, and Hamill (2003) used distorted sine waves with a known phase relationship to present data that suggested that calculating CRP without normalizing the data on a phase plane produced erroneous results. Even when two sine waves with a frequency other than $0.5 / \pi$ were tested, incorrect CRP values were obtained without normalization. Another reason for normalizing the data on a phase plane is to center the trajectory on the origin (Hamill et al., 2000). In their analysis, Kurz and Stergiou (2002) used phase angle definitions of $0° \le \varphi \le 180°$ and $0° \le \varphi \le 90°$, which have been shown to produce questionable CRP results (Wheat et al., 2003). Additionally, not normalizing the data affects the variability of CRP. As Heiderscheit (2000) indicated when highlighting the reasons why nonsinusoidal data affect variability in CRP, the proximity of a data point to the origin of the phase plane can directly influence the calculated variability in coordination. Two data points at a fixed distance exhibit a greater difference in phase angle the closer they are to the origin of the phase plane (figure 9.3). This suggests that when the data on phase planes are not normalized, high variability is observed in segments with small amplitudes. More work using both circular statistics and suitable definitions of component phase angle is required to determine the effects of different normalization techniques on calculations of CRP and variability in CRP.

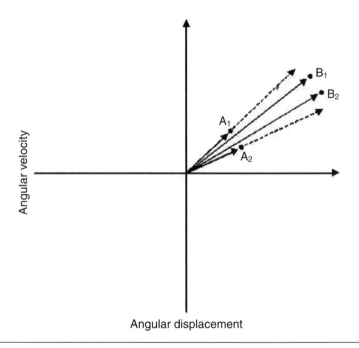

FIGURE 9.3 Data points are influenced by their proximity to the origin. Data points A_1 and A_2 have a greater difference in phase angle than do data points B_1 and B_2, even though the points in each pair are the same distance apart.

CRP has many advantages in quantifying both coordination and variability in coordination. First, because angular velocity is included in the calculation of the component phase angles, CRP contains temporal—in addition to spatial—information (Hamill et al., 1999; Hamill et al., 2000), which gives a higher-dimensional and more detailed analysis of the behavior (Hamill et al., 1999). Additionally, the inclusion of angular velocity data might make CRP a more sensitive measurement of variability in coordination (Wheat, Mullineaux, Bartlett and Milner, 2002) than other techniques. However, a higher derivative (angular velocity) in the calculation propagates any errors—whether they are due to movement of the skin marker, to the recording system, or to any other source—in the displacement data. It may also introduce a greater error into the CRP data, which may then be interpreted as increased variability. Several authors (Burgess-Limerick et al., 1991; Stergiou, Scholten et al., 2001) have reported that CRP is advantageous since there is evidence suggesting that receptors exist within muscles and tendons that control both the position and velocity of the respective body segment (McCloskey, 1978). Finally, another advantage of CRP is that it continuously measures coordination and variability in coordination throughout the entire movement. CRP and variability in CRP can therefore be calculated for different phases of the gait cycle for example (Hamill et al., 1999; Heiderscheit et al., 1999; Stergiou et al., 2001a; Stergiou et al., 2001b). This is particularly useful because of changing functional demands on the lower extremity throughout the stride cycle (Heiderscheit et al., 2002).

There are also limitations to calculating CRP. A fundamental limitation is the assumption that the time histories of the joint motions are sinusoidal. Clearly, this is not the case for some joint motions during some activities. However, in some cases centering the phase-plane trajectory on the origin by using a normalization procedure makes the time histories more suitable. As mentioned previously, the issue of whether or not the data on a phase plane need normalizing is a contentious one and requires further clarification. Also, there are techniques that effectively transform the data so that they have a more sinusoidal time history. Relative Fourier phase, for example, essentially transforms the data into the frequency domain and discards any frequencies other than the fundamental frequency. When the data are reconstructed in the time domain, the displacement trace is suitable for CRP calculations can be conducted. In their study on coordination between the pelvis and thorax during pathological walking, Lamoth et al. (2002) justified this approach because "movements of the pelvis are affected by forceful contacts between the feet and the support surface . . . which induce oscillations affecting the phase progression of the pelvis rotation" (p. 112). In other words, Lamoth et al. were arguing that oscillations other than those at the fundamental frequency are not relevant to the coordination of the pelvis and thorax. However, when applying this technique to other coordinative structures, care should be taken to not disregard potentially relevant information. Another possible problem with CRP that has been raised by other authors (Tepavac and Field-Fote, 2001; Mullineaux and Wheat,

2002) is that it is hard to relate to conceptually. This is mainly a problem for practitioners trying to interpret the type and nature of the relationship between joints and body segments. If the magnitude of variability in coordination is of interest, this is not so much of an issue.

Vector Coding Techniques

Numerous vector coding techniques have been introduced to quantify the data in relative motion plots and the variability in angle–angle trajectories (e.g., Whiting and Zernicke, 1982; Sparrow et al., 1987; Tepavac and Field-Fote, 2001; Heiderscheit et al., 2002). These techniques stem from the early work of Freeman (1961), who devised a chain-encoding technique to quantify an angle–angle curve. The procedure involves using a superimposed grid to transform the angle–angle trajectory into digital elements (see figure 9.4). Subsequently, a chain of digits that are based on the directions of the line segments formed by the frame-to-frame intervals between two consecutive data points is created. The chain of digits approximates the shape of the original analog curve. Integer chains from two different cycles are then cross-correlated to obtain a recognition coefficient, which is the peak value of the cross-correlation function. This technique has been used in studies of locomotion (Hershler and Milner, 1980; Whiting and Zernicke, 1982). However, as Tepavac and Field-Fote (2001) suggested, a flaw with this technique is that it converts data on the ratio scale to the nominal scale, risking the loss of important information and limiting the types of statistical analysis that can be applied. Also, a moti-

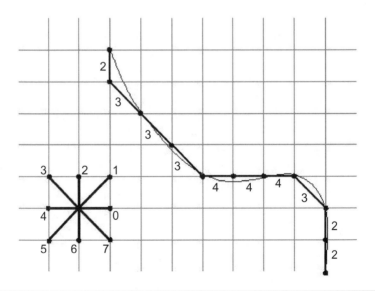

FIGURE 9.4 Freeman's (1961) chain-encoding technique.

vation behind Freeman's (1961) technique, computer efficiency, is no longer applicable owing to advances in computer hardware and software technology such as increased processor speeds and more sophisticated statistical analysis packages (Sparrow et al., 1987).

Another problem with this technique is that it requires the data points to be equally spaced. Sparrow et al. (1987) recognized that data are not always equally spaced in human movement and proposed a revised cross-correlation formula that takes into account the length of the frame-to-frame interval. However, Tepavac and Field-Fote (2001) identified two problems with the technique of Sparrow et al. (1987): (1) the two trajectories of interest must have an equal number of data points, and (2) it can only compare two trajectories at a time (multiple cycles must be compared in pairs).

Tepavac and Field-Fote (2001) revised the technique to address the above limitations. The authors presented a vector-based coding scheme that keeps data on a ratio scale for the quantification and analysis of relative motion. Field-Fote and Tepavac (2002) suggested that the technique provides an alternative to relative phase analysis. The technique was designed to help practitioners interpret the data, because these practitioners are more likely to think of movement in terms of joint angles and not phase values. In a way similar to that of Sparrow et al. (1987), Tepavac and Field-Fote (2001) identified the direction and magnitude of the frame-to-frame intervals on the angle–angle trajectories and calculated the magnitude and direction of the vector connecting the two points of the relative motion plot. However, as opposed to using pair-wise comparisons and cross-correlations, circular statistics were used to calculate the standard deviation of the direction of the vector at each frame-to-frame interval ($a_{i,\,i+1}$). This means that the variability in the angular component of the angle–angle trajectory can be calculated at each frame-to-frame interval for multiple cycles. The variability in the magnitude of the frame-to-frame vector was also calculated ($m_{i,\,i+1}$). Finally, the overall variability of the angle–angle trajectories was measured by simply finding the product of $a_{i,\,i+1}$ and $m_{i,\,i+1}$ ($r_{i,\,i+1}$) and was called the coefficient of correspondence. Field-Fote and Tepavac (2002) contended that this revised technique is mathematically equivalent to that of Sparrow et al. (1987). These three separate measurements mean that when using the vector coding algorithm (Tepavac and Field-Fote, 2001) it is possible to separately analyze a relative motion plot by its shape, the lengths of the frame-to-frame intervals, or the frame-to-frame vector deviation (a combination of shape and magnitude). Field-Fote and Tepavac (2002) used their vector coding technique to assess the consistency or variability of the coupling between the hip and knee in patients with incomplete spinal cord injury. These authors studied the patients over multiple cycles of treadmill walking performed both before and after a time of training. They used only the measurement of shape to assess variability, presumably because they thought changes in magnitude (changes in the range of motion at each joint from cycle to cycle) do not significantly affect the cycle-to-cycle variability relative to the shape changes in this population.

Both Hamill et al. (2000) and Heiderscheit et al. (2002) proposed subtle alternatives to the technique of Tepavac and Field-Fote (2001). These alternatives were presented as modifications to the method of Sparrow et al. (1987). In both techniques a coupling angle was defined as the orientation of the vector (relative to the right horizontal) between two adjacent points on the angle–angle plot (see figure 9.5). This is similar to the measurement of shape by Tepavac and Field-Fote (2001).

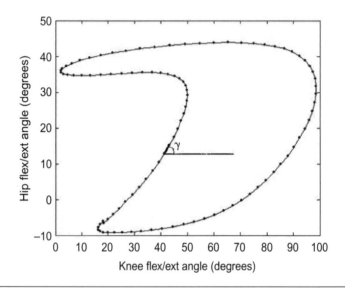

FIGURE 9.5   An illustration of the calculation for a coupling angle from an angle–angle plot.

The variability in the coupling angle over multiple cycles was then calculated at each frame-to-frame interval using circular statistics. However, no measurement was made of the magnitude of the frame-to-frame vectors, which may represent a limitation of this technique. This method of vector coding was also used by Heiderscheit et al. (2002) to compare variability in joint coordination during treadmill running in participants with and without patellofemoral pain.

The advantages of this technique, or collection of vector coding techniques, include no requirement for normalization (Hamill et al., 2000) which maintains the true spatial information in the data. This seems especially advantageous when using the technique of Tepavac and Field-Fote (2001), which incorporates a measurement of both the shape and magnitude of the angle–angle trajectories. Additionally, Field-Fote and Tepavac (2002) contended that vector coding techniques are more suitable than other methods such as relative phase analysis because "clinicians . . . are more likely to think of movement in terms of joint angles as opposed to phase values" (p. 710). The notion that vector coding is easier to relate to than relative phase seems reasonable. However, the output data from these techniques are not joint angles but the directions and magnitudes of frame-to-frame vectors, which may still be hard to understand conceptually.

A potential disadvantage of vector coding techniques is that they provide only spatial information, with no regard to temporal information (Hamill et al., 2000), which may limit the sensitivity to variability in coordination. Also, Heiderscheit et al. (2002) suggested that there is a potential problem with vector coding at times when joint motions change direction. Clark and Phillips (1993) hypothesized that these times of movement reversal are critical in the study of movement coordination, as are the apparent increases in variability in coordination (Ghez and Sainberg, 1995; Heiderscheit et al., 2002). However, as Heiderscheit et al. (2002) noted, during periods of movement reversal there is minimal joint displacement, and thus there is a cluster of data points on the relative motion diagram. The apparent increase in variability in coordination may simply be an artifact of the greater proximities of consecutive data points and the inherently greater sensitivity to slight changes in displacement.

Other Techniques

Techniques other than relative phase and vector coding have been used to quantify the coordination and variability in coordination between two body segments or joints. Two techniques that have received varying coverage in the literature are cross-correlations (Amblard et al., 1994) and normalized root mean squared differences (NoRMS: Sidaway et al., 1995).

Cross-correlations have been used to measure changes of coordination in an elite javelin thrower over 5 years (Morriss, 1998), assess changes in coordination during the learning of a task simulating skiing (Vereijken, van Emmerik, Whiting, and Newell, 1992; Whiting and Vereijken, 1993), monitor the acquisition of coordination during handwriting (Newell and van Emmerik, 1989), examine the effects of practice on coordination during dart throwing (McDonald, van Emmerik and Newell, 1989), and analyze the differences in intralimb coordination between expert and novice volleyball players performing a serve (Temprado, Della-Grast, Farrell and Laurent, 1997). Cross-correlations are based on the assumption that a linear relationship exists within segments or joints. However, it is not assumed that these segments or joints move in synchrony throughout the movement (Mullineaux, Bartlett, and Bennett, 2001). By introducing time lags into the data—shifting data from one segment forward or backward in relation to the data of another segment by a given number of data points—it is possible to find high correlations in two segments between which there is a constant time lag (Mullineaux et al., 2001). Amblard et al. (1994) suggested that cross-correlations are particularly relevant for analyzing human movement, as there are often time lags between coordinated segments.

Cross-correlation appears to be similar to DRP, as the lag time from cross-correlation, if expressed relative to the oscillation period, indicates the phase relationship between the two segments (Temprado et al., 1997). However, determining whether the relationship is a phase lag or a phase lead can be problematic (Amblard et al., 1994). Advantages of cross-correlation include that no normalization procedure is required if the data are linear and, similar to DRP, no further manipulations are required other than what are normally carried out in the calculation of joint angles. However, if the data are nonlinear, a transformation procedure such as a log–log transformation is required to linearize the data (see Snedecor and Cochran, 1989). Nonetheless, if the coefficient of cross-correlation is still small after the transformation (there is still no linear relationship between the segments of interest), cross-correlations are unsuitable. Another disadvantage of the technique is that it provides only one measurement per movement cycle.

Sidaway et al. (1995) presented NoRMS, a technique for measuring the consistency or variability of several angle–angle trajectories. By measuring the resultant distance between the angle–angle coordinate of a curve and the angle–angle coordinate of the mean curve at each instant, a root mean square difference is calculated at each point in time. These values are averaged across the entire trial and subsequently normalized with respect to the number of cycles and the excursion of the mean plot using the equations presented by Sidaway et al. (1995) which were reduced by Mullineaux et al. (2001) into the following:

$$NoRMS = 100 * \left(\frac{\sum_{j=1}^{k} \sqrt{\sum_{i=1}^{n} \left(\overline{x}_A - x_{Ai} \right)^2 + \left(\overline{x}_B - x_{Bi} \right)^2} \Big/ n_j}{R} \right) \qquad (9.4)$$

where A and B denote the two variables of interest, k is the number of cycles, n is the number of data points, R is the resultant excursion of the mean angle-angle curve over the entire cycle, $\overline{\chi}$ is the mean position of a given variable at the ith data point and χ is the position of a given variable at the ith data point on the jth cycle.

Sidaway et al. (1995) suggested that multiplication by 100 is used to make the resulting scores more manageable. However, the authors highlighted that, because linear statistical techniques are used on directional data, joint angles need to be greater than $0°$ and less than $360°$ and that the technique is not valid should joints, in an unusual situation, rotate through $360°$. Sidaway et al. (1995) also suggested that it is more appropriate to express joint angles in relative terms to avoid neutral joint positions.

The NoRMS technique appears to offer a measure of the variability in angle–angle traces that takes account of changes in the magnitude and shape of the plots. However, it gives no indication of the coordination between the segments of interest. Furthermore, there are some issues that need to be considered before using the NoRMS technique. Firstly, NoRMS in the form outlined by Sidaway et al. (1995) only provides one measure of coordination variability over the entire duration of the movement of interest. This might limit the use of the technique to analyse the variability in coordination during movements in which changes in the functional demands of the task over its duration may alter the magnitude of the variability during different phases; e.g., throughout the stance period of running (Heiderscheit et al., 2002). Moreover, the stage of the calculation during which the average cycle root mean square is divided by the resultant excursion of the mean angle–angle curve (see equation 9.4) appears to be similar to dividing the standard deviation by the mean value during the calculation of the coefficient of variation. Mullineaux (2000) stated that normalising data to the mean is appropriate if the means of the two sets of measurements are similar in size but it should not be done if the means are dissimilar as the results can be misleading. Therefore, in some instances where resultant excursions of the mean angle–angle curves are different between data sets under investigation, NoRMS may be inappropriate in the form presented by Sidaway et al. (1995). This technique has received little attention in the biomechanics and motor control literature.

Summary

There are advantages and disadvantages associated with all the techniques outlined in this chapter, but ultimately the choice of technique depends on the research question and the activity under scrutiny. Problems exist when applying relative phase techniques to nonsinusoidal data. However, when using vector coding techniques there are also issues surrounding the interpretation of variability in coordination during the reversal of the joint motion. Cross-correlations are unsuitable if the relationship between segments and joints is not linear. NoRMS might be misleading or indeed inappropriate for answering some research questions. Furthermore, Wheat et al. (2002) found that CRP and vector coding (Tepavac and Field-Fote, 2001) produced contradictory results for variability in coordination during certain times in the stance phase in running. These inconsistencies may result from the limitations discussed in this chapter, and further work is required to substantiate these preliminary findings. Finally, as Hamill et al. (2000) suggested, before choosing a particular technique, the researcher should be aware of the benefits and limitations of each and appreciate which are most suited to the movement or activity of interest.

Part IV

Variability Across the Life Span

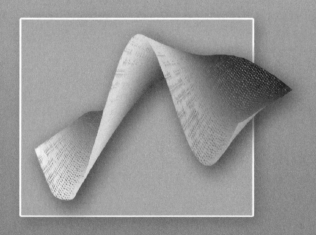

Chapter 10

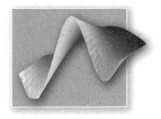

Functional Variability in Perceptual Motor Development

Geert J.P. Savelsbergh, PhD, John van der Kamp, PhD, and Karl S. Rosengren, PhD

Editors' Overview

This chapter shows how constraints shape emergent patterns of coordination during motor development and demonstrates how analysis of the structure of movement variability over time provides potentially interesting insights into the exploratory behavior of children. Variability is seen as a functional process that permits children to use adaptive behaviors to satisfy the typical task constraints they face as developing organisms. The interaction of constraints pertaining to the individual, the task, and the environment influences the coordination solution that emerges for each child during goal-directed activity. From this perspective, individual development is best viewed as a messy, noisy, and nonlinear process characterized by jumps, regressions, and discontinuities. Despite the interindividual variability observed in patterns of coordination such as reaching to grasp, the movement behavior of children adheres to the use of body-scaled ratios between key action spaces (e.g., objects to be grasped or surfaces to be climbed) and effector dimensions (e.g., moments of inertia of grasping limbs or tools to use). Variability of motor patterns supports the active, exploratory behavior that permits children to perceive the affordance of key objects, surfaces, and implements in the environment. A model is presented to explain how children pick up information for action, using the key ideas of Bernstein's (1967) stages of learning in a context of motor development.

Darwin (1877) and Preyer (1888) were the first to report detailed observations of infant behavior. However, more systematic research on motor development began with the work of Gesell (1929, 1946), McGraw (1935), and Shirley (1931) (for an excellent historical overview see Pick, 2003) in the 20th century. The major contribution of these pioneering efforts was establishing the so-called milestones of development such as reaching, grasping, sitting, crawling, and walking. The description of these milestones resulted in motor development being viewed as a rather rigid and gradual unfolding of postures and movements that was mainly attributed to the general maturation of the central nervous system. From a perspective of neural maturation, the development of movement coordination was a gradual unfolding of predetermined patterns (from cephal to caudal and proximal to distal) in the central nervous system and an increasing cortical control over lower reflexes. In such a depiction, it was forgotten that simple actions such as postural stabilization and reaching are based on an enormously complex apparatus that achieves and maintains coordination among thousands of sensory and motor neurons and musculoskeletal units. Developmental processes are not strictly linear but are often characterized by discontinuities, jumps, instabilities, and regressions (Savelsbergh, van der Maas, & van Geert, 1999).

In an ontogenetic context, ascribing behavioral achievements to something as vague and all-encompassing as neural maturation fails to capture the complexities of the processes involved (Savelsbergh, 1993). Therefore, the theoretical paradigm for this chapter is based on the work of Bernstein (1967), Gibson (1979), Newell (1986), and Kugler, Kelso, and Turvey (1982). In this perspective, the development of movement coordination is brought about by changes in the constraints imposed on the system of the organism and the environment. At certain developmental times, particular constraints may act as rate-limiting factors in the emergence and mastering of new actions.

A key aspect that is often overlooked in the emergence and mastering of new actions is variability. The goal of this chapter is to discuss the role of variability and to illustrate its functionality with respect to the development of perception–movement coordination. In the section, "Functional Coupling of Perception and Movement: Constraints," we introduce our theoretical framework, which is the functional coupling of information and movement in perception–motor development and the role of constraints in this coupling. In the next section, "Variability in Early Infant Reaching," we provide an illustration of intra- and intervariability in the emergence of reaching. In the section, "Functional Variability and Exploration," we discuss the functionality of variability. In the final section, "Variability and Selection in the Coupling of Information and Movement," we present a developmental model for the functional coupling between information and movement, in which variability plays a key role.

Functional Coupling of Perception and Movement: Constraints

The study of coordination in movement is highly influenced by the writings of Bernstein (1967), who formulated one of the central issues in motor coordination: the problem of degrees of freedom. He argued that the complex and nonlinear interactions among the different components of the movement apparatus (i.e., muscles, tendons, joints) make controlling each of these components impossible. Therefore, the very large number of individual degrees of freedom has to be coordinated. Hence,

> the coordination of movement is the process of mastering redundant degrees of freedom of the moving organ, in other words, its conversion to a controllable system. (Bernstein, 1967, p. 127)

The problem of coordination has been approached differently depending on the theoretical perspective of the researcher. For instance, Gibson's (1979) direct perception approach (also called ecological psychology or the theory of ecological optics) emphasizes the role of perceptual information in the coordination of action. *Direct* refers to the fact that objects, places, and events in the environment can be perceived without cognitive mediation to make perception meaningful. In contrast, information about objects, events, and places is unambiguously specified by the change or persistence of optical patterns in the environment. The core idea is that perceptual information guides action and that action generates perceptual information. In other words, the task-specific organizations of the action system (i.e., coordinative structures) generate perceptual information that attunes these coordinative structures to the specifics of the task (Turvey, 1990). The infant or child has to learn to pick up and select the information that tailors the action in a specific task. Therefore, researchers in development search for the (changes of) information infants and children use to guide their actions.

One of the main concepts in Gibson's (1979) approach is affordance. An affordance expresses the relationship between perceiving and acting:

> The affordances of the environment are what it offers the animal, what it provides or furnishes, either for good or ill. The verb to afford is found in the dictionary, but the noun affordance is not. I have made it up. I mean by it something that refers to both the environment and the animal in a way that no existing term does. It implies the complementarity of the animal and the environment. (p. 127)

Affordances relate to the possibilities for action of an organism in a particular environment. Therefore, they relate to the perceiver's potential action system. This implies the use of body-scaled information and not absolute metric information (e.g., meters, kilograms) for perceiving. *Body-scaled* means that the pattern of coordination is determined by the ratio between a metric of the action space and a metric of the actor (body dimension). For an actor climbing stairs, the pattern of coordination is specified by the ratio between the tread height (action space) and the length of the actor's leg (metric of the actor) (Warren, 1984). In more in general terms, perceiving and acting are guided by body-scaled ratios, which should be similar over individual differences in body dimensions. Therefore, changes in development due to physical growth should not affect the perception of affordances. That is, during development children remain attuned to similar body-scaled ratios without needing new learning or reorganization of the action system (van der Kamp, Savelsbergh, & Davis, 1998; Pufall & Dunbar, 1992). In the section, "Functional Variability and Exploration," we use this concept of affordance to discuss the relationship between exploration and functional variability. As stated, the theoretical paradigm for this chapter is based on the work of Bernstein (1967), Gibson (1979), Newell (1986), and Kugler, Kelso, and Turvey (1982). In this paradigm, coordination in movement develops through changes in the constraints imposed upon the system of the organism and its environment. Particular constraints may act as rate-limiting factors in the emergence and mastering of new actions. A classic example stems from the research of Thelen et al. on the development of leg movements (Thelen, Fisher, & Ridley Johnson, 1984). These researchers found that when 8-week-old infants were held upright, the stepping movements they displayed at a younger age disappeared. However, when the infants were lying supine, they performed kicking movements that were kinematically similar to the earlier observed stepping movements. Moreover, when the same infants were held upright in water, the stepping pattern reemerged. If its disappearance was simply due to cortical inhibition, as in traditional explanations, why would the cortex inhibit movements in the upright posture but not in the supine posture? Thelen et al. explained the disappearance of newborn stepping movements as a consequence of the disproportionate growth of leg muscles and fat tissues. Specifically, during this time of development infants acquire fat faster than muscle mass, which leads to relatively less muscle force. The stepping movement (task) is a consequence of the interaction between organismic constraints (body proportions) and environmental constraints (orientation to the gravity vector) and is not uniquely determined by constraints of neural maturation.

Savelsbergh and van der Kamp (1994) made similar observations when studying reaching. These researchers manipulated the orientation of infants with respect to gravity by reclining the infant's seat by 0°, 60°, or 90°. Depending on the infant's age, biomechanical demands sometimes played a large and sometimes a rather insignificant role in reaching. Only the reaching of 3- to 4-month-olds was affected by body orientation. Subsequent research by Wimmers, Savelsbergh, van der Kamp, and Hartelman (1998) stressed the importance of organismic constraints in the development of reaching. These authors found that the change from reaching to reaching with grasping during the first 6 mo of life is characterized by a discontinuous phase transition. It was shown that the change is best described with a model of cusp catastrophe in which arm weight and circumference (organismic constraints) and body orientation (environmental constraint) significantly contribute to the control parameters that lead the system through the transition.

In a more recent experiment, van Hof, van der Kamp, and Savelsbergh (2002) examined how the development of crossing the midline is interwoven with the development of bimanual reaching. Previously, it was held that the development of crossing the midline is uniquely determined by the maturation of hemispheric specialization (Provine & Westerman, 1979) or by the maturation of spinal tracts (Morange & Bloch, 1996). Van Hof et al. longitudinally observed 12-, 18-, and 26-week-old infants reaching for two balls (3 and 8 cm in diameter) at three positions (ipsilateral, midline, and contralateral). With age, the infants increasingly adapted the number of hands they used to the size of the object. The number of reaches crossing the midline of the body increased with age. Furthermore, most of the midline crossings were part of two-handed reaches for the large ball and occurred at or after the onset of bimanual reaching. This research strongly suggests that crossing the midline emerges in the context of bimanual reaching. It was concluded that the need to use two hands to grasp a large ball in a contralateral position induced midline crossing. Hence the development of crossing the midline does not exclusively depend on organismic constraints (e.g., the maturation of hemispheric connections), but on their interaction with environmental constraints (e.g., object size).

There is clear empirical evidence that constraints act as rate-limiting factors on the emergence of motor abilities. A small change in one of the constraints (e.g., change in the ratio of fat to muscle or change in object size) can lead to large changes in the pattern of coordination. Changes in development brought on by changes in the interaction between environmental and organismic constraints lead to inter- and intraindividual variability. This variability is central to the developmental process. The next section illustrates that small changes in constraints can influence variability in the emergence of reaching in early infants.

Variability in Early Infant Reaching

One of the most striking features in motor development is the appearance of the well-known milestones such as the onset of reaching. The ubiquity of these milestones has led some researchers to conclude that development follows a fixed sequence and timetable. In the last decade, empirical evidence has become available to refute a strict timetable (Largo, Molinari, Wber, Comenale, & Duc, 1985; Darrah, Redfern, Maguite, Beaulne, & Watt, 1998), especially with respect to reaching (Thelen, et al., 1993; Wimmers, Savelsbergh, Beek, & Hopkins, 1998; Corbetta, & Thelen, 1996). As argued in the section, "Functional Coupling of Perception and Movement: Constraints", the influence of environmental constraints on the observed coordination of arm movements has been supported by experimental work. It has been shown that the orientation of the body to the gravitational vector (i.e., sitting versus supine) affects the number of spontaneous arm movements in neonates (Kawai, Savelsbergh, & Wimmers, 1999), the quality and quantity of grasping behaviors in 3- and 4-month-old infants (Savelsbergh & van der Kamp, 1994), and the amount of uni- versus bimanual reaching in 6-month-old infants (Rochat, 1992).

Although environmental constraints greatly influence reaching, there are also differences in the kinematic trajectories of reaching among individual infants

(Thelen et al., 1993; Konczak, Borutta, Topka, & Dichgans, 1995; Out, van Soest, Savelsbergh, & Hopkins, 1998), though over the long run all healthy infants develop a well-coordinated reaching pattern. Wimmers and Savelsbergh (2001) assessed variability in the development of reaching by shifting the emphasis by fixed time based behavior to the dynamics of the observed behavior. These researchers studied the development of reaching at the behavioral level by examining the variability in the frequency of reaching among infants. They did this in order to identify the rate-limiting factors (constraints) that contribute to the (variability in the) emergence of reaching.

In the study by Wimmers and Savelsbergh, 10 infants were observed weekly: 9 from 8 to 24 wk and 1 from 10 to 24 wk. A stick or a rattle was presented to the infant at chest level at a distance of about 2/3 of the length of the infant's arm, as measured from the midline of the body. Trial duration was kept constant at 1 min, and within a trial multiple reaches could be made. A reach was scored when one of the hands came within 5 cm of the object or contacted it (Wimmers et al., 1998). The following arm measurements were obtained to investigate whether or not they contribute to the developmental process (Kawai et al., 1999; Savelsbergh, & van der Kamp, 1994; Thelen et al., 1984; Wimmers, Savelsbergh, van der Kamp & Hartelman, 1998): arm length; arm circumference; arm volume; arm weight, which was taken as the sum of the estimated masses of the upper and lower arms based on the regression equations of Schneider and Zernicke (1992); and arm ponderal index (API), which is 100(arm weight / arm length^3). To index the amount of learning, the cumulative frequency of reaches for each infant was calculated.

Figure 10.1 shows the frequency of reaching per minute for each individual. These time series were regressed against time and time squared. The overall analysis of the means showed significant differences among the infants. The calculated Z scores among the different pairs of infants showed that 9 infants differed significantly with 3 or more other infants. This finding led the researchers to conclude that infants differ significantly (intersubject variability) from each other with respect to the mean incidence of reaching and in the overall developmental pattern. This is in line with previous studies on the development of reaching at a kinematic level (Thelen, et al., 1993; Konczak et al., 1995), which showed that depending on their initial states, infants found different solutions to bring the hand into contact with an object.

A forward regression analysis was applied to each developmental trajectory (Wimmers & Savelsbergh, 2001). The analysis indicated that arm weight and the cumulative reaching frequency were the most significant contributors to the regression model. In half of the cases, arm weight and circumference were the relevant variables for the observed developmental trajectory. In the other half, the cumulative variable was the relevant variable. It was argued that both variables (arm weight and circumference) reflect changes in the ratio between muscle power and fat, as was observed in the kicking study of Thelen et al. (1984). The cumulative variable in the analysis serves as an indicator for learn-

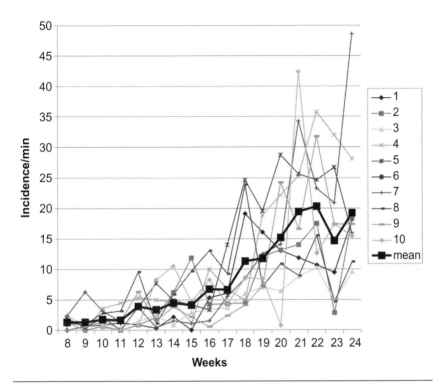

FIGURE 10.1 The number of reaches per minute for each of 10 infants.
Adapted from Wimmers and Savelsbergh 2001.

ing. The rationale behind using this variable is that the increase in the number of contacts made with the object likely increases the intention and desire to contact that particular object for exploratory purposes (Thelen, 1995).

The findings of the study by Wimmers and Savelsbergh emphasize that small changes in the environment or context may affect developmental trajectories (Wimmers et al., 1998; Van der Maas & Molenaar, 1992).

Functional Variability and Exploration

The relationship among affordances, sudden changes in the observed pattern of coordination, and increases in variability can be illustrated by an experiment of van der Kamp et al. (1998). The purpose of the experiment was to find evidence that during childhood, grasping is scaled to the body (see the section, "Functional Coupling of Perception and Movement: Constraints") and thus remains invariant during development. The basic idea is that a small object affords grasping with one hand, while a large object requires two hands. As in Warren's (1984) study on stair climbing, it was hypothesized that a change in the ratio between object size and hand size would cause a transition from one- to two-handed reaching. In order to examine this hypothesis, children aged 5, 7, and 9 were required to grasp and lift 14 cardboard cubes of different sizes (2.2, 3.2, 4.2 . . . 16.2 cm in diameter). Every cube was lifted four times. Video recordings were analyzed frame by frame and scored qualitatively for one-handed and two-handed grasps. Figure 10.2a shows the mean percentage of two-handed grasps for the three age groups. The older the children, the lower was the occurrence of two-handed grasps (63%, 54%, and 45% for ages 5, 7, and 9, respectively). Moreover, the older the children, the larger were the cubes they grasped with one hand. From the theoretical approach advocated in the section, "Functional Coupling of Perception and Movement: Constraints," it is hypothesized that the detected differences in the grasping behavior among the age groups were due to the increase of hand size with age. The observed differences in reaching were expected to disappear when the size of the hand was taken into account. That is, when the ratio of object size to hand size was considered, differences were expected to disappear, which would confirm the body-scaling phenomenon. To examine whether or not the observed grasping follows body-scaled patterns, the data from figure 10.2a are replotted using an independent axis of cube size / finger span in figure 10.2b. In figure 10.2b the curves for the different age groups are more congruent and intersect more often, suggesting the use of body-scaled information (Warren, 1984; Newell, Scully, McDonald, & Baillargeon, 1989). Thus, when data were scaled to hand size, differences in prehension among the three age groups disappeared. In addition, the shift from one-handed to two-handed grasping occurred at the same ratio of cube size to hand span for all three age groups. How about the variability? When the data are grouped with respect to the transition point, that is, the change from one-handed to two-handed grasping, an increase in variability is found at that point (figure 10.3). In addition, when the averages of the standard errors within subjects for each group were scaled to the transition cube, increased variability around the transition point was again found. Thelen and Smith (1994) suggested that variability around a transition is a prerequisite for jumping to a qualitatively new level of behavior. In their view, variability is highly functional because it provides the infant and child with possibilities for exploration, that is, with opportunities to discover qualitatively different solutions, such as switching from one-handed to two-handed grasping.

The ratio between hand size and object size is probably only one of many aspects that determine the variability of the observed patterns of movement. For instance, the role of visual anticipation in variability should also be considered. In contrast to grasping stationary objects, grasping moving objects requires not only coordination among the eyes, head, arms, and fingers but also anticipation because the moving objects are within reach for only a limited time (Savelsbergh et al., 1991, 1993, 1997). It is suggested in the literature that anticipation behavior depends strongly on the level of development (for instance, the level of coordination between reach and grasp). It has been reported that 9-month-

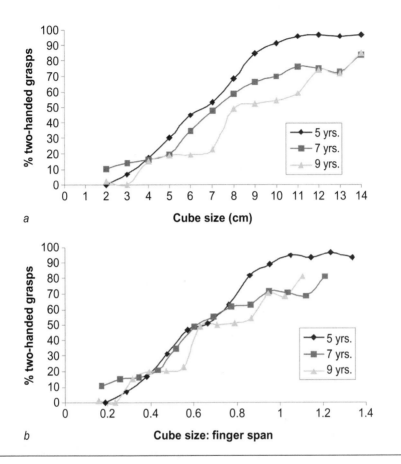

FIGURE 10.2   Mean percentage of two-handed grasps as a function of *(a)* cube size and *(b)* ratio of cube size to finger span.
Adapted from Van der Kamp, Savelsbergh, and Davis 1998.

old healthy infants successfully anticipate moving objects, with 100% grasping (Savelsbergh et al., 1997), while preterm infants are only capable of doing so around 10 to 12 mo (Van der Meer, Van der Weel, Lee, Laing, & Lin, 1995). This suggests an influence of the maturation of the nervous system (organismic constraint). These changes in anticipation behavior and thus prospective control, could also be responsible for variability in the observed coordination between reaching and grasping. Furthermore, high variability in real time could lead to an earlier transition in anticipation behavior in developmental time, while a constant low variability over weeks of observation could lead to a relatively late transition on the developmental timescale.

The relationship between exploratory behavior and affordances is emphasized by the direct perception approach. In order to detect an affordance, we

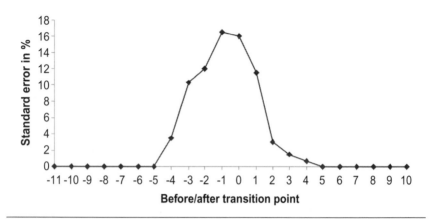

FIGURE 10.3　Mean within the standard error of the percentage of bimanual grasps normalized to the transition point.
Adapted from Van der Kamp, Savelsbergh, and Davis 1998.

must pick up the information specifying the particular affordance (Michaels & Carello, 1981). According to E. Gibson (1988), affordances have to be discovered with the aid of the perceptual systems and exploratory behavior. Michaels and Carello (1981) stress the active nature of exploratory behavior:

> Exploration (attention) is not an unconscious sifting-through and subsequent rejection of most inputs: It is directed control of what will be detected. (Michaels & Carello, 1981, p. 70)

In the eyes of these authors, exploration is an active and directed process that reveals affordances. Actively exploring the environment reveals information and so affordances become apparent (van der Kamp & Savelsbergh, 1994). During development, organismic constraints (depth vision, muscle power, and so on) change very quickly and therefore the exploratory possibilities change dramatically. For instance, when infants start crawling, the number of action possibilities increases, which leads to the discovery of new information and the detection of new affordances. Furthermore, by exploratory activities, infants become more sensitive to relevant information that guides their actions.

A study by Adolph and coworkers (Adolph, Eppler, & Gibson, 1993) demonstrated this relationship between exploration and affordance. In their study, walkers and crawlers were encouraged to ascend and descend walkways with slopes of 10°, 20°, 30°, and 40°. The findings showed that the exploratory activities of the subjects related to locomotion abilities. For instance, on descending trials, walkers switched from walking to sliding. Also, they touched and hesitated most before descending the 10° and 20° slopes, and they explored alternative means for descent by testing different sliding positions before leaving the platform. Crawlers hesitated most before descending the 30° and 40°

slopes, and they did not test alternative sliding positions. The experiment nicely demonstrated the relationship among locomotion capability, the perception of affordances (walkable or not), and exploratory activity in infants.

The relationship between variability and behavior was demonstrated in a study on learning to crawl conducted by Adolph, Vereijken, and Denny (1998). In their study, they examined the effects of age, body dimension, and experience on the development of crawling before walking. Several patterns of crawling were identified, namely, "army" belly crawling, "inchworm" belly crawling, standard hands-and-knees crawling, and "bear" crawling. These patterns were defined as the combinations of body parts used for propulsion and balance. The researchers were particularly interested in the emergence of new behavior, so they focused on the emergence of new patterns (patterns not previously seen). The belly crawlers showed higher variability than the hands-and-knees crawlers. Our interpretation of this finding is that belly crawling is a relatively inefficient and ineffective manner of locomotion. Thus, belly crawlers are constantly searching for better crawling solutions. For the hands-and-knees crawlers, there is less need to search for better solutions because this type of crawling is relatively effective. Evidence of its effectiveness can be seen in the fact that newly walking infants often adopt a hands-and-knees crawl in order to move swiftly from one location to another. A key aspect of the development of locomotion is that as an optimal crawling solution is discovered, variability decreases.

In conclusion, from this perception-action point of view, the emergence of motor milestones is not just a consequence of the maturation of the nervous system but is due to the changing interaction between organismic and environmental constraints. New perception–action couplings are discovered and new patterns of stable action are acquired by exploration. Hence, action is developed through exploration, that is, the process of repeatedly producing (slightly) different movements or experimenting with different musculoskeletal organizations (Goldfield, Kay, & Warren, 1993) whereby infants learn how to coordinate and control their action systems. The infants perceive information (proprioceptive, visual) produced by their movements and discover how they can use this information to guide their movements. As previously argued, exploratory behavior (visible by an increase in variability) is especially prominent during transitions. This was nicely shown by Thelen in her earlier ethological studies (1979) on rhythmic behaviors like kicking, rocking, arm waving, and banging in natural settings. She showed that these behaviors occurred most frequently around transitions where new behaviors emerged. Rocking on hands and feet, for example, emerged just before the onset of crawling. This rocking might represent the infant's exploration of his action capabilities and the (proprioceptive) information it produces. Exploration eventually leads to a new pattern of stable action (crawling). Through exploring the perception–motor work space, the infant discovers how perception and action are coupled.

Variability and Selection in the Coupling of Information and Movement

In the section, "Functional Coupling of Perception and Movement: Constraints," we argued that information and movement are tightly coupled. In the section, "Functional Variability and Exploration," we maintained that variability enables greater flexibility (exploration possibilities) in information–movement couplings and provides the opportunity to select from a larger set of responses. Thus variability increases the likelihood of performing successfully. It is functional and enables successful adaptation. Savelsbergh and van der Kamp (2000) proposed a model that describes different information–movement couplings from a perspective of skill acquisition, in which variability, degrees of freedom, and constraints are key players. This model can be applied to development (Rosengren & Savelsbergh, 2003).

Three stages in learning can be discerned from Bernstein's concept of degrees of freedom: freezing, freeing, and exploiting the degrees of freedom (McDonald, Van Emmerik, & Newell, 1989; Vereijken, Whiting, & Beek, 1992; Steenbergen, Marteniuk, & Kalbfleisch, 1995). A recent study by Ledebt (2000) illustrated these three stages in the development of walking. She studied the changes in the posture and movement of the arms in relation to the width of step in infants just starting to walk. She found that the arms were held in a fixed posture during the first 10 wk (freezing). A freeing of this fixed posture correlated with a decrease in the width of the infant's step. The emergence of arm movements occurred when the control of balance improved (exploiting). While at first toddlers avoid arm movements during walking to reduce the degrees of freedom, later in the exploiting stage they use arm movements to help counterbalance forces arising from the pelvis.

We consider the development and learning of information-movement couplings to be analogous to the sequence of freezing, freeing, and exploiting the degrees of freedom. Analogous to the freezing of degrees of freedom, the learning process starts with the emergence and strengthening of a coupling between information and movement (figure 10.4a). Within a certain set of constraints (e.g., body dimension, locomotion surface), a particular coupling between information and movement emerges, which fits the task requirements (e.g., moving forward). With repetition the coupling strengthens. In other words, the movement is tuned to information (e.g., rocking during crawling). As such, the coupling strength enhances the probability that this coupling reoccurs under a similar set of constraints. This tuning eventually eliminates other potential couplings and increases the stability of the pattern (and decreases the variability). However, when in this early phase of learning the particular set or interaction of constraints changes, the coupling is disturbed and the action breaks down. An alternative coupling between information and movement is not available or is too weak to be successful. More practice is required to strengthen an alternative coupling specific for the new set of constraints.

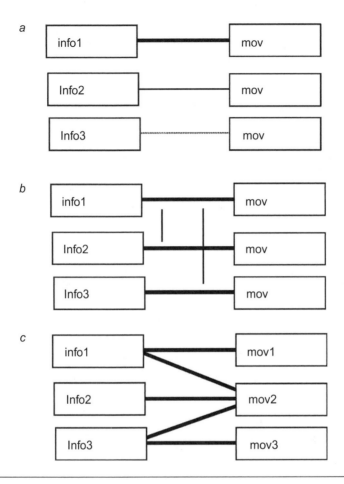

FIGURE 10.4 The stages of learning. *(a)* In strengthening, the coupling between information (info1) and movement (mov) strengthens during practice, while the coupling between Info2 or Info3 and mov does not. *(b)* In freeing, the subject can jump from one strong coupling to another. *(c)* In exploiting, information (info1) can be used for different actions (mov1 and mov2), and different perceptual information (Info2 and Info3) can be used for the same movement (mov2).

Adapted from Savelsbergh and Van der Kamp 2000.

The second stage involves freeing different information–movement couplings (figure 10.4*b*). Practice and experience under different sets of constraints eventually lead to a whole repertoire of possible information–movement couplings for a certain task (e.g., the descending of a slope by walking or crawling). Hence, if certain constraints change, the actor accesses another available coupling without needing to learn it from scratch. Moreover, in contrast to the early stage of learning, a change of constraints does not lead to a complete breakdown of the action. Skilled performance can be characterized by the ability to exploit different information-movement couplings (figure 10.4c). Because the child has a whole repertoire of these couplings, she can exploit the information that is available under a certain set of constraints. That is to say, information (e.g., locomotion surface) may be tuned to one movement (e.g., crawling), but it may also be exploited for another movement (e.g., walking) that is characteristic of a newly emerging coupling.

What about variability? We argue that variability is highly functional in at least two ways. First, a change from one information–movement coupling to another coupling is similar to the change from one pattern of coordination to a qualitatively different pattern. As argued in the section, "Functional Variability and Exploration," variability provides opportunities for exploration that are essential for shifting from one pattern to another. Second, in the early freezing stage, children select one of multiple sources of information that enable them to successfully perform the task at hand. But their performance is not necessarily perfect due to variability. Variability in the available sources of information increases the possibilities of establishing or selecting a coupling. This selection requires ongoing exploration of information. It is determined by the interaction of constraints and is not an internal process. In the freezing stage, the observed variability in behavior decreases, and the third stage is characterized by stability in the pattern of coordination and by the ability to exploit as well as use different information couplings.

Conclusions

From the current constraint-led perspective, development and learning are considered as establishing and further refining couplings between information and movement. It is argued that the process of coupling information and movement consists of a sequence of mutually overlapping phases. Variability is of the utmost importance, as it increases the possibility of achieving successful couplings. In this process of coupling, various constraints can act as rate-limiting factors that lead to selection, and a change in one constraint can change the overall pattern of coordination (e.g., lead to a new information–movement coupling). Around changes in the patterns of coordination, there is greater variability, which increases the possibilities to explore and search for optimal solutions. Variability is central to both learning and development, as it enhances movement opportunities. Indeed, variability makes development and learning possible!

Chapter 11

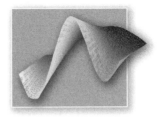

Aging and Variability in Motor Output

Evangelos A. Christou, PhD, and Brian L. Tracy, PhD

Editors' Overview

This chapter continues the focus on development across the life span by examining the influence of aging on the variability of motor performance. Variability of motor output has been traditionally measured by evaluating the subject variability within a single trial or among different trials. Data on movement accuracy of younger and older adults are presented and require careful interpretation due to complexity. Many studies show a mixed picture on the differences between older and younger adults in controlling the force and accuracy of movements. In particular, the speed of the required movement response seems to be a critical constraint on the magnitude of the intertrial variability shown in older adults for variables such as reaction time and the smoothness of the movement trajectory. From a practical perspective, research has indicated that physical fitness activities may benefit fluctuations of force outputs in older adults. The mechanism for such performance enhancements remains unclear but it seems likely that increased motor learning may increase the accuracy of motor responses. The implication is that training emphasizing stability of coordination and skill could still benefit older adults in tasks requiring them to maintain strong and steady muscle contractions.

Older adults often exhibit an inability to move smoothly and accurately. Even healthy older individuals display increased kinematic variability during functional movements when compared with younger individuals (Grabiner, Biswas, & Grabiner, 2001; Hortobagyi & DeVita, 1999; Williams, 1998), and they prefer to slow down to eliminate errors and loss of balance (Hortobagyi & DeVita, 1999; Schultz, Alexander, & Ashton-Miller, 1992). The reduced ability of older adults to control the force or timing of a muscle contraction (motor output) can produce a more variable trajectory of the limb and can impair accuracy in movement,

The authors would like to thank Dr. Roger Enoka for comments on a draft of this chapter.

199

leading to instability, loss of balance, and declining function (Enoka, 1997; Schultz et al., 1992).

The variability of the motor output is usually quantified as the fluctuations in force or acceleration (variability within a trial) or as the variability around a target among several trials by the same subject (variability from trial to trial) (Christou & Carlton, 2001). Recently, Harris and Wolpert (1998) demonstrated that the accuracy of goal-directed movements directly relates to the magnitude of the fluctuations in the motor output. Although no direct link has been established between increased kinematic variability and fluctuations in the motor output in older adults, reorganization in the aging neuromuscular system could influence the control of the motor output and consequently the accuracy of movements.

Neurophysiological changes that accompany aging include the death of cortical motor neurons (Eisen, Entezari-Taher, & Stewart, 1996) and spinal alpha motor neurons (Masakado et al., 1994; Roos, Rice, & Vandervoort, 1997) as well as the slowing of the signal transmitted from the corticospinal and reflex pathways to the motor neurons (Henderson, Tomlinson, & Gibson, 1980). These changes may alter the motor command and consequently alter the precision of the motor output. Furthermore, the motor command can be altered by changes in the properties of the motor unit. Because the motor unit is the final common pathway to the muscle, alterations in the size or discharge of motor units that occur with aging can contribute to a more variable output (Enoka & Fuglevand, 2001). For example, when spinal motor neurons are lost with aging, the remaining motor units reorganize to innervate more muscle fibers and consequently there are fewer and larger motor units in the muscle (Roos et al., 1997). The remaining motor units exert a greater twitch force than is exerted in younger adults (Masakado et al., 1994). Although controversial (Semmler, Kornatz, Miles, & Enoka, 2002), current evidence suggests that older adults exhibit a greater variability in the discharge rate of motor units that significantly contributes to increases in fluctuations of muscle force (Laidlaw, Bilodeau, & Enoka, 2000) and acceleration (Kornatz, Christou, & Enoka, in press).

Variability in motor output has been studied in young and healthy individuals for about a century (Fullerton & Cattell, 1892). Although fluctuations due to pathological tremor (typically examined in the frequency domain) associated with aging have been studied for decades (McAuley & Marsden, 2000), the variability of motor output exhibited by healthy older adults in the time domain has received attention only recently (Galganski, Fuglevand, & Enoka, 1993). Several studies have provided evidence of the impaired ability of older individuals to control force output, particularly at low levels of force (Burnett, Laidlaw, & Enoka, 2000; Christou & Carlton, 2001; Galganski et al., 1993; Hortobagyi, Tunnel, Moody, Beam, & DeVita, 2001; Keen, Yue, & Enoka, 1994; Laidlaw et al., 2000; Laidlaw, Kornatz, Keen, Suzuki, & Enoka, 1999; Semmler, Steege, Kornatz, & Enoka, 2000; Tracy, Mehoudar, Ortega, & Enoka, 2002). The effect of age on variability in motor output, however, is not consistent across force levels, limbs, experimental tasks, and contractions. This chapter examines the influence of aging on variability in the motor output of single joint movements and discusses neurophysiological changes that may contribute to altered motor performance.

Older Adults Do Not Always Exhibit Greater Variability in Motor Output Within a Trial

When an individual attempts to match a target force or displacement velocity, the outcome of the muscular contraction always fluctuates around the requirements of the task (figure 11.1, *a-b*). The fluctuations of the motor output within a trial requiring isometric or anisometric contraction are quantified as the variability within a trial. For isometric contractions, subjects are asked to exert a constant force and match a horizontal target line for a specified time (Christou & Carlton, 2001; Tracy et al., 2002). The fluctuations in force during isometric contractions increase as a function of mean force (Burnett et al., 2000; Christou & Carlton, 2001; Christou, Grossman, & Carlton, 2002). Because younger adults are stronger than older adults, the coefficient of variation (CV) of force is used to normalize the fluctuations (Burnett et al., 2000; Christou & Carlton, 2001; Christou, Grossman et al., 2002; Laidlaw et al., 2000; Tracy & Enoka, 2002). For anisometric contractions, subjects are typically asked to match a target line moving at a constant velocity while they lift various loads. The variability in motor output is quantified as the fluctuations in acceleration or position. In contrast to the fluctuations in isometric contractions, the fluctuations do not increase significantly with the weight of the load lifted (Christou, Shinohara, & Enoka, 2003; Christou, Tracy, & Enoka, 2002). Thus it is more appropriate to compare the performance of younger and older adults by using the standard deviation of acceleration or position (Christou et al., 2002).

Generally, older adults exhibit a greater CV of force as compared with younger adults during isometric contractions of the first dorsal interosseus (figure 11.2*a*). This increased variability in force for older adults appears to be consistent for force levels lower than 20% MVC (Burnett et al., 2000; Galganski et al., 1993; Keen et al., 1994; Laidlaw et al., 2000; Semmler et al., 2000). However, when performing isometric contractions with the elbow flexors (figure 11.2*b*), younger and older adults exhibit similar fluctuations in force at all levels of force (Graves, Kornatz, & Enoka, 2000). Furthermore, the findings on the knee extensors appear to be mixed. Tracy and Enoka (2002) found a greater CV of force for sedentary older adults as compared with younger adults at low levels ranging from 2% to 10% MVC but not at 50% MVC. Christou and Carlton (2001) observed no significant differences in the CV of force between physically active younger and older adults in contractions ranging from 5% to 90% MVC (figure 11.2*c*). Two other studies with significantly different experimental protocols compared the variability in force at an absolute level of force in younger and

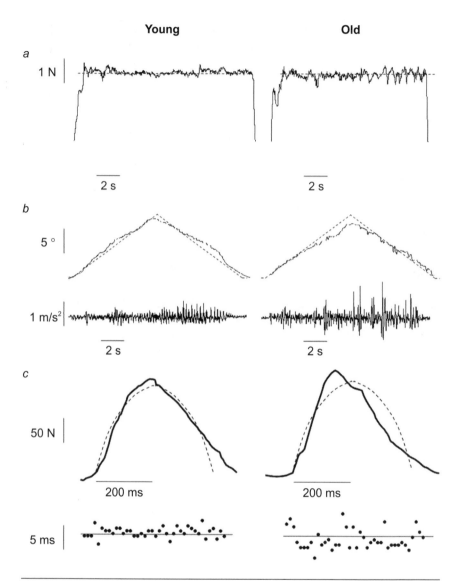

FIGURE 11.1 Representative data for younger and older individuals performing three tasks. *(a)* Fluctuations in force during a low-intensity (5% maximum voluntary contraction, or MVC), constant isometric contraction of the first dorsal interosseus muscle. *(b)* Position (top trace\solid line) and acceleration (bottom trace) during shortening (ascending limb) and lengthening contractions (descending limb) while lifting a light load with the same muscle (5% 1-repetition maximum, or 1RM). *(c)* A single trial in which subjects attempted to match a force-time parabola (top\solid line) while repeatedly and rapidly contracting the knee extensors. The variability of the time to reach peak force around the mean time in 40 discrete contractions is shown at the bottom of *(c)*.

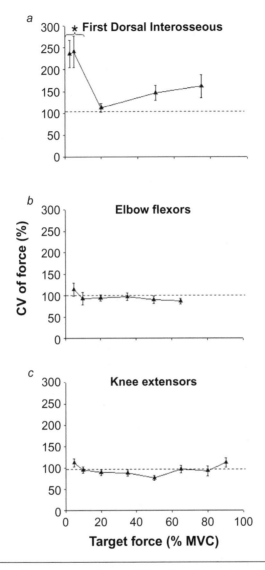

FIGURE 11.2   The fluctuations in force exhibited by older adults during isometric contractions with the *(a)* first dorsal interosseus (Burnett et al., 2000), *(b)* elbow flexors (Graves et al., 2000), and *(c)* knee extensors (Christou & Carlton, 2001). The fluctuations in force are presented as the CV of force exhibited by older adults relative to that exhibited by younger adults, or (CV in old / CV in young) × 100. Values greater than 100% indicate greater variability in older adults. The * indicates statistically significant differences.

older adults and reported no significant differences (Hortobagyi et al., 2001; Schiffman & Luchies, 2001).

Numerous studies have examined the effect of age on the fluctuations of motor output during shortening and lengthening contractions. Collectively, the findings suggest that the motor output of older adults is more variable during lengthening than during shortening contractions. For example, when older individuals use the first dorsal interosseous to slowly abduct and adduct the index finger at a constant velocity, the fluctuations in displacement (Laidlaw et al., 2000) and acceleration (Burnett et al., 2000) are greater than those in younger adults, especially during lengthening (figure 11.3a). Similarly, the fluctuations in wrist acceleration during contractions with the elbow flexors were greater in older adults as compared with younger adults, especially during lengthening contractions (Graves et al., 2000) (figure 11.3b). These differences, however, were only significant at loads lower than 15% of the maximum load (1RM) (Christou et al., 2002).

Numerous findings also indicate that fluctuations in motor output are not always greater for older adults. For example, younger and older adults exhibit similar fluctuations in isometric force while performing a precision pinch grip (Cole & Beck, 1994; Cole, Rotella, & Harper, 1999). Similarly, fluctuations in motor output have been reported to be comparable between younger and older adults lifting or lowering loads with the elbow flexors (Tracy et al., 2002) and knee extensors (figure 11.3, b-c) (Tracy & Enoka, 2002). Even the studies that reported greater fluctuations in older adults moving light loads indicated that the fluctuations in displacement and acceleration at heavier loads appear to be similar or even lesser for older adults (figure 11.3, a-b) (Burnett et al., 2000; Christou et al., 2002; Graves et al., 2000; Laidlaw et al., 2000). Furthermore, older adults exhibited significantly lower fluctuations in acceleration as compared with younger adults when lifting and lowering a constant load (15% of the maximum) at various speeds (Christou et al., 2003).

The ability of older adults to exhibit similar or even lower fluctuations in motor output when compared with younger adults may be explained by the following possibilities. First, the amplitude of the fluctuations in movements of single joints does not influence the accuracy of the limb trajectory and thus cannot explain the higher kinematic variability typically observed during functional movements in older adults. Second, the amplitude of the fluctuations significantly influences the accuracy of the limb trajectory, but this effect is greater in older than younger adults. Recently we found that in both younger and older adults, the greater were the fluctuations in acceleration, the lower was the accuracy of movement (Christou et al., 2003). This result was suggested previously by Harris et al. (2000). However, in older adults the accuracy of movement was reduced more with lower fluctuations in acceleration (see figure 11.4). This finding suggests that younger adults can perform as accurately as or more accurately than older adults with fewer constraints imposed on their performance by the fluctuations in motor output.

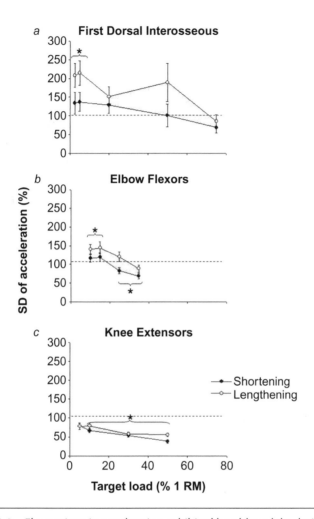

FIGURE 11.3   Fluctuations in acceleration exhibited by older adults during short-ening and lengthening contractions with the *(a)* first dorsal interosseus (Burnett et al., 2000), *(b)* elbow flexors (Graves et al., 2000), and *(c)* knee extensors (Tracy et al., 2002). The fluctuations in acceleration are presented as the SD of acceleration exhibited by older adults relative to younger adults, or (SD in old / SD in young) × 100. Values greater than 100% indicate greater variability in older adults. The * indicates statistically significant differences.

Various findings indicate that the magnitude of fluctuations in acceleration varies for younger and older adults depending on the muscle group being tested, the intensity of the contraction, and the task. Although older adults exhibit lower fluctuations in acceleration, particularly during high-intensity contractions, the amplitude of the fluctuations appears to more greatly impair the accuracy of movement in older adults.

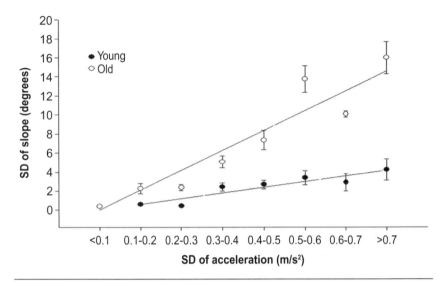

FIGURE 11.4   The association between the fluctuations in acceleration (grouped in bins of SD of acceleration) and the accuracy of reproducing the target slope (SD of slope) in younger and older adults. For both groups the accuracy of reproducing the target was significantly impaired with increases in the fluctuations in acceleration. This impairment was significantly greater in older adults as compared with younger adults.

Older Adults Exhibit Greater Variability in Motor Output From Trial to Trial

When an individual repeatedly attempts to match a target, the motor output varies around the target (see figure 11.1c). The variability around the target is quantified as the trial-to-trial variability, and it is often assessed during brief contractions that minimize the role of sensory feedback (Carlton & Newell, 1993; Cordo, Carlton, Bevan, Carlton, & Kerr, 1994) and allow inferences about the motor program (the descending command and excitation of motor neurons). Typically the subjects attempt to match a prescribed force-time parabola (figure 11.1c). Variability in the peak force, the time-to-peak force, the force-time integral (impulse), and the duration of the force-time integral is measured (Carlton & Newell, 1993; Christou & Carlton, 2001; Christou & Carlton, 2002). Like variability within a trial, the variability in peak force and impulse increases with the mean force. Because the mean force produced at each submaximal target force (% MVC) is usually greater for younger adults, trial-to-trial variability is quantified with the CV, whereas the variability in timing (time-to-peak force and impulse duration) is quantified with the SD.

Compared to the number of studies that have examined variability in motor output within a trial, there are fewer studies that have compared trial-to-trial variability in younger and older adults. For example, one study compared variability in motor output in younger and older adults within a trial and across trials (Christou & Carlton, 2001). The variability within a trial was assessed with constant isometric contractions of the quadriceps, whereas the trial-to-trial variability was assessed with a rapid isometric contraction of the quadriceps (the time-to-peak force = 200 ms) as the subjects repeatedly attempted to match a force-time parabola. The younger and older adults exhibited a similar CV of force from 5% to 90% MVC during the task requiring constant force (see figure 11.2c), whereas the older adults exhibited a significantly greater CV of peak force during the rapid, discrete task (see figure 11.5a). Furthermore, the older adults exhibited the most variability in the temporal characteristics of movement (time-to-peak force, impulse duration) when attempting to reproduce the force-time parabola (see figure 11.5b).

Trial-to-trial variability appears to be even greater in older adults during anisometric contractions, especially when the goal is to match the target force and timing during lengthening contractions. Three findings demonstrate the impaired ability of older adults to repetitively perform anisometric contractions. First, when younger and older adults contracted the knee extensors on an isokinetic device and aimed for targets of peak force ranging from 20% to 90% MVC, older adults exhibited significantly greater variability in peak force, impulse, time-to-peak force, and impulse duration (figure 11.5c) (Christou & Carlton, 2002). The ability of older adults to produce a repeatable temporal outcome was substantially impaired during lengthening (as compared to shortening) contractions (figure 11.5d). Second, when younger and older subjects contracted the first dorsal interosseous while lifting and lowering a constant load (15% of 1RM) at six different velocities (0.03-1.16 rad/s), older subjects exhibited greater trial-to-trial variability only during the fastest velocity (figure 11.6a) and during lengthening contractions (Christou et al., 2003). Speed of movement appears to be critical, and current findings (Tracy et al., 2002) indicate that the trial-to-trial variability in slowly moving the index finger at a constant velocity is similar for younger and older adults at loads ranging from 5% to 50% of the maximum (figure 11.6b). Third, in studies that compared the ability of younger and older adults to rapidly aim with the arm, the older adults exhibited trajectories that were less smooth (Yan, 2000), and they exhibited greater trial-to-trial variability for the reaction time (Yan, Thomas, & Stelmach, 1998).

The overall findings suggest that older adults exhibit greater trial-to-trial variability than younger adults during isometric and anisometric contractions with various muscle groups. The impaired ability of older adults to reproduce the motor outcome appears to be influenced *only* during rapid contractions and to be amplified during lengthening contractions.

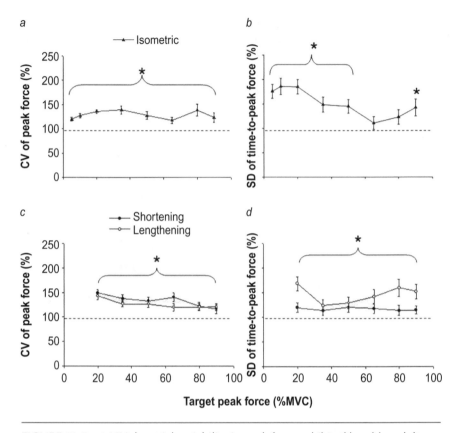

FIGURE 11.5 *(a)* Trial-to-trial variability in peak force exhibited by older adults performing isometric contractions with the knee extensors (Christou & Carlton, 2001). *(b)* Trial-to-trial variability in time-to-peak force exhibited by older adults performing isometric contractions with the knee extensors (Christou & Carlton, 2001). *(c)* Trial-to-trial variability in peak force exhibited by older adults performing anisometric contractions with the knee extensors (Christou & Carlton, 2002). *(d)* Trial-to-trial variability and time-to-peak force exhibited by older adults performing anisometric contractions with the knee extensors (Christou & Carlton, 2002). Trial-to-trial variability is presented as the CV of peak force and the SD of time-to-peak force exhibited by older adults relative to younger adults, or (SD in old / SD in young) × 100. Values greater than 100% indicate greater variability in older adults. The * indicates statistically significant differences.

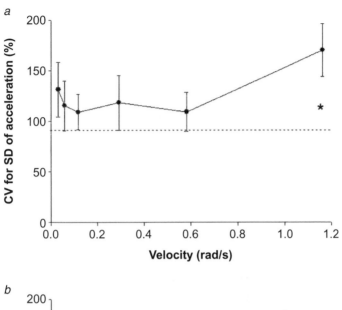

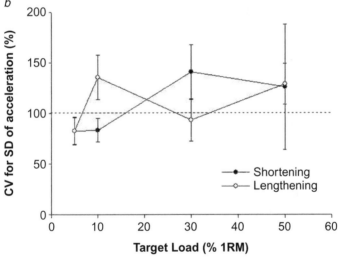

FIGURE 11.6　Trial-to-trial variability of fluctuations in acceleration exhibited by older adults in using the first dorsal interosseus to lift *(a)* a constant load (15% of 1RM) at six different velocities (Christou et al., 2001) and *(b)* various loads (5%-50% of 1RM) at a constant velocity (0.05 rad/s) (Tracy et al., 2002). The trial-to-trial variability is presented as the CV for the SD of acceleration exhibited by older adults relative to younger adults, or (SD in old / SD in young) × 100. Values greater than 100% indicate greater variability in older adults. Older adults were significantly (*) more variable than younger adults only at the fastest velocity (1.16 rad/s).

Physical Training Attenuates the Variability of Motor Output in Older Adults

The loss of muscle strength with age is a well-characterized phenomenon (Vandervoort, 2002). Two observations suggest that maintaining physical fitness and muscle strength may be associated with lower fluctuations in force in older adults. First, highly active older adults exhibit fluctuations in force that are similar to those of active younger adults when exerting constant forces (5%-90% MVC) with the knee extensors (Christou & Carlton, 2001), whereas sedentary older adults appear to exhibit greater fluctuations than those exhibited by younger adults when using the knee extensors to produce contractions of low force (Tracy & Enoka, 2002). Second, 12 wk of strength training with heavy loads (80% MVC) improved the ability of sedentary older adults to perform steady isometric contractions with the first dorsal interosseous muscle (Keen et al., 1994) (figure 11.7*a*).

Recently, however, improvements in the strength of the first dorsal interosseus in older adults have been disassociated from improvements in the variability of motor output. For example, older adults improved the strength and steadiness of the first dorsal interosseous while training with light (10% MVC) or heavy

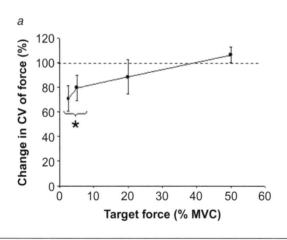

a

(continued)

FIGURE 11.7   The effects of training on variability in motor output in older adults. The effects of strength training on the fluctuations in force are shown for the *(a)* first dorsal interosseus (Keen et al., 1994) and *(b)* knee extensors (Tracy et al., 2001) at relative target forces (% MVC). The effect of tai chi on the fluctuations in force for the knee extensors at absolute target forces is shown in *(c)* (Christou et al., 2003). The change in the variability of motor output by older adults is presented as the fluctuations in force (SD or CV) exhibited after training compared with before training, or (pretraining / posttraining) × 100. Values lower than 100% indicate attenuation of the variability in motor output that occurred with training. The * indicates statistically significant differences.

loads (80% MVC) (Laidlaw et al., 1999). Furthermore, new evidence suggests that older individuals who trained with a load equal to 10% of 1RM for 2 wk improved their abilities to perform steady shortening and lengthening contractions with the first dorsal interosseus (Kornatz et al., 2005). This training was followed with 4 wk of training with a heavy load (70% of 1RM), and although the additional training improved the strength of the first dorsal interosseus, it had no effect on the fluctuations in acceleration.

In addition to the findings on the first dorsal interosseus, there are findings showing that strengthening the knee extensors is also not associated with decreasing fluctuations in the motor output. Results from two longitudinal studies, one conducted for 12 wk (Bellew, 2002) and the other for 16 wk (Tracy 2001), suggest that strength training the knee extensors in healthy sedentary older adults does not reduce fluctuations in motor output (see figure 11.7b).

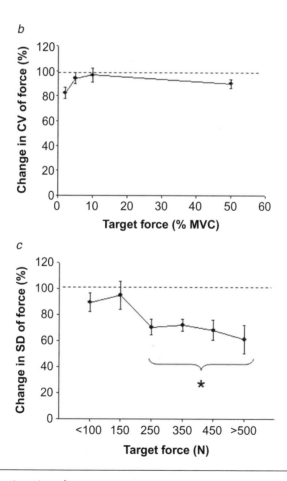

FIGURE 11.7   *(continued)*

Further support for an effect of motor learning and not strength training comes from a study in which older adults improved their abilities to match a constant force of 25 N following low- or high-intensity strength training (Hortobagyi et al., 2001).

Numerous studies have examined the effect of training protocols requiring skill improvement on the consistency of motor output. In one study, subjects learned to roll two metal balls clockwise and counterclockwise in their palms using independent and coordinated movements of their fingers (Ranganathan, Siemionow, Sahgal, Liu, & Yue, 2001). While this training protocol did not improve strength, it reduced the fluctuations in force during a low-intensity pinch (<20% MVC) and improved the ability of individuals to use their hands to accurately displace a small object. Furthermore, tai chi, a form of exercise that does not significantly load muscles in the upper body, resulted in lower variability in motor output and improved accuracy of arm movements in older adults (Yan, 1999). Similarly, when older adults trained with tai chi for 16 wk, both muscle strength and fluctuations in force improved in the knee extensors (Christou, Yang, & Rosengren, 2003) (figure 11.7c). Nonetheless, strength improvements were not associated with improvements in fluctuations in force.

Strength training with light or heavy loads appears to improve the ability of older adults to produce stronger and steadier contractions when the primary mover of the limb is a single muscle (i.e., the first dorsal interosseous). For movements that are controlled by multiple muscles, however, attenuation of the variability in motor output appears to occur with training that does not emphasize strength but rather muscle coordination and skilled movement.

Changes in the Nervous System Alter Variability in Motor Output

A number of neurophysiological changes occur with aging that can alter the motor program and the variability of motor output. Such changes include neuronal death in higher centers, death of the motor neurons in the spinal cord, and subsequent remodeling of motor units in the muscle.

One major observation is that older adults consistently exhibit greater fluctuations during low-intensity contractions (<10% of maximum). Fluctuations in motor output occur because the motor command does not elicit a fused tetani in all activated motor units, and thus force fluctuates around a mean value. Only a few low-threshold motor units are recruited during low-intensity contractions. It has been hypothesized that with aging, small motor units innervate more muscle fibers (this reorganization occurs because of the deaths of large alpha motor neurons in the spinal cord), an arrangement that produces greater twitches and impairs the ability of older adults to produce steady low forces (Roos et al., 1997). Experimental findings indicate that the motor unit force that is contributed to the total force in older adults is greater compared with that of younger adults. However, the greater contribution to total force by the small motor units is not responsible for the greater variability in force exhibited by old adults during low-intensity contractions (Keen et al., 1994). Computer simulation suggests that the synchronized discharge of motor units can also increase fluctuations in force (Yao, Fuglevand, & Enoka, 2000). Experimental evidence, however, suggests that motor unit synchronization is not associated with the greater fluctuations observed in older adults (Semmler et al., 2000). There is evidence that the only adaptation at the level of the motor units that can contribute to the greater fluctuations is greater variability in the discharge rate of the motor units (Kornatz et al., 2005; Laidlaw et al., 2000).

When high-intensity contractions are compared to low-intensity contractions, the fluctuations in motor output appear to be similar or even lower for older adults. The contribution of individual motor units to the total muscle force is less during high-intensity contractions (Fuglevand, Winter, & Patla, 1993). Therefore, the impaired ability of older adults to regulate the forces exerted by individual motor units is only observable at low levels of force and in small muscles. Furthermore, in older adults, during low-intensity lengthening the fluctuations in the motor output are amplified when compared with the fluctuations in shortening contractions. This increase in variability observed during lengthening contractions may relate to the finding that there are fewer active motor units and lower discharge rates during lengthening than during shortening contractions (Christou, Shinohara, & Enoka, 2001; Christova & Kossev, 2000; Kossev & Christova, 1998). For example, a lower mean discharge rate of motor units is associated with increased variability in the discharge (Person & Kudina, 1972; Piotrkiewicz, 1999). In addition, both simulation (Taylor, Steege, & Enoka, 2000) and experiments found that increased variability in the discharge rate of the motor units was associated with increased fluctuations in motor output (Kornatz et al., 2002; Laidlaw et al., 2000).

The minimum variance theory (Harris & Wolpert, 1998) suggests that the functional significance of the amplitude in fluctuations of motor output is that greater fluctuations reduce the accuracy of movement. Interestingly, this relation differs for younger and older adults. For example, we found that the greater are the fluctuations in acceleration, the lower is the accuracy of movement in both younger and older adults; however, the fluctuations in acceleration impaired the accuracy of movement more in older adults than younger adults (Christou et al., 2003). From this observation the question arises: Why do fluctuations in motor output impose a greater effect on movement accuracy in older adults as compared to younger adults?

There is experimental evidence that older adults coactivate the antagonist muscle more than do younger adults when abducting the index finger (Burnett et al., 2000; Spiegel, Stratton, Burke, Glendinning, & Enoka, 1996). Although the *normalized fluctuations* in motor output were not significantly correlated with the increased coactivation of the antagonist muscle (Burnett et al., 2000), simulations of muscular contractions suggest that coactivation of the agonist and antagonist muscles can attenuate fluctuations in force (Seidler-Dobrin, He, & Stelmach, 1998). Coactivation of the antagonist muscle can potentially decrease fluctuations in acceleration by stiffening the joint (Hogan, 1985; Karst & Hasan, 1987). Nonetheless, increased coactivation in older adults can impair the ratio and timing of activation in the agonist and antagonist muscles (Darling, Cooke, & Brown, 1989) and consequently impair the ability of an older individual to accelerate the limb segment and accurately match a target velocity. It is possible that the greater impairment in movement accuracy that occurs even in older adults displaying similar or lower fluctuations relates to the higher coactivation of the antagonist muscle, particularly at faster velocities.

Voluntary rapid contractions represent the descending command along with the excitation of the motor neuron pool (motor program), because the motor output from the spinal cord is modified the least by peripheral feedback (Cordo et al., 1994). The ability of older adults in comparison to younger adults to duplicate a contraction appears to be more variable only during fast movements (figure 11.6). Because older and younger adults often exhibit similar variability during slower movements, the neural impairment in older adults *may* be not in the motor neuron pool but rather in the higher centers. There is evidence suggesting that loss of cortical motor neurons begins as early as 50 y (Eisen et al., 1996), and thus deficits in cortical areas can significantly limit planning, executing, and regulating the motor command (Willott, 1999). In addition, decreases in transmissions from the corticospinal and reflex pathways to the motor neurons (Henderson et al., 1980) might also reduce the effectiveness of the motor command. Similarly to the variability within trials, the trial-to-trial variability of the motor output appears to be amplified during lengthening contractions in older adults. It is possible that the impaired descending command in older adults is more noticeable when fewer motor units act during a contraction (Christova & Kossev, 2000; Kossev & Christova, 1998; Sogaard, Christensen, Jensen, Finsen, & Sjogaard, 1996).

Finally, physical training in older adults appears to attenuate fluctuations in motor output by improving motor learning. The disassociation between improvements in strength and improvements in variability is shown by the similar improvements in variability achieved with low- or high-intensity strength training of the first dorsal interosseous (Laidlaw et al., 1999; Kornatz et al., 2002) and of the knee extensors (Hortobagyi et al., 2001). Furthermore, longitudinal studies found that strength training the knee extensors improved strength but did not improve fluctuations in motor output (Bellew, 2002; Tracy, 2001). In contrast, training protocols that emphasize muscle coordination and skill improved the consistency of motor output in various muscle groups (Christou, Yang, & Rosengren, 2003; Ranganathan et al., 2001; Yan, 1999). Although it is unclear whether altered coordination of the synergist muscles can reduce fluctuations in force, it is possible that the timing of activation in the synergist muscles and appropriate coactivation of the antagonist muscle can improve movement accuracy (Seidler-Dobrin et al., 1998).

Summary

Older adults often exhibit greater variability in motor output during voluntary contractions. The fluctuations within a trial appear to be higher in older adults only for contractions of a very low intensity; nonetheless, fluctuations with a similar amplitude may impose a greater constraint in the accuracy of movements in older adults than in younger adults. Findings from the few studies that have examined variability in motor output from trial to trial indicate that older adults exhibit greater variability during very fast and lengthening contractions. There is evidence that physical training in older adults can reduce the fluctuations in the motor output. This attenuation in variability appears to relate to improvements in muscle coordination and not to improvements in strength. Considering these findings, we propose that in healthy older adults the amplified variability in motor output is a consequence of the altered discharge characteristics of the motor units and the altered muscle coordination imposed by an impaired motor command to the motor neuron pool.

Part V

Variability Within Subsystems

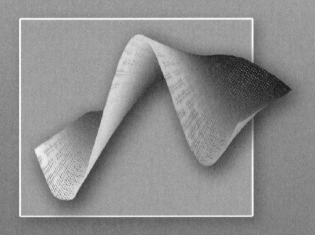

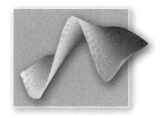

Chapter 12

Mechanical Properties of Muscles Reduce Performance Variability

Alberto E. Minetti, MD

Editors' Overview

This chapter demonstrates the power and elegance of mathematics in analyzing a computer simulation of the relationships between flexors and extensors in a joint complex. This simulation showed how covarying these relationships can reduce the amount of information needed for controlling the movement system over time. Formal support is provided for the hypothesis that self-organization can explain the coordination of degrees of freedom at the level of muscles. A reduction in the control problem for the movement system is hypothesized, since covariation of simulated activation levels of flexors and extensors helps stabilize joint angles in an attractor while the overall movement amplitude helps set joint stiffness for a particular angle. Two mundane physical activities, arm wrestling and drop jump landing, are discussed to highlight the role of variability at the mechanical level of analysis. The data can be interpreted as demonstrating how the CNS, in maintaining stable performance outputs according to specific intentions, exploits self-organization at the level of muscle characteristics. This position on variability contrasts starkly with theories of motor control that suggest that variability is tolerated within a bandwidth so that it does not contribute to noise in the motor system that might interfere with task performance.

Most of the literature on the normal actions of muscles concentrates on positive work and power production, but there are situations in which the fixative and stretching roles of muscles are very important. The first role is associated with the need to stiffen a given joint, while the second is crucial when we wish to slow a movement.

The ability to fix and stiffen a joint relates to the control of antagonist muscle groups, such as the biceps and triceps brachii in a tennis strike (figure 12.1) or the medial and lateral rectus muscles in moving the eyeball (figure 12.2). In both cases, a successful performance is linked to the quickest and most accurate action, and we could wonder about the complexity of the control system in setting up the reciprocal action of antagonist muscle groups. In particular, a question that about half of this chapter addresses is: Do muscle properties help the neural control system reduce the complexity and increase the effectiveness of such actions? The part of the central nervous system devoted to controlling antagonist muscles is structured, both at the cortical and spinal levels, as a

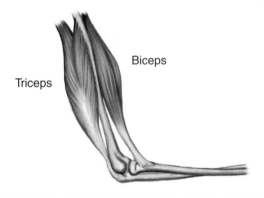

FIGURE 12.1　Two main muscles of the upper arm work against each other to stiffen the elbow joint during action such as a tennis strike.
© Human Kinetics

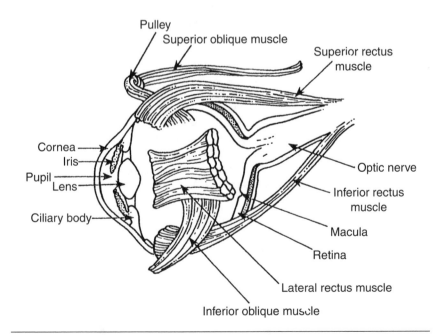

FIGURE 12.2　The reciprocal muscles in the eyeball work against each other to move and fix the glance to a new position.

complex neuronal network (see figure 12.3) in which inputs from the motor cortex and local sensors are integrated to produce a smooth and calibrated action in many different situations.

We also know that muscle responds differently to the same neuronal activation, depending on the length and speed or load of the given muscle. Particularly, there is an optimal length at which the maximum (isometric) force is produced. Maximum force is generated when the muscle is stretched, while during shortening the force decreases with increasing speed. Because of these mechanical characteristics, it is reasonable to hypothesize that two antagonist muscles, one of which shortens while the other lengthens, can reach a stable configuration even with very simple patterns of activation. In this chapter, a computer simulation of arm wrestling is used to show that there are theoretical reasons to confirm such a hypothesis (Minetti, 1994).

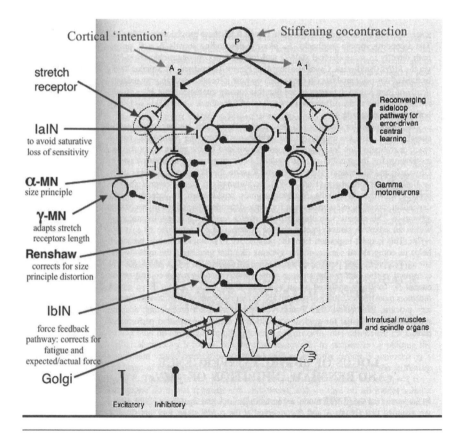

FIGURE 12.3 The currently known neuronal structures responsible for controlling a pair of antagonist muscles. Pathways from cortical areas, spinal (inter)neurons, and muscle and tendon sensors are integrated to calibrate muscle contraction.

Reprinted, by permission, from K.M. Newell and D. Corcos, How spinal neural networks reduce discrepancies between motor intention and motor realization. In *Variability and motor control*, edited by D. Bullock and J.L. Contreras-Vidal (Champaign, IL: Human Kinetics), 203.

The second half of this chapter discusses another aspect of how musculo-skeletal arrangement affects the variability of motor performance. By considering the drop landing as being affected only by the timing in the activation of the knee extensors, it is shown that different scenarios (safe and controlled, safe and uncontrolled, and unsafe landings) emerge, even without taking into account the complexity of the control system (figure 12.3). The computer simulation provides the results of an otherwise unfeasible experiment identifying the three scenarios (and their critical boundaries) (Minetti, Ardigò, Susta, and Cotelli, 1998).

Arm Wrestling

In order to simulate the action of two antagonist muscles, the model of two arm wrestlers was used. Figure 12.4 shows how such an example offers complete symmetry in the relationships between actuator force and length (obtained from Winters & Stark, 1985) and force and velocity characteristics. The two competitors in the left-hand scenario of figure 12.4 have to flex their forearms (as in normal arm wrestling) while the others on the right-hand side have to extend their forearms to win. This second situation was introduced to account for nonsuperimposable relationships in reciprocal force and length of the two actuators.

In describing how the two muscles relate to each other, we started with the second example. Figure 12.5a shows how the diagrams of force versus length and force versus speed for each competitor can be represented by a single 3-D surface where the force (vertical) axis is shared by the two relationships; force versus length and force versus speed. To be consistent, the 3-D surfaces for the two competitors should be oriented so as to account for one muscle stretching when the other is shortening, and this reciprocal orientation also applies to the speed axis. Then the surfaces can be layered in a single 3-D graph (figure 12.5b), in which the mutual relation between the two surfaces is more evident. There are values of speed and length in which the two surfaces display the same force (the isoheight sigmoidal boundary between A and B) and other zones where one of the competitors is stronger than the other. If we imagine that subjects (muscles) A and B are always maximally active by starting from an optimal initial condition (of length and speed), the dynamics of the resulting movement are determined by the difference in the forces of the two surfaces. The zero-speed line (in bold) shows the points where the dynamics can stop if the two forces coincide, and this happens (in the displayed configuration) in the middle of the horizontal plane (with a stable point) and in two other conditions (with unstable points) (see figure 12.5b).

Since, when only looking to figure 12.5b, it is difficult to imagine the whole variety of scenarios, a computer simulation has been designed. A program was written (using software by LabView, National Instrument Incorporated, United States) to calculate the dynamics trajectories in the horizontal plane of

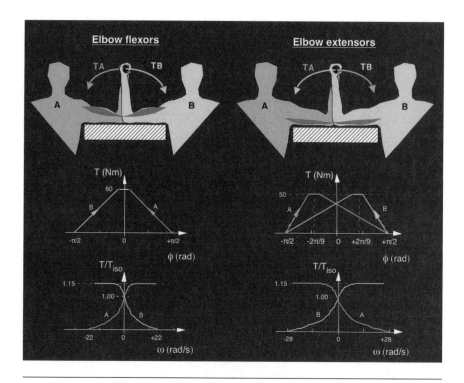

FIGURE 12.4   Two arm wrestlers flexing (left column) and extending (right column) their forearms are depicted to mimic the effect of antagonist muscles acting across a single joint (in a single body). The graphs, taken from Minetti (1994), reflect the muscle characteristics of the biceps and triceps brachii as found in the specific literature. Plots of torque versus angle and torque versus angular speed replace plots of force versus length and force versus velocity in order to account for the angular nature of the performance.

Reprinted from *Journal of Theoretical Biology,* Vol 169, A.E. Minetti, Contraction dynamics in antagonist muscles, pg. 295-304, Copyright 1994, with permission from Elsevier.

figure 12.5*b* (called the phase plane) for many pairs of speed and length. This simulation corresponds to allowing our arm wrestlers to start competing from different positions and with different initial speeds (positive, negative, and zero) and to observing the outcome of the fight.

Figure 12.6 shows the dynamics for a configuration similar to the right-hand column of figure 12.4 (depicting the elbow extensors). The mechanical characteristics of the muscle are illustrated at the borders of the inset graph (which is enlarged in figure 12.6*b* for sake of clarity), representing the outcome of the simulation. Along the line of isometric contraction (solid horizontal line) at which speed = 0 rad/s, three interesting points are marked. Point 1 (0, 0) represents an attractor, or a point where several trajectories in the phase plane tend to converge. At this position, where there is a big basin of attraction, a perturbation in angle or speed difference does not affect the final result

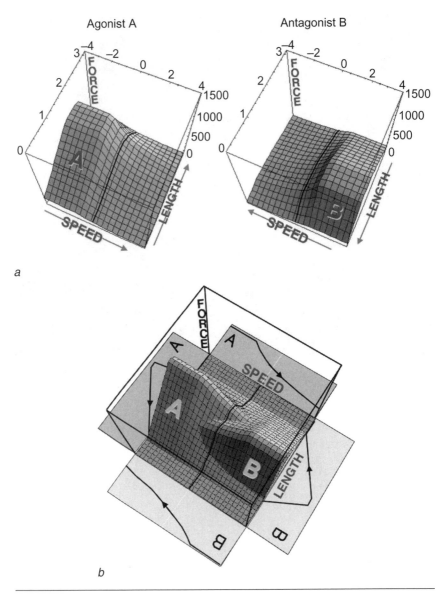

FIGURE 12.5 *(a)* The relationships shown in the right-hand column of figure 12.4 (for the elbow extensors) are summarized in a single 3-D graph in which the ordinate is shared. For the two graphs to be superimposable, when muscle A is short, muscle B must be long and when muscle A is shortening, muscle B must be lengthening. This means reverting the horizontal axes for one of the two muscles. *(b)* On the layered 3-D graph, the zones of angle and angular speed where one of the muscles is stronger than the other are clearly delimited by the sinusoidal boundary between the two surfaces.

Reprinted from *Journal of Theoretical Biology,* Vol 169, A.E. Minetti, Contraction dynamics in antagonist muscles, pg. 295-304, Copyright 1994, with permission from Elsevier.

(0, 0). Differently, points 2 and 3 are repulsors since a trajectory starting from them remains at these points forever, but an infinitesimal perturbation causes a departure toward attractors. Point 1 can also be considered as a condition of stable equilibrium and points 2 and 3 as conditions of unstable equilibrium, as represented in the lower right corner of figure 12.6a. Regions near points 2 and 3 tend to converge to point 1 or to zones 4 and 5, which also can be considered as attractors. As a consequence, the regions near points 2 and 3 are quite uncertain with respect to the final result of the competition, which can only be point 4 (A wins), point 1 (draw), or point 5 (B wins). In this example the size of the basin of attraction of point 1 is much greater than the other two basins at zones 4 and 5 so that we can predict a prevalence of draw outcomes (basins are shaded in different gray tones in figure 12.6a).

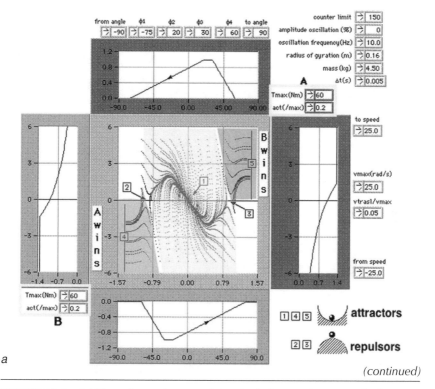

a

(continued)

FIGURE 12.6 *(a)* The software framework in which the simulations took place. Around the inset graph, the relationships between torque and angle and between torque and angular speed are represented. The shaded areas differentiate the basins of attraction. *(b)* Enlargement of inset in *(a)*. The arrows show the time course of the different dynamics. The basins of attraction, or in other words, the initial conditions leading to point 1 (draw) or to zones 4 (A wins) or 5 (B wins), are immediately apparent. Points 2 and 3 represent repulsors, or conditions of unstable equilibrium in which the slightest deviation would move the dynamic away.

Reprinted from *Journal of Theoretical Biology*, Vol 169, A.E. Minetti, Contraction dynamics in antagonist muscles, pg. 295-304, Copyright 1994, with permission from Elsevier.

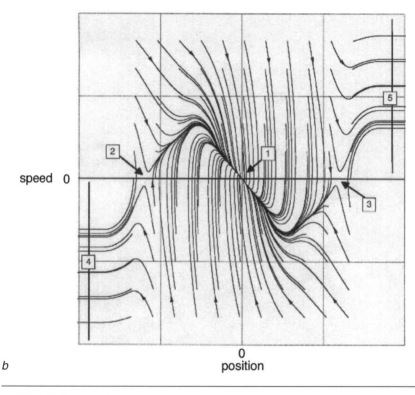

speed 0

0
position

b

FIGURE 12.6   *(continued)*

In figure 12.6, the reciprocal arrangement of the relationship between torque and angle, we can change the shape and size of the basin of attraction by modifying the activation level of one muscle. For example, figure 12.7 shows the same reciprocal arrangement between the two muscles, but muscle A is activated at twice the level of muscle B. Here the central attractor is located near to the left repulsor, and their closeness indicates a greater opportunity for muscle A to win (as expected), since a little perturbation from that point (while stable) makes the system cross the uncertainty zone and move toward the left attractor. In figure 12.7, the basin of attraction for A to win is greater, while the one for B to win is smaller than in figure 12.6. An important message from these dynamics is that a position within a certain range of movement can be rapidly reached and kept stiff (at a stable equilibrium) only by changing the ratio between activation levels (and not the time courses) of antagonist muscles. This process could save a lot of information in the control of complex movements involving stabilization of multiple joints because you need to change just the activation level and not the time course of it, which could be constant.

Whether making changes in a single muscle or in both muscles, by adjusting the shape and the reciprocal position of the curves for torque versus angle, the torque and speed characteristics, the maximum muscle torque, or the neuromuscular activation, we obtain dynamics displaying only attractors, only repulsors, or combination of both. In figure 12.8, a simulation where different torque and angle relationships have been input (at the same activation level), there are just two attractor zones and one central repulsor point.

Finally, figure 12.9 shows the effects of a sinusoidal tremor induced in the contraction of the two muscles. The resulting trajectories do not partition the phase plane into clearly delimited areas, and this increases the indeterminism of the final outcome of the cocontraction.

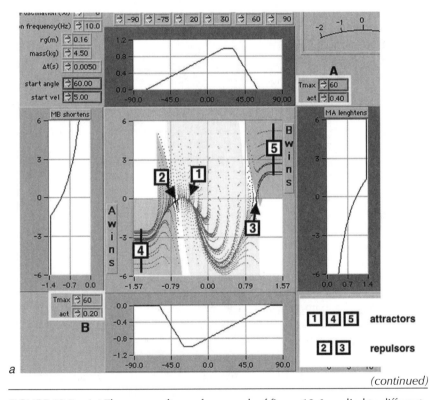

(continued)

FIGURE 12.7   *(a)* The same software framework of figure 12.6 applied to different activations for the two muscles. Opponent A is twice as strong as opponent B and this affects the resulting phase plane. The basin of attraction for A to win increases in size and the attractor point (marked with 1) is positioned so that a little perturbation of the system (a little extra force, for instance) favors subject A. *(b)* Enlargement of inset in *(a)*. Point A is an attractor while R refers to repulsors, i.e., unstable equilibrium points.

Reprinted from *Journal of Theoretical Biology,* Vol 169, A.E. Minetti, Contraction dynamics in antagonist muscles, pg. 295-304, Copyright 1994, with permission from Elsevier.

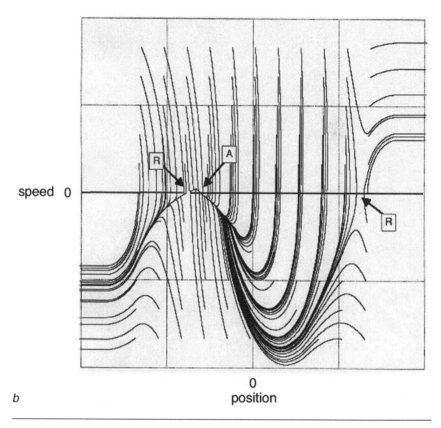

FIGURE 12.7 *(continued)*

The take-home message from these simulations is the following:

1. Despite the complexity and the related variability of the neuromuscular system, simulations of antagonist and agonist muscles show that joint stability can rely on mechanical muscle characteristics only.

2. The relationships between force and length and between force and speed, specularly arranged for the two muscle groups, potentially allow you to quickly reach and maintain a wide range of joint angles just by only setting different levels of activation.

3. Depending on the shapes of the curves of force versus length and on the time course of neural activation, some unstable situations can occur in which even a small perturbation causes a catastrophic drift toward one of the opponents.

For further detail on this topic, see Minetti (1994).

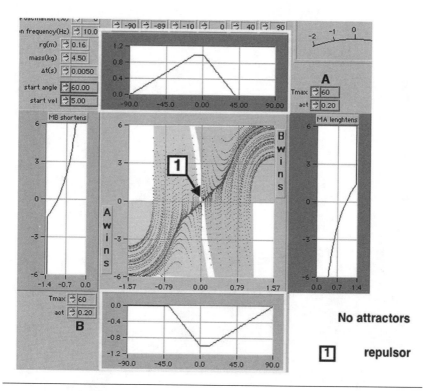

FIGURE 12.8   The same software framework of figure 12.6, but with different torque and angle characteristics. Stiffening of the joint can occur, but the joint is quite unstable. A minimum perturbation causes the system to collapse on one side (i.e., one of the two subjects will win).

Reprinted from *Journal of Theoretical Biology,* Vol 169, A.E. Minetti, Contraction dynamics in antagonist muscles, pg. 295-304, Copyright 1994, with permission from Elsevier.

Variability in Drop Landing

To evaluate the variety of potential performances in landing from drops of different heights and how musculoskeletal timing affects the overall outcome (in terms of maximum negative power and landing dynamics), a theoretical model of landing was designed (Minetti et al., 1998). The need for simulation came from realizing that we could not ask subjects to risk their safety during increasingly tough experiments. We found that very different scenarios in performance are possible, even when dropping from a constant height, with different timing in muscle activation. Thus there is some dependence on initial conditions.

We used an approach similar to the one used for studying antagonist muscles dynamics. Here, the only opposing force is gravity, the subject is described by a simple two-segment model representing the lower limbs, the overall mass is concentrated on the hip, and the only actuator is the knee extensor. The knee

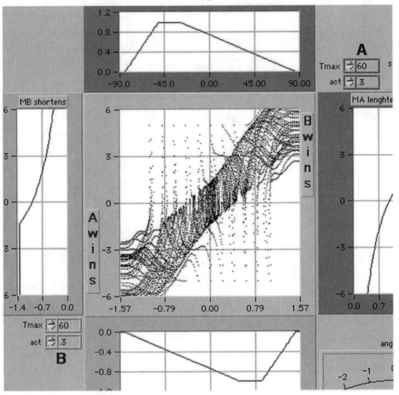

FIGURE 12.9 The same software framework of figure 12.6, but with a tremor simulated by a sinusoidal perturbation of the forces in the two muscles.

Reprinted from *Journal of Theoretical Biology,* Vol 169, A.E. Minetti, Contraction dynamics in antagonist muscles, pg. 295-304, Copyright 1994, with permission from Elsevier.

extensor is modeled as a torque generator with mechanical characteristics like those of muscles, with realistic relationships between torque and angle (obtained from Winters and Stark, 1985) and between torque and angular speed (see figure 12.10). The modeling constraints set the maximum torque of the actuator at a given level. If the required performance exceeds this level, the muscle is supposed to lengthen. Exceeding the maximum torque of the actuator could happen on jumps from remarkable heights, resulting in an unsafe landing. In trying to closely approach reality, we included in the model a torsional spring located at the ankle level in order to simulate the tissue resistance at extreme foot dorsiflexion that prevents further lowering of the center of mass of the body.

Figure 12.11 shows the mechanical characteristics of the knee extensors as used in the simulation. The 3-D surface on the left-hand side, similar to what was illustrated for antagonist muscle A in figure 12.5*a,* deals with force, angle,

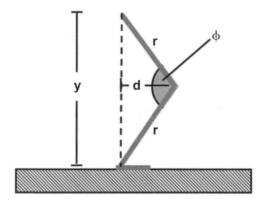

FIGURE 12.10   Stick diagram of the model used to simulate the drop jump.

Reprinted, by permission, from A.E. Minetti et al., 1998, "Using leg muscles as shock absorbers: Theoretical predictions and experimental results of human drop landing," *Ergonomics* 41(21): 1171-1791. Http://www.tandf.co.uk.

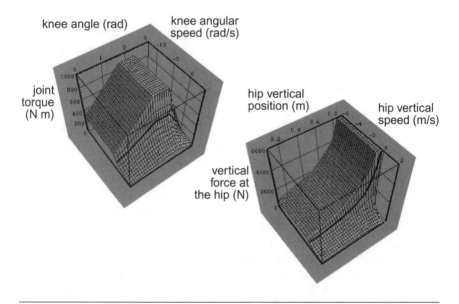

FIGURE 12.11   In the graph on the left, the torque of the knee joint is represented as a function of both the knee angle and angular speed (corresponding to the relationships between force and length and between force and speed in the knee extensors) when muscles are fully activated. In the graph on the right, the vertical ground reaction force, produced by the knee extensors, is shown as a function of the vertical position and speed of the hip. In both graphs the highlighted (bolded) curve on the 3-D surface denotes the isometric contraction (condition of zero speed).

Reprinted, by permission, from A.E. Minetti et al., 1998, "Using leg muscles as shock absorbers: Theoretical predictions and experimental results of human drop landing," *Ergonomics* 41(21): 1171-1791. Http://www.tandf.co.uk.

and angular speed. It needs to be transformed into linear terms to contrast the opposing force (gravity). The 3-D surface on the right-hand side is the equivalent of the one on the left-hand side once the different moment arms of the knee at different angles are taken into account.

Before discussing the results from the simulation of drop landing, some notes about how to read a phase-plane diagram are needed. Obviously, when the speed is negative, the displacement has to decrease and the overall direction (vector) points to the lower left or right corner of the plane according to acceleration or deceleration, respectively. Conversely, for positive speeds the trajectory vector is always ascending and points to the upper right or left corner of the plane according to acceleration or deceleration, respectively. The overall message is that closed trajectories crossing the zero-speed line move counterclockwise (if speed is represented in the abscissa). Also, constant force is represented as a parabola in the phase plane. A body moving under the effect of only gravity (a negative force) shows a downward parabola that starts at different ordinates depending on the initial height of the drop. Conversely, a body moving under the effect of only a positive (upward) force shows an upward parabola, with the dynamics following the descending or ascending limb according to the initial speed (negative or positive, respectively).

The stick diagram on the right-hand side of figure 12.12 depicts dropping from a given height, touching the ground, and starting to flex the knees up to body crushing into the ground. The sketch reflects the ordinate (the vertical) position of the hip. The subject cannot touch the ground before the hip has reached a position below 0.9 m, the length which corresponds to the fully extended leg. The diagram on the bottom of figure 12.12 represents the vertical speed of the hip, with negative speeds illustrating descending. During flight, the only force acting on the subject is gravity, and the dynamic is a downward arch of a parabola in the negative side of the abscissa. The choice of a given curve depends on the drop height, which is measured from the ground to the feet. Drop heights are indicated in the upper area of the graph in figure 12.12. When the hip is lower than 0.9 m, the final performance depends on the timing of muscle activation (maximum activation is supposed to occur from then onward). For example, when following the downward parabola labeled 1.5 m (meaning that the subject started falling from a feet height of 1.5 m), the timing of activation can be crucial. If the subject switches on his muscles early, the dynamics curve changes and starts moving to the right (into the light gray region) until it reaches the vertical line indicating zero speed, where the movement can stop (if muscles are deactivated). If a small delay in activation occurs, the hip keeps on descending on the parabola and abandons that curve in the blue region, where the curves pointing to the right represent the hip reaching zero speed when the hip is in a much lower vertical position. Recovering from a risky jump is made possible by the spring incorporated into the ankle structures (connective tissue, ligaments, and so on). In the case of a longer delay in muscle activation, the hip dynamics leave the downward parabola in the dark gray zone, where all the deceleration curves that are pointing right never reach

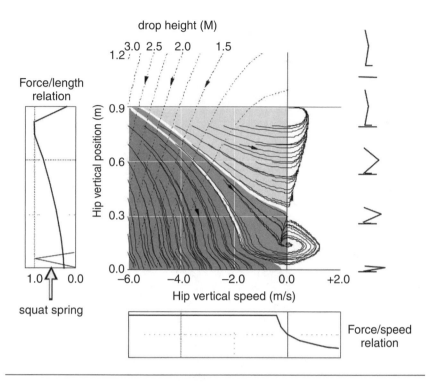

FIGURE 12.12   The phase plane represents all of the possible landing dynamics of a subject (*m* = 70 kg, *Tmax* = 500 N·m) falling from different heights. The three shaded zones correspond to landing dynamics that are safe and controlled (light gray), safe and uncontrolled (medium gray), and unsafe (dark gray).

Reprinted, by permission, from A.E. Minetti et al., 1998, "Using leg muscles as shock absorbers: Theoretical predictions and experimental results of human drop landing," *Ergonomics* 41(21): 1171-1791. Http://www.tandf.co.uk.

the zero speed. This corresponds to a very unsafe landing, with damage done to musculoskeletal structures.

According to the final outcome, we could say that the three shaded zones correspond to safe and controlled, safe and uncontrolled, and unsafe landings. It is apparent from figure 12.12 that depending on the height of the drop landing, the opportunities to decide the destiny of the landing are wider or narrower. Sometimes a delay of a few milliseconds can transform a safe landing into an unsafe one, and this is an example of dependency on initial conditions. The model prediction and the experimental data obtained by integrating the signal coming from a dynamometric platform showed very good agreement, particularly after the initial muscle contraction was able to take up the slack in the chain of actuators (Minetti et al., 1998), as illustrated in figure 12.13.

The same simulation can be extended to represent deviation from the average human. People with the same mass and stronger knee extensors or with the same strength and higher mass should show very different dynamics with

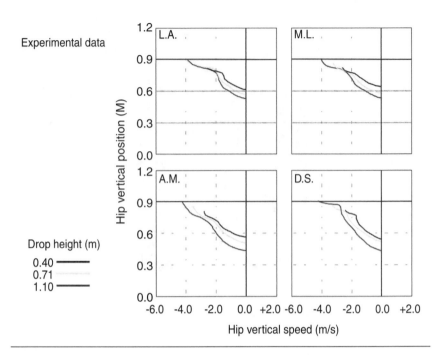

FIGURE 12.13   The experimental speed and the position of the center of mass are represented in the phase plane (the axes units and ticks spacing are the same as those in figure 12.12). Each panel shows a different subject landing from the three imposed heights.

Reprinted, by permission, from A.E. Minetti et al., 1998, "Using leg muscles as shock absorbers: Theoretical predictions and experimental results of human drop landing," *Ergonomics* 41(21): 1171-1791. Http://www.tandf.co.uk.

respect to what is shown in figure 12.12. The dynamics of the two described extremes, representing the *athlete* and the *obese*, respectively, are illustrated in figure 12.14. The left-hand graph tells us that athletes are less affected by the initial conditions since the outcome is only partitioned between safe and unsafe landings, with a much more extended zone for safe ones. The situation for the obese subject (right-hand graph) is opposite. The safe landing (controlled and uncontrolled) is greatly reduced when compared to figure 12.12, which corresponds to a reduced choice about the heights from which to land and the successful performance. From figures 12.12 and 12.14 it can be observed that for control subjects, the maximum suggested drop height is about 2.0 m, while for athletes and obese subjects it is 3.0 and 1.0 m, respectively.

Apart from being a tool to investigate the diversity of scenarios in experimentally unfeasible maneuvers such as the drop landing, the phase plane reserves additional potential. The simulation showed that if constant (and maximal) activation is applied, a consistent dynamics can be obtained. The next question is: What if the drop height, the visual constraints, the subjective preparation and reaction to impact, the type of descent, and the contribution of antagonist

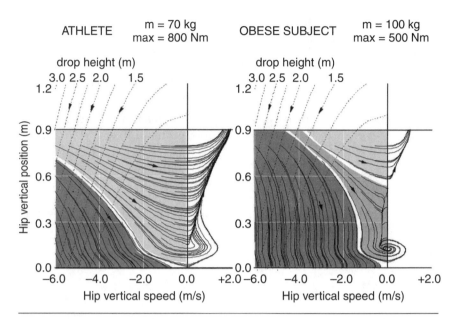

FIGURE 12.14   The same representation of figure 12.6 shown for different subjects. Simulations of the landing dynamics in athletes (*Tmax* = 800 N·m, *m* = 70 kg) and obese subjects (*Tmax* = 500 N·m, *m* = 100 kg) are illustrated in the left and right graphs, respectively.

Reprinted, by permission, from A.E. Minetti et al., 1998, "Using leg muscles as shock absorbers: Theoretical predictions and experimental results of human drop landing," *Ergonomics* 41(21): 1171-1791. Http://www.tandf.co.uk.

muscles change to modulate the input from the musculoskeletal apparatus to the central nervous system (figure 12.3), so that the muscle activation is no longer constant? Sensors, like tendon organs and muscle spindles, continuously inform the central nervous system about the status of the actuator and the forces involved. The phase-plane dynamics could potentially reveal deviations in motor control from a reference simulation.

Conclusions

The aim of this chapter was to illustrate how a variety of motor outputs can originate just from an interaction between agonist and antagonist and from a given musculoskeletal arrangement fighting against gravity, when no real neural control is introduced as an input to the model. Depending on the particular motor act, neural modulation is expected to simplify or increase the complexity of the final output.

The illustrated simulations may be used to reach a different goal. Rather than producing a winner (virtual arm wrestling) or the quickest deceleration (drop landing), we could be interested in, say, the softest possible landing. In that case the model could provide the optimal pattern of muscle activation in order to fulfill the new goal (Minetti et al., 1998).

This chapter has

- introduced a new way to graphically represent musculoskeletal dynamics,
- described simple but realistic models of human motor performances and the predictions associated with the assumption of maximum muscle activation, and
- shown how a different configuration or initial condition can affect the overall dynamics.

It is suggested that the value of the phase plane extends beyond just answering biomechanical questions.

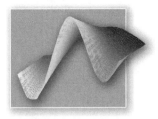

Chapter 13

Cellular and Molecular Basis of Heterogeneity in Contractile Performance of Human Muscles

Carlo Reggiani, PhD and Susan Bortolotto, PhD

Editors' Overview

The levels of analysis addressed in this chapter are cellular and molecular. It is argued that skeletal muscles are engines, and like all engines, they exhibit variability in performance as conditions change. The chapter describes how the nervous system is involved in the activation of motor units in muscles and in their frequency and rate of discharge over more extensive timescales of human motor performance. The regulation of muscle function by the nervous system is not only quantitative. Most muscles contain motor units that demonstrate different properties such as capacity for force development and resistance to fatigue. These variations can be exploited by muscle through a selective recruitment process, which enhances functional behavior. Despite great structural homogeneity in the composition of the protein base of all vertebrate muscle, nervous systems can exploit organismic (structural) constraints, such as diversity among populations of motor units and variability in types of muscle fibers, to support specialized performance in a variety of movement tasks. The cellular and molecular basis of functional diversity in muscle fibers has been observed in variations in biochemical synthetic reactions, in the production of energy for work, in short- and long-term muscle regulatory mechanisms, and in the role of muscle proteins called isoforms. Small adaptations in the amino acid sequences of proteins can lead to great functional diversity in the muscle properties captured by a wide range of isoforms (a single protein can have up to 60 isoforms in some mammals).

S keletal muscles are living engines that produce mechanical energy from chemical energy, and myosin is the molecular motor responsible for this energy transduction.

Skeletal muscles are employed in a variety of mechanical tasks. Different muscles in the body fulfill specific tasks. For example, the contraction of the wrist flexors and the finger flexor support the light and fast touch of the pianist's finger on the keyboard, whereas the strong leg quadriceps extend the leg when the football player kicks the ball more than 50 m. The same muscle can also be employed in extremely different tasks. For example, the adductor pollicis can be used to thread a fine needle as well as to grasp a bar and contribute to supporting the whole body weight. Finally, when the performance of corresponding muscles is compared in different animal species, the diversity of functional tasks is surprising. For example, in all mammals the soleus and gastrocnemius muscles extend the ankle and support the body weight in static and dynamic conditions even though the body weight can vary by almost 100,000 times when comparing a mouse and an elephant.

The control of muscle performance is in the hand of the nervous system. During a movement the motor centers decide how many motor units (a motor unit is a group of muscle fibers innervated by a motor neuron) must be activated and at which frequency of action potential discharge they must be activated. Inside each motor unit, the force developed increases in relation with the discharge rate (force–frequency relation), and inside a muscle, the higher the number of motor units are activated, the greater is the force. The regulation, however, is not only quantitative. With the exception of some muscles that are composed of only one type of motor unit, muscles consist of motor units with different properties. Force development, power output, time course of contractile responses, and resistance to fatigue all vary from one motor unit to another. Thus, by recruiting (selectively activating) motor units with the more appropriate properties, a given muscle can behave in different ways in relation to the functional task that is required.

The diversity among motor units, discovered in the 1960s (Henneman, Clamann, Gillies & Skinner, 1974; Burke, Levine & Zajac, 1971), can be categorized into at least three main types:

- S, or slow motor units, develop little force with a slow time course, and are very resistant to fatigue.
- FF, or fast-fatiguing motor units, develop high force with a fast time course but quickly become fatigued.
- FR, or fatigue-resistant motor units, fall between the other two groups in force development and fatigue resistance.

The basis of this diversity is localized in the differing muscle fibers composing the motor unit.

When observing the fine structure of the muscle using electron microscopy, the similarity between muscle fibers in all animal species is remarkable. The sarcomeric structure is highly conserved in all muscle fibers of all vertebrates. The same holds true for the molecular architectures of the sarcomeric muscles, in that all muscle fibers of all animal species are virtually composed of the same proteins. Only some quantitative features such as fiber thickness vary in an obvious way. In contrast, when muscle fibers are dissected from the muscles and their functional properties are analyzed, a large diversity can be observed in their mechanical power output, speed of shortening, and resistance to fatigue in prolonged contractions.

What is the basis of this functional diversity? In spite of their structural homogeneity, muscle fibers are functionally heterogeneous because they are composed of different isoforms of the same proteins. Isoforms are two or more proteins whose slight differences in amino acid sequence determine distinct functional properties. Virtually all muscle proteins can exist in two or more isoforms; extreme examples are troponin T (fast), which in each mammalian species may be produced in 64 isoforms obtained by alternative splicing of the same gene (Breitbart & Nadal-Ginard, 1986, 1987), and myosin, which is a hexamere (composed by 2 myosin heavy chains, or MHCs, and 4 myosin light chains, or MLCs) that may be produced in at least 60 isoforms (Pette & Staron, 1997).

In the following sections we briefly review the variability of contractile properties among muscle fibers and delineate their molecular basis. Also, we briefly look at how the nervous system can exploit this variability during motor performance and how nervous stimulations, mechanical loads, and hormonal factors can modulate the fiber heterogeneity over the long term.

Functional and Molecular Heterogeneity of Muscle Fibers

The diversity among muscle fibers involves many aspects of muscle structure and function. Virtually any functional parameter in a population of human muscle fibers shows a large and continuous range of variability. Three examples of functional parameters are shown figure 13.1. The first parameter, the time required to reach peak tension (panel A), depends on the rate of calcium release and reuptake by the sarcoplasmic reticulum and on the rate of force generation during actin–myosin interaction. The second parameter, SDH activity (panel B), is an enzymatic activity directly related to the production of ATP. The third parameter, maximum shortening velocity (panel C), is determined by the rate of actin-myosin interaction and ATP hydrolysis and is a major determinant of the ability to generate mechanical power.

As figure 13.1 suggests, the molecular heterogeneity implicated in the functional heterogeneity extends from intracellular calcium kinetics to biochemical pathways for energy production and chemomechanical energy conversion in the myofibrils. The molecular diversity is based on gene regulation, which occurs through two main mechanisms:

1. Qualitative mechanisms produce the many muscle proteins that exist as isoforms. Isoforms can derive from the same gene through alternative

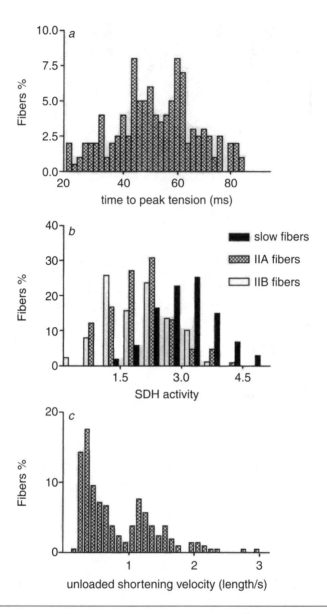

FIGURE 13.1 Examples of diversity among human muscle fibers. Panel A shows the distribution of the contraction times (time from stimulus to peak tension) of fiber bundles from the biceps brachii. Panel B shows the distribution of SDH activities of single fibers from the tibialis anterior; fibers are divided in three groups according to their ATPase activities. Panel C shows the distribution of maximum shortening velocities of single fibers from leg muscles (vastus lateralis, soleus, and tibialis anterior). The three peaks probably correspond to slow and fast IIA and fast IIX fibers.
Adapted from Bottinelli and Reggiani 2000.

splicing or from different genes of the same family (isogenes). Replacing isoforms represents a first mechanism to generate diversity among muscle fibers.

2. Quantitative mechanisms are differential expressions of the same gene. Many genes can be up- and down-regulated independently of each other, depending on factors such as mechanical load, pattern of neural discharge, hormones, and so on. The proportions among the products of these genes are therefore modified and new functional or structural features appear.

The number of possible combinations generated by the two mechanisms described above is limited by constraints set by structural requirements or by rules of expression which define preferential associations among isoforms. For this reason the number of possible combinations is reduced and some more frequent phenotypes of muscle fibers appear. Identifying these frequent phenotypes, generally indicated as fiber types, becomes a preliminary step to studying the diversity in muscle fibers.

The fact that distinct fiber types exist is best demonstrated by the conditions under which fiber transformations take place. In prenatal development, fiber types emerge during the three waves of myoblast fusion typical of human muscles (Draeger, Weeds & Fitzsimons, 1987). Before 20 wk there is no detectable difference among fibers. Later, around 1 y postnatal, when all the fibers are fully differentiated, the adult phenotypes can be identified by their specific ATPase staining and enzymatic histochemistry. In addition, the fiber phenotype can be further altered during postnatal life when, due to variations in the pattern of neural discharge, the mechanical load, and the hormonal stimulation, structural and functional features of the muscle fibers are changed.

In spite of the asynchrony produced by the different thresholds and turnover rates of the various muscle proteins, it is possible to observe that muscle fibers move from one phenotype to the other (transition between fiber types). This movement implies the existence of rules that coordinate the expression of various genes and modulate various functions (energy production, energy consumption, calcium metabolism, and so on) in muscle fibers. Fiber type transformations have been studied in greater detail in animals, particularly in small mammals such as the rat or rabbit, and have been recently well reviewed by Pette and Staron (1997). Several data are also available on the plasticity of muscle fiber in humans (for example, plasticity induced by training or disuse), and these data substantially confirm what is already known from animal studies.

Functional Characterization of Human Muscle Fiber Types: Contractile Properties

As mentioned earlier, motor units differ in their contractile properties. Some are stronger and faster when contracting and some are weaker and slower. This property of motor units closely reflects the properties of the muscle fibers that belong to the motor unit and can be studied in vitro after dissection. Needle or surgical biopsies provide the tissue samples from which single muscle fibers can be dissected. The biopsy sample is immersed in a skinning solution containing a high concentration of potassium propionate and EGTA, and it is then divided in small bundles (Bottinelli, Canepari, Pellegrino & Reggiani, 1996). From these bundles, segments of single fibers are dissected under a stereomicroscope, the membranes are made permeable with a detergent (such as Triton X100), and the fibers are mounted in the experimental apparatus for an in vitro determination of contractile and energetic properties. Fibers are directly activated with the appropriate concentration of calcium, and they then develop tension or shorten, consuming ATP as the energy source. Once the functional analysis is done, single fibers are tested by SDS-PAGE (and in some cases by Western blot) for the MHC isoform composition. MHC isoforms are preferably used as molecular markers of the types of fibers and are used to classify skeletal muscle fibers for several reasons. They are the most abundant proteins of muscle fibers and are the major determinant of both the rate of ATP consumption and mechanical performance (for example, mechanical power output). They are also responsible for the sensitivity of myosin ATPase to alkali or acid preincubation, the feature generally used for fiber typing in muscle histochemistry in neurological diagnostic protocols (Guth & Samaha, 1969; Brooke & Kaiser, 1970). If MHC isoforms are adopted to classify fibers, groups with specific functional characteristics can be delineated. In adult human muscles, five types of fibers can be identified by their MHC isoform composition: slow and fast IIA, fast IIB or IIX, mixed I-IIA, and mixed IIA-IIX.

Figure 13.2 shows tracings of isometric contractions of a fast and of a slow fiber in vitro along with the simultaneous recording of ATP consumption. Average values of the isometric tension *(Po)* and rate of ATP consumption *(Ao)* are reported in table 13.1.

If the fibers are allowed to shorten against various loads during contraction, the force-velocity curve can be obtained. From force and velocity the mechanical power developed by the fiber can easily be calculated. Representative force-velocity curves and power-velocity curves of the three main types of fibers are displayed in figure 13.3. The diversity in maximum shortening velocity can reach as much as 4 times (i.e., the fastest fibers are 4 fold faster than the slowest), and the difference in peak power can be even higher.

Several studies (Bottinelli, Schiaffino & Reggiani, 1991; Bottinelli, Betto, Schiaffino & Reggiani, 1994; Bottinelli, Canepari, Pellegrino & Reggiani, 1996) have shown that the rates of ATP consumption during isometric contraction and the rates of maximum shortening velocity and peak power during active shortening are directly determined by the isoform of MHC present in the muscle fiber.

The amount of force developed during isometric contraction is proportional to the concentration of calcium in the medium perfusing the fibers. Figure 13.4 shows pCa-tension curves, which are used to describe the sensitivity of the

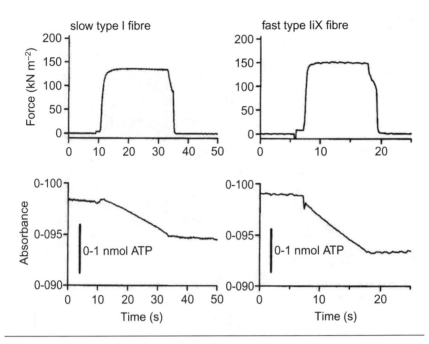

FIGURE 13.2   Experimental recordings of tension development and ATP consumption during isometric contractions of slow and fast fibers.

Adapted from Stienen, Kiers, Bottinelli, and Reggiani 1996.

TABLE 13.1   Average CSA, *Po, Ao,* and Tension Cost* in Single Human Fibers of Vastus Lateralis, Determined in Vitro at 20 °C

	CSA (μm²)	*Po* (mN/mm²)	*Ao* (mM ATP/s)	*Po / Ao*
Type I fibers	9278	114	0.10	0.87
Type IIA fibers	7922	136	0.27	1.98
Type IIX fibers	6294	171	0.41	2.39

* = *Po / Ao* is measured in pmol/mN·mm·s

Data from Stienen et al., 1996.

contractile system to the calcium (Ca). Differences both in slope (less steep in type I than in type II) and in position along the abscissa are visible.

The isoforms of regulatory proteins (tropomyosin and troponin C, T, and I) in the fiber determine the slope and the position of the pCa-tension curve (Schachat, Bronson & McDonald, 1985; Danieli Betto, Betto & Midrio, 1990; Bottinelli, Coviello, Redwood, Pellegrino, Maron, Spirito, Watkins & Reggiani, 1998).

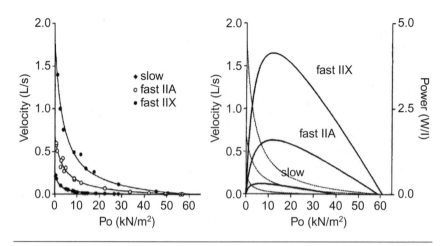

FIGURE 13.3   Force-velocity and power-velocity curves of the three main types of fiber in human muscles, determined in vitro at 12 °C.
Adapted from Stienen et al. 1996.

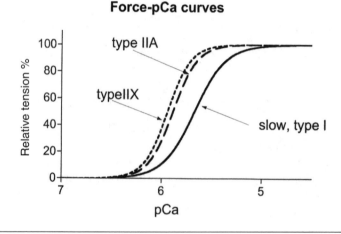

FIGURE 13.4   Tension versus pCa for the three main types of fiber in human muscles, determined in vitro.

Heterogeneity of Electrophysiological Properties and Excitation–Contraction Coupling in Human Muscle Fibers

The speed of the contractile cycle is markedly different among fibers and motor units, and this difference (and not the diversity in maximum shortening velocity) gives origin to the notion of slow and fast motor units. The time required to reach peak tension shown in panel A of figure 13.1 varies from 20 to 80 ms in human biceps brachii. The contractile speed directly relates to the major calcium-regulating membrane system, the sarcoplasmic reticulum. In fast fibers, calcium is released faster and in larger amounts and is also taken up more efficiently. Direct evidence that calcium transients differ in slow and fast fibers comes from studies on animal muscle fibers conducted with fluorescent indicators (Eusebi, Miledi & Takahashi, 1980; Fryer & Neering, 1989). Although similar evidence is not available for human muscle fibers, experiments with voltage clamps on cut fibers show a larger and faster calcium transient in fast fibers (Delbono, O'Rourke & Ettinger, 1995). The molecular basis of the diversity lies firstly in the fractional volume of the sarcoplasmic reticulum. An inverse relation between the volume of the terminal cisternae and the time required to reach peak tension has been shown by Kugelberg and Thornell (1983). Two isoforms of the calcium pump are present: the SERCA1 typical of fast fibers and the SERCA2 typical of slow fibers (Lytton, Westlin, Burk, Shull & MacLennan, 1992). The density of the calcium pump is higher in fast fibers than in slow fibers (Everts, Andersen, Clausen & Hansen, 1989), and differences in density are also present between fast IIX and fast IIA fibers (Salviati, Betto, Danieli Betto & Zeviani, 1984).

In relation to the different speed of the contractile cycle and the resistance to fatigue, the discharge rate of the motor neurons is much higher in fast motor units than in slow motor units. Continuous recordings of motor units show that slow motor units are active for longer times at low frequency whereas fast motor units are active in bursts of short duration at higher frequency (Monster, Chan & O'Connor, 1978; Hennig & Lomo, 1985, in rat muscles). Thus, in addition to the other aspects of heterogeneity in the contractile response described in the previous sections, muscle fibers are different in their excitability and ability to follow the rate of motor neuron discharge. The functional demands the rates of motor neuron discharge place on the membrane properties of muscle fibers are very different. Slow fibers must be able to generate action potentials during prolonged firing at a low rate without losing their excitability despite the accumulation of potassium in the extracellular space and particularly in the T-tubules. In contrast, fast fibers (especially IIX fibers) need to quickly recover excitability after each action potential, but they do not need to maintain excitability for long times, as discharge in fast motor units occurs in short bursts of high frequency (Henneman, Clamann, Gillies & Skinner, 1974; Monster, Chan & O'Connor, 1978; Bawa, Binder, Ruenzel & Henneman, 1984).

In human muscles the resting potential does not show significant differences between the two fast types of fiber, but it is less negative in slow fibers (Ruff 1996; Ruff & Whittlesey 1992, 1993a). The membrane capacitance and resistance per unit area seem similar in both fast and slow fibers (Ruff & Whittlesey, 1992). Whereas in neurons the ionic conductance across the membrane is dominated by potassium, in muscle fibers 70% of the membrane conductance is due to chloride (Bretag, 1987) and only 30% is due to potassium. There are at least two isoforms of chloride channels expressed in muscles: the voltage-gated chloride channel (ClC1), which is muscle specific and important for fiber repolarization after action potential, and the ubiquitous ClC2 (Pusch & Jentsch, 1994). There is no available evidence of heterogeneous expression of chloride channels in different fiber types.

Sodium (Na) channels also play a central role in determining the excitability of muscle fibers. Excitability of the membrane is determined by the number of Na channels and the fraction of inactivated channels. The density of Na channels is greater in fast fibers than in slow fibers in humans (Ruff & Whittlesey, 1992) and in other mammals (Caldwell, Campbell & Beam, 1986). In each fiber, the density of the Na current is higher at the border of the end plate than away from the plate (Ruff & Whittlesey, 1993b), thus ensuring that an action potential is triggered every time the release of acetylcholine produces an end plate potential. This decrease in Na current that occurs away from the end plate is reported as being much lower in slow fibers than in fast fibers (Ruff & Whittlesey, 1992). Even though no local differences (close and away from the end plate) have been found in the voltage dependence of the activation and inactivation processes (Ruff, 1996), there are differences in the inactivation processes between slow and fast fibers (Ruff & Whittlesey, 1993a). These differences may be relevant for keeping fiber excitability during repetitive firing.

Metabolic Heterogeneity of Human Muscle Fibers

One of the most notable diversities among single muscle fibers deals with fatigue resistance. Motor units are divided between being fatigable and fatigue resistant, and this property depends on the characteristics of the muscle fiber. Muscle fatigue can be defined as a decrease in force development that follows repeated contractions. The decrease in force is determined by the accumulation of by-products from the chemical energy supply, such as inorganic phosphate, lactate, and hydrogen ions (for a review see Westerblad, Allen, Bruton, Andrade & Lannergren, 1998).

The energy necessary for contractile activity is provided by the hydrolysis of ATP to ADP and Pi. ADP is then resynthesized to ATP from PCr through the creatine kinase reaction. PCr is the molecular form of stored chemical energy and is produced from creatine and ATP. ATP in turn is synthesized from gly-colytic processes in the sarcoplasma and from oxidative phosphorylation in the mitochondria. Glycolytic processes are the initial stages of glycogen and glucose metabolism, and they lead to pyruvate or lactate production. Pyruvate, fatty acids, and ketone bodies provide a supply of acetyl-CoA, which is the substrate for the mitochondrial oxidative processes. During contractile activity, lactate, Pi, and hydrogen ions may accumulate in muscle fibers and trigger the decrease in contractile performance called fatigue.

Muscle fibers can better resist fatigue if they can promptly resynthesize ATP and if they can avoid lactate accumulation with a fast catabolism of pyruvate to lactate and then to water and carbon dioxide through mitochondrial oxidative processes. In simplified terms, resistance to fatigue is associated with active mitochondrial energy production.

The metabolic heterogeneity of muscle fibers was first observed with the histochemical determination in muscle cryosections of the enzymatic activities of glycolytic (LDH) and mitochondrial oxidative (SDH, COX, NADH) processes (Ogata & Mori, 1964; Padykula & Gauthier, 1967). In the muscles of small mammals, three fiber types were classified: S, or slow-twitch oxidative; FOG, or fast-twitch oxidative-glycolytic (S and FOG are both based on enzymatic activities of oxidizing aerobic substrates); and FG, or fast-twitch glycolytic (Barnard, Edgerton, Furukava & Peter, 1971; Peter, Barnard, Edgerton, Gillespie & Stempel, 1972). In combining the stimulation of a single motor unit with the histochemical analysis of enzymatic activity, it was found that

1. the fibers belonging to the same motor unit have identical metabolic properties, and

2. the enzymatic properties of the fibers can be correlated with resistance to fatigue, in that slow motor units with fatigue resistance are composed of SO fibers while fast motor units that have fatigue resistance or that are fatigable are composed of FOG and FG fibers, respectively (Burke, Levine & Zajac, 1971; Burke, Levine, Tsairis & Zajac, 1973; Kugelberg, 1973; Nemeth, Pette & Vrbova, 1981).

Some studies, however, show variability even within a motor unit, and the gradients relate to the position of the fiber within the muscle (Kugelberg & Lindgren, 1979; Larsson, 1992). On the other hand, the variability of enzymatic properties along the length of individual muscle fibers seems to be small (Pette, Wimmer & Nemeth, 1981).

Microchemical methods allow the determination of substrate concentrations and enzyme activities in single muscle fibers (Essen, Jansson, Henriksson, Taylor & Saltin, 1975; Lowry, Kimmey, Felder, Chi, Kaiser, Passoneau, Kirk & Lowry, 1978; Reichmann & Pette 1982). The distribution of the enzymatic activities determined in single fibers shows broad ranges of variation, in which some peaks corresponding to groups of fibers with comparable activities are detectable (Reichmann & Pette, 1982) (see panel B in figure 13.1). Determining more than one enzymatic activity in the same fiber reveals direct correlations among enzymatic activities of the same pathways and inverse correlations between glycolytic and aerobic-oxidative enzymatic activities (see figure 13.5) (Rosser & Hochamba, 1993).

The picture emerging from enzymatic determination in single human muscle fibers shows that the anaerobic power, or the rate of ATP generation through the glycolytic pathway, is 50% to 90% of the total power generated (anaerobic

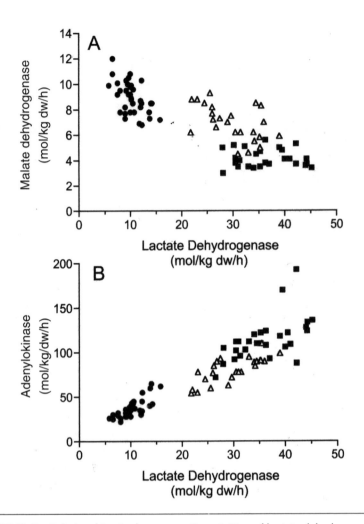

FIGURE 13.5 Relationships in the enzymatic activities of lactate dehydrogenase, malate dehydrogenase, and adenylokinase in individual human muscle fibers. In each fiber the enzyme activities were determined and the fiber was classified as type I (filled circles), fast IIA (empty triangles), and fast IIX (filled squares). Note the diversity among fiber types and the large variability inside each type.
Adapted from Bottinelli and Reggiani 2000.

+ aerobic). The rate of aerobic-oxidative ATP production in the mitochondria is about 30% higher in slow fibers than in fast fibers (Essen et al., 1975; Lowry et al., 1978), whereas the rate of the anaerobic-glycolytic pathway is much faster (5-10 times) in fast fibers than in slow fibers (Greenhaff, Soderlund, Ren & Hultman, 1993). The difference becomes relevant when compared with ATP consumption during contraction. In slow fibers the rate of ATP consumption (by myosin and ionic pumps) during contraction is estimated to be around 6 mmol/kg/s, and this rate can be completely accounted for by ATP regeneration through aerobic-oxidative processes. In contrast, the rate of ATP consumption in fast fibers during maximal contraction is much higher (18-27 mmol/kg/s), and it cannot be covered by the total metabolic (aerobic + anaerobic) power of the fiber. This observation helps explain why slow but not fast fibers can cope with prolonged and repeated contractile activity without undergoing fatigue (for further discussion see Sahlin, Tonkonogi & Soderlund, 1998; Bottinelli & Reggiani, 2000).

Plasticity of Human Skeletal Muscles

The picture of heterogeneity in muscle fibers that emerges from the previous sections implies two questions deserving answers: how interfiber diversity is generated and maintained and what advantage is given to muscles by the interfiber diversity.

The fiber composition of a given muscle can change significantly under the influence of physiological and pathological factors. This changeability is referred to as muscle plasticity. It appears that muscle plasticity and diversity allow the muscle to respond to a wide range of mechanical demands. Factors that have been found to determine or regulate muscle plasticity include mechanical demands, neural activities, hormonal outputs, and pathological conditions such as diabetes and muscular diseases (Heene, 1975).

Optimization of Muscle Performance by Selective Recruitment

The diversity in muscle fibers can be best exploited if motor neurons can select which muscle fibers are convenient to activate for a given motor task. Fast and slow, weak and strong, and fatigable and fatigue-resistant fibers are available in each muscle, and the most suitable for a given task can be recruited. According to Henneman's size principle (Henneman et al., 1974; Bawa et al., 1984), motor units are recruited in a stereotypical way: those that are slow and fatigue resistant (S) are recruited for movements that require low speed and force (standing and walking), those that are fatigue resistant (FR) are recruited for movements requiring higher speed and force (running), and those that are fast and fatiguing (FF) are recruited only for the fastest and strongest movements (jumping). As S motor units are the least fatigable and the weakest and FF units are the most fatigable and the strongest, the size principle has long been considered a way for smoothly accumulating force during contraction and for optimizing fatigue. Interestingly, as S motor units are made of type I fibers, FR motor units of type IIA fibers, and FF motor units of type IIX fibers, recruiting according to the size principle also optimizes power and efficiency.

Whether or not the size principle holds in all conditions, and especially in humans, is largely debated (Desmedt & Godaux, 1977; Kanda, Burke & Walmsley,1977; Thomas, Schmidt & Hambrecht, 1978; Nardone, Romano & Schieppati, 1989). Significant modifications in the size principle have been suggested. The idea that motor units can be organized into groups recruited in order during a motor task, that is, into task groups, has been introduced (Chanaud, Pratt & Loeb, 1991). It has also been suggested that a task group does not necessarily correspond to a muscle but can dynamically change for subtle changes in the motor task and can even span different muscles in the same group (Calancie & Bawa, 1990; Cope & Pinter, 1995). Task groups can account for the observation that in some cases within a muscle FR or FF motor units can be recruited and small S motor units can remain silent. The size principle holds that motor units are recruited in the order of S > FR > FF within a defined task group if not within a muscle. Finally, real exceptions to the size principle not accounted for by the existence of task groups have been shown during eccentric contractions (Nardone et al., 1989).

Conclusions

The muscle fibers of human skeletal muscle are very heterogeneous in their functional properties and molecular structures. This heterogeneity can be detected in all aspects of muscle contractile activity and is aimed to optimize motor performance and minimize fatigue. Mechanisms for motor control inside the nervous system learn how to best exploit the diversity in muscles and motor units. Differences in fiber composition of muscles, differences in motor unit composition of muscles, as well as the ability of the nervous system to optimally organize the activation of fibers and motor units will then determine the interindividual diversity in muscle performance.

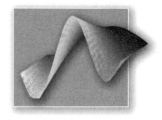

Chapter 14

Self-Organizing Brain Dynamics and Movement Goals

Walter J. Freeman, MD

Editors' Overview

This chapter emphasizes the dominant role played by self-organizing dynamics in the brain that conceives goals as images of future possibilities and directs actions of the body to realize those goals. In order to achieve this, the brain must situate itself and its body in space and time through the action-perception-assimilation cycle. That cycle implements and embodies the process of intentionality by which the brain predicts the sensory consequences of its own actions and learns from them. The philosophical lineage of this concept can be traced through 2,500 y of theorizing to Tomaso d'Aquino's conception of intentionality as a process deeply embedded in and controlling the brain and body in relation to the environment. The main focus of the chapter is on internally constructed brain dynamics. In more recent years, intelligence has been biologized and distanced from that which is conceptualized for logical machines. Actions are viewed as embedded in cycles of intention, action, perception, and assimilation by which the finite brain explores the infinite world. By acting, the brain thrusts its body into the future space-time of the world while predicting the sensory consequences. By perceiving its actions and their results, remembering them, and comparing them with its predictions and goals, the brain learns how to act effectively in future environments. The embodied brain alters itself by changing its synaptic connections. The internal goal states and their sensory and motor implementations are constructed through chaotic dynamics. This construction introduces intrinsic variability into all movements. The loop is completed to show how the embedded brain, aided by its plasticity, acts to shape individual differences in processes such as perception and action.

This work was supported by grant MH06686 from the National Institute of Mental Health. An earlier version of this chapter was published as "Perception of time and causation through the kinesthesia of intentional action" in *Cognitive Processing* (Freeman, 2000b).

A widespread practice in the study of brains and in writing textbooks about them is to divide their main functions into sensory, motor, and associational, cognitive, or higher. Textbooks then describe these mechanisms by starting with sensation and quickly exiting into reflex movements of the spine and brain stem with perhaps a nod to the motor cortex and cerebellum, while leaving higher functions including voluntary movements to the last chapters. Yet by operational definition, reflexes are stereotypic patterns of movement with very low variance and with little or no contribution from the forebrain, while much greater variability is encountered in the performance of voluntary actions that do involve the forebrain. Attempts to describe voluntary actions in terms of a hierarchy of reflexes have not met with success. My aim in this chapter is to take a new approach by beginning in the middle. The observable fact is that most movements made by animals and humans are directed toward achieving future states, the definitions for which are primarily formed within their brains. The movements are clearly constrained by the innate capacities and properties of the animal and human bodies and by the environments in which the bodies are physically located and exercised, but the structures of the movements over time clearly indicate the shaping of the move-ments toward ends that have been created within the brains and bodies. In the 17th century, Thomas Hobbes (1651) adapted the word *voluntary* into English from the Thomist Latin *volere* in order to distinguish reflexes and the actions deriving from the will. Volition was unequivocally assigned to the cerebrum by a then eminent neuroanatomist who left his name on the circle of arteries at the base of the brain, Sir Thomas Willis (1664, 1683). The commonly used *voluntary* does little to address the mechanisms by which goals are created within brains, and indeed the term was coined in a religious context when the growth of scientific and engineering knowledge about machines made it necessary to distinguish between machinelike deterministic behaviors (reflexes from Newtonian reflections) and those engendered by the Cartesian soul.

The derivation of a fresh approach can be undertaken by looking back in time 2,500 y or more to philosophical debates about the core cognitive process of perception, of whether it follows directly from sensation or is a consequence of motor action. I propose that this question has a biological answer. The critical debates about the nature of observation took place in ancient Greece among the followers of Plato and Aristotle. Platonic doctrine held that percep-tion is passive and that the world exists as a collection of imperfect copies of ideal forms. The task of the senses is to collect impressions of the forms from examples, and the work of the intellect in the brain is to deduce the ideals. Plato taught this scheme with the metaphor of a cave. Sunlight on the ideal objects cast shadows on the walls, and the senses imprinted these shadows into the eyes and brain as the basis for reasoning by the soul. Aristotelians held that perception is active. The observer acts in the world transitively by probing, cutting, and burning to acquire the forms of objects and intransitively to comprehend the nature of the forms by logic and induction—these are the processes of abstraction and generalization. Accordingly, the actively moving heart was the seat of comprehension instead of the motionless brain, which served merely to cool the hot blood.

The Platonic view dominates in modern times. Descartes succeeded in establishing mathematics as the foundation of neuroscience but failed to biologize brain dynamics. He conceived that the soul, residing in the body like a pilot in a boat, takes charge of the bodily machine by controlling the flow of nerve spirits from the brain through the nerves into the muscles, inflating the muscles to make them contract. Physiologists in Italy and the Netherlands quickly showed that muscles do not increase in volume when they shorten in length and that the ends of cut nerves do not give off bubbles of nerve spirit when they are stimulated. Willis swept the problem under the rug by adopting the term *voluntary* to cover for the soul. Kant (1781) then revolutionized Platonic doctrine by postulating that the ideal forms are not in the world but are in the human mind and that the world is only indirectly accessed through the impressions that objects make on the senses, from which the intellect constructs representations of the objects by making comparisons with its storage of forms. These forms and comparisons are all that the observer can know; the observer cannot know the *Ding-an-sich,* or the world in itself.

Cartesian-Kantian doctrine flourishes today in cognitive science because representationalism is at the heart of the logical machines—the computers—that serve for many people as the instantiation of true intelligence and the early harbinger of the coming termination of the age of trans-biological dominance. In this passive view, time is represented in our minds by the image of segments forming a straight line. The line is broken into the steps of binary digits and is measured by the basic cycle of a central processing unit (CPU). The components in our bodies and brains that correspond to the CPU are the biological clocks that imperfectly and unreliably give us the time of day or the season of the year and that express their output in volleys of action potentials, which neurobiologists refer to as *units* when observing them with microelectrodes inserted into brains. Space is represented by a cognitive map in the hippocampus of the medial temporal lobe, and locations are thought to be read out by the place cells' discharges that signify to an animal its location in the map.

Aristotelian doctrine evolved independently and in parallel to the Platonic view. It was resurrected from Arabic translations and transformed in the 13th century by Tomaso d'Aquino (1272), whose mission was to make it compatible with the Christian concept of free will. He did this by distinguishing between his concept of the human will and the Aristotelian concept of intention as biological destiny, which Tomaso believed humans shared with other animals. The key concept in his approach to the biology of humans was the unity of the individual, which maintained around itself an impenetrable boundary. In modern times we can compare this boundary to the digestive system, which breaks down consumed substances before they are admitted into the body as elementary chemicals, and to the immune system, which rejects from the body any substance that has a structure differing from that of the self. The sense organs also break down forms of objects into patterns of action potentials on the two-dimensional sheets of receptors in the nose, eyes, and skin. To the extent that the neural pathways carrying the action potentials into the brain have a topographic order between receptors and cortex, there is a persistence of spatial as well as temporal information about sensory stimuli in these transmissions, but the action potentials are not copies of the inputs.

Tomaso conceived of sensation in similar terms as the effect on the sense organs of material events that are unique in their ultimate details and therefore not knowable, anticipating Kant's *Ding-an-sich*. Unlike Kant he did not postulate preexisting eternal forms, but he instead transcended Aristotle by conceiving of the imagination, by which the mind creates forms with abstraction and generalization over the unique, transient, and unknowable minutiae of sensory events. In a bold move, he conceived that intentionality is a process by which the self thrusts its body into the world and through taking action gives itself the basis for learning about the world. It learns by changing its body structure, the relationship of the body to the world, and (we now believe) its internal neural connectivity to assimilate to the world, thereby coming to know the world. No forms (we now say *information*) cross the boundary of the self. Instead, the self creates expectations that are hypotheses about the world and tests them by action in the world. All that brains can know are the forms of the hypotheses and the results of the tests.

This idea in microcosm describes the scientific method in modern times. Thomist doctrine survives as a relic in surgery, where wound healing is said to be by first intention leaving a clean scar or by second intention using the copious flow of pus. This usage captures the original biological nature of intentionality as the maintenance and elaboration of the unity and wholeness of the self, in contrast to the cognitive view of central images, thoughts, and beliefs that represent in the brain (or computer) objects and events in the world and also in contrast to the psychology view of intent of future action that is instigated and guided by purposes and motives.

Where physiology has failed to keep up with philosophy is in dealing with the imagination, by which future states are created in brains and expressed as goals to be pursued by intentional actions. In the past two decades the necessary theory and analytical tools for understanding brain dynamics have been made available through developments in the field of nonlinear dynamics. This chapter introduces some elementary conceptions in both neuroscience and neurodynamics for organizing a program of research into the structures and variances of goal-directed intentional behaviors. In terms of dynamics, these behaviors are best understood as patterns of movements in time and space that require an underlying concept of the biological basis for apprehending space and time. The most important feature of the patterns of central neural activity is the chaotic dynamics by which the patterns form. Chaos has the capacity to create information. The information that sensory cortices create in response to stimuli replaces the information brought by the senses.

Limbic Contributions to Intentional Action

Biological intelligence emerged and evolved in the context of brutal warfare: Eat or be eaten. Living in a rich organic stew, our ancestors moved in search of molecules that were sloughed off by predators and prey. The ability to move gave animals a competitive advantage over plants, but the advantage came at a price. In order to track a sequence of molecules toward a potential source of food or away from a dangerous sink in some other maw, an animal had to navigate in space and time and to predict the directions, distances, and travel times from its present site to significant future locations. These neural capacities are apparent in the organization of even the simplest vertebrate forebrain (Herrick, 1948), that of the tiger salamander (figure 14.1). Each of the two hemispheres consists of an anterior third devoted to sensation, mostly olfactory, a lateral third devoted to motor functions, and a medial third devoted to the capacities that are required for the spatiotemporal guidance of movements. This medial third is the recognizable forerunner of the hippocampus, which in vertebrates ranging through reptiles and mammals to humans is essential for forming memories and remembering places, that is, for temporal orientation, and for orientation of action in space. O'Keefe and Nadel (1978) designated this capacity as a cognitive map, after the concept developed by Tolman (1948), though Hendriks-Jansen (1996) and others have concluded that this process of orientation does not depend on a table or chart, so the term is metaphorical. These authors propose that animals (and robots) do not literally have maps in their heads but instead have the capacity to flexibly and site-specifically direct their behavior in space-time.

The simplest living example, found in salamanders (see figure 14.1), reveals three essential components: the sensory cortex, including the olfactory bulb

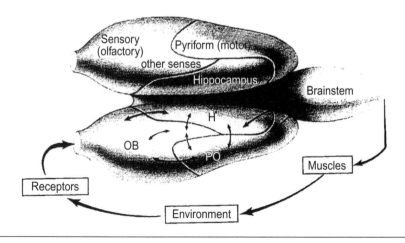

FIGURE 14.1   The forebrain is the organizing focus of intentionality in vertebrates.

(OB); the motor cortex, including the pyriform cortex (PC); and the association cortex, labeled here as the hippocampus (H), which is symmetrical in the two hemispheres. The arrows indicate that transmissions between parts go in both directions. The basic architecture of these parts endures through the evolution of brains in mammals and humans as the limbic system. In most vertebrate brains the limbic system is dominated by olfaction, but in human brains the limbic system is overgrown in the way an ancient town is transformed by its modern suburbs without losing its core role and street plan. The limbic system is like the downtown center of a city; the neocortical add-ons in mammals are like vast suburbs that can and do cooperate directly but that cannot function adequately without the hub.

Olfaction is an excellent paradigm for the study of intelligence, partly because the elements are so clear and partly because the sense of smell was the first to achieve sophistication, becoming both the final arbiter of success in finding food and the prototype for perception through the other senses. The environment in which it functions is an infinitely complex mix of chemicals. Very few molecules in the mix lead to edible substances, and those few are subject to aging, chemical combinations with other substances, and the vagaries of odor masking. The olfactory receptors in the nose are extremely numerous and exquisitely sensitive in order to capture odorant molecules. Each receptor is broadly tuned to an indefinite range of substances, as the receptors must be in order to deal with the incredible richness of the olfactory environment (Freeman, 2001), but each receptor is usually tuned to a narrow range of concentration of each odorant. A single odorant sample excites a selection of receptors that forms a spatial pattern of neural activity in the lining of the nose. That pattern is transmitted by axons into the cerebrum, where it is registered as another spatial pattern of activity by the microscopic neurons that are driven by the afferent volley. The sensory patterns on successive sniffs are never the same, because turbulence in the nose randomly distributes odorant molecules. This exemplifies the Thomist concept of the unknowability of individual sensory events. Neural mechanisms are required in the brain for abstraction and generalization for identifying odors from such evanescent and nonreproducible bursts of action potentials.

Neural mechanisms are provided by the cortex, including the olfactory bulb in the case of odorant stimuli. The spatial pattern of cortical neural activity driven by receptor input is the end of sensation and the beginning of perception. What happens is that the afferent volley of microscopic action potentials from the receptors destabilizes the sensory area of the cortex into which it is injected, and the cortex transits from a basal receiving state of expectancy to a self-organized transmitting state (Freeman, 1991, 1995). This new state leads to a novel pattern of activity that is generated by the entire sensory area. Whether or not the individual cortical neurons fire, all of them participate, because patterns require both high and low intensities of activity. This pattern, being mesoscopic (Freeman, 2000a), has the properties of a mean field that the neurons contribute to and are regulated by. The form of the spatial pattern depends on the intracortical synaptic connections, which have been shaped through learning from past experience.

The olfactory area can only generate spatial patterns from connections that were modified during an experience with a limited number of odorants. Each mean field is a construction of the cortex that is simultaneously transmitted to both the motor area of the cortex and the hippocampal formation along with the sensory-driven activity pattern. However, owing to the way in which the cortical pathways are organized, it is the mean field that is effectively received by target areas, while the sensory-driven activity pattern that triggered the transition in the cortical state is attenuated by transmission through the output pathway of the cortex (Freeman, 2000a). This pathway, the lateral olfactory tract, is not topographically organized. It is a divergent-convergent projection in which each transmitting neuron broadcasts its pulses and each receiving neuron picks up pulses from widely distributed transmitting neurons. The pathway operates to perform a spatial integral transformation on the bulbar output, which selects for the spatially coherent signal created by the bulb and smoothes the sensory-driven action potentials that lack spatial coherence.

The reason the brain works this way is that the environment is far too complex to be defined as a finite collection of images or representations. Kant was correct in surmising that a human or other animal cannot know the world as it truly is, owing to the infinity of particles of matter and the still greater infinity of ways these particles can be assembled. But Kant was wrong in supposing that in the brain there are ideal odorant representations that are primary forms from which complex odors are made, as colors are made from red, green, and blue. Odorant receptors have been shown by genetic engineering to number in excess of 1,000, which is too great to serve as a meaningful alphabet. Brains can only know what they have learned to hypothesize, including the results of their behavioral testing. These hypotheses are modified and refined through experience (Freeman, 1995).

Neurodynamics of Chaos in Perception

Odorant identification provides an instructive example of the way humans generalize from particulars. The mesoscopic cortical pattern triggered by sensory input is transmitted to other parts of the brain, whereas the microscopic sense data are not. This constitutes a necessary adaptation of finite biological intelligence to an infinite world through selectively transmitting only the essential finding of the hypothesis testing. Recordings of the patterns of mean-field activity of the other sensory areas, including the visual, auditory, and somatosensory cortices, support this principle (Freeman and Barrie, 1994; Barrie, Freeman and Lenhart, 1996; Ohl, Scheich and Freeman, 2001). Further evidence is found in the counterintuitive fact that the human brain is in the head. Because it has a mass of 1.5 kg, it would have far better protection in the chest than when attached by a slender stalk to the top of the body. The explanation is that the sensory receptors for events at a distance are located in the head. These receptors are exceedingly numerous. The retina, actually an integral part of the brain, has about 100 million. The 100 million chemical receptors in each nostril send their axons directly into the brain. The axons from these receptors are very small in diameter in order to provide for dense packing, and since length is proportional to diameter, they must be short. In the retina, the great reduction in the number of axons occurs in the strong convergence of rods and cones into ganglion cells from 10^8 down to 10^6. Olfactory receptor axons converge to mitral cells from 10^8 down to 10^5 in the olfactory bulb. These high convergence ratios imply a massive loss of information early in sensory processing.

In both cases the immense number of receptors is necessary to capture the photons and molecules that come from locations far removed from the body. The capture results in the formation of exceedingly complex spatial patterns of excitation in the arrays of receptors. This complexity owing to enormous information content does not apply to further transmissions, because the main task of the cortex is to reduce the information load by abstraction and generalization. Thus it sends messages only about classes and not about unique events, as messages on classes need far fewer transmitting neurons. Each sensory area broadcasts its abstracted output to many other parts of the forebrain. The divergence implies that selectivity in information transfer is achieved by the tuning of the receivers rather than the transmitters. Such broadcasting is facilitated if all transmitters and receivers are located in relative proximity, which is achieved by the topological organization of the forebrain, as is illustrated in figure 14.1.

Why are the eyes, nose, and ears in the head and not in the chest? The answer is obvious; these sense organs are directed in space at the front end of the animal so that they are optimally oriented toward desired targets during looking, sniffing, and listening. These activities can be performed more flexibly and efficiently when the organs are placed in the head instead of in the body. These three senses differ from other senses such as touch, taste, and muscle sense in that light waves, sound waves, and chemicals carried by convection currents in the air and water come from locations far from the body. They provide early warnings of the locations of prey and predators, which give the brain time to receive stimuli, identify and classify them, determine their meanings and locations in space, and devise suitable plans of action. Within the blanket of space-time surrounding our bodies that is provided by the distance receptors, it is the power of prediction that has fueled the intellectual arms race and paced the evolution of biological intelligence.

Conjoining of Time and Space Through Action

Action under guidance by odors is complicated by the fact that the odorant molecules carry no information about the spatial locations of their origins. The location can only be formed in the brain of the pursuer in the following way. A hungry animal captures the scent of food, creates the element of an olfactory percept, and holds it momentarily. It moves, creates a second sample, and determines whether the second is stronger or weaker than the first. This difference has no meaning unless the animal retains knowledge of where it was on taking the first sample and where it moved to for taking the next, because those two locations direct which way to go next. Knowledge of place depends on combining visual and auditory percepts with those from the olfactory system and also from the somatosensory cortex that provides proprioceptive input concerning what movements the body has made in the interim between samples. These contributions from all sensory systems are combined into a multisensory pattern before they are delivered into the hippocampus. Here in the hippocampus integration takes place over elapsed time and over the accumulated experience (with spatial locations) that is manifested in so-called "place cells" (Wilson and McNaughton, 1993). Place cells fire selectively when animals occupy particular sites in their customary spatial fields of behavioral action. It is the hippocampus, or more accurately, the collection of neural structures that comprises the hippocampal formation in the medial temporal lobe, that is essential for constructing the space-time regulatory system that orients search movements through the environment. These requirements for space-time orientation for searching actions are met by systems that are commonly referred to metaphorically as a cognitive map and a short-term memory.

Yet deeper meaning lies in space-time orientation. Before each act of observation leading to perception, there emerges in this core neural complex a pattern of activity that establishes what sensory input an animal seeks, and why that input is needed. Perception is the process by which the brain uses the body to engage the environment and to assimilate itself in accordance with the sensory results of its own actions. This is the process that Tomaso described with his theory of intentionality. The pattern of neural activity that underlies intentional action is expressed in two ways. One is by actualizing a sequence of motor neuron firings that moves the muscles to carry the body into goal-directed behaviors. The other is by sending neural messages from the medial temporal cortex to all of the primary sensory areas. These messages, called "corollary discharges" by Roger Sperry (1950) and "reafference" by von Holst and Mittelstaedt (1950), prepare areas receiving sensory input for the consequences of the intended actions and, in particular, sensitize them for the construction of perceptual patterns should the expected stimuli turn out to be present. The process underlying purposive action is intention. The predictive process of "preafference" (Kay and Freeman, 1998) is observable in the behavioral state of attention, in which a person or other animal focuses the several sensory systems in the expectation that intended actions and their forthcoming stimuli will occur as time elapses.

Neither intention nor attention requires awareness of the actions or stimuli. On the contrary, most of our intentional behaviors unfold habitually and without awareness, and those most important to us occur in states of intense concentration, when the mind is so focused on the sequence at hand, whether in sport, military action, prayer, love, or creation of art, that awareness is deferred until the process has reached closure. When we do become aware of intention, we experience the outcome of the intent to act, the action, and the sensory consequences at the time the brain is updated to the current learning. It is this elementary sequence from an act of observation leading to perception that provides the basis for consciousness. Here is where our conception of causality enters. We experience our actions as causing sensory input. More specifically, we experience the preafferent intent to act and the ensuing constructions of the sensory cortices as cause and effect. Everything that we learn and know comes through hypothesis testing, which Merleau-Ponty (1945) described as achieving "maximum grip" through his "intentional arc," and which Jean Piaget (1930) described as "the cycle of action, assimilation, and adaptation" that we learn, as other animals do, in the sensorimotor stage of early development, long before we become adept in the use of language. Thelen and Smith (1994) have extensively developed these insights in the context of dynamic systems theory. Causality is very closely tied to our perception of time because it takes place through actions in the perceptual time and space of ourselves and others like ourselves.

Linear Causality Versus Circular Causality

The intentional cycle of intent, action, assimilation, and adaptation takes us to the center of the web of perceptual being, where we encounter the spider of causality (Freeman, 1995). The problem of understanding causality in the warp and woof of the material and spiritual worlds has concerned philosophers for millennia. Ineluctably, causality is bound to the concept of time in both of its usual meanings. On the one hand, *to cause* means to bring on an effect or to precipitate some state of affairs by acting as an agent. We refer to usage in the sense of acting as an agent as *linear causality*. The criterion by which we apply the term is the strict temporal order between the antecedent cause and the subsequent effect. No effect can precede a cause, but every cause is an effect of a preceding cause. In this way we build linear chains of cause and effect to describe processes we observe in ourselves and in the world. On the other hand, *to cause* means to explain an observed relationship without invoking an agent. We call this usage *circular causality*, and here we allow simultaneity in the bidirectional flow of influences, which are not merely very fast, but which transcend time and space and become nonlocal in being conjoint.

Linear causality is very congenial to humans in thinking about the world because it mirrors the intentional arc of Merleau-Ponty (1945): I act (cause), therefore I perceive (effect). An example is Piaget's somatomotor phase of development, in which we learn to experience ourselves as an agent and we extrapolate that agency not only to other people but to animals and objects in the world. The passive view of perception with its accompanying concept of the reflex is built with causal chains. A stimulus (the * in figure 14.2) carries information to a sensory receptor, causing a cascade of molecular events that transduces the stimulus and encodes the information the stimulus contains into a train of action potentials. The train triggers a series of relays through the spinal cord, thalamus, and cortex by which the information is processed into a passive representation of an object. The image of the object is transmitted to the frontal lobes, where it initiates identification, classification, and selection of the proper action. Then the causal chain of upper (cortical) and lower (spinal) motor neurons and muscles effects the action, which becomes the cause of proprioceptive feedback through other causal chains. By repeated extrapolation, the entire life of an animal and its brain can be modeled, in principle, by deterministic causal chains.

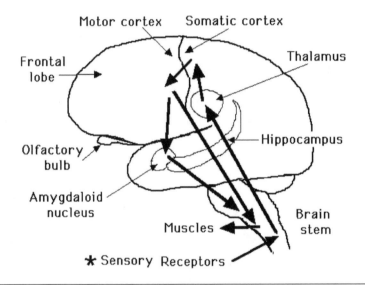

FIGURE 14.2   The view of perception shared by materialists and cognitive scientists is that of perception as a passive process.

Perception begins when a stimulus gives information that is transduced by sensory receptors into a burst of neural activity that cascades through the brain stem and thalamus into a sensory cortex, here somatic receptors transmitting to the somatic cortex. The * marks where passive perception starts. In the somatic cortex, information processing binds the activity of detector neurons into the representation of an object. The representation is either stored in a local network of neurons or is retained and compared with other representations of previous stimuli that were stored and are now retrieved. The best match is sent by stages to the frontal lobes, where an appropriate response is selected. The motor cortex sends a command through the brain stem and spinal cord to the muscles. There are several noteworthy side loops. One upward loop, through the reticular formation in the brain stem and thalamus, produces arousal and selective attention. Another loop through the cerebellum fine-tunes behavior. One of the downward loops is through the amygdala, which provides emotional tones from its repertoire of fixed patterns of action and its controls on the secretion of emotionally specific neurohormones in the brain stem.

Circular causality is foreign to humans to the point of mystification. Yet the active view of perception is drenched in it. The first place that circular causality appears is in the genesis of an intentional state in the core structures of the forebrain (the * in figure 14.3). In the forebrain, the interaction of a myriad of neurons grouped into populations leads to a global transition that is expressed in a large-scale pattern of neural activity. The circularity is apparent in the fact that the neurons create the global pattern while at the same time the pattern constrains and shapes the activities of the individual neurons. There is no way that the actions among the individual neurons can be reduced to linear chains. We see circular causality when the volley of action potentials following a stimulus destabilizes a sensory cortex and triggers a state transition leading to a mesoscopic, mean-field pattern of activity. These kinds of phase transitions have been observed in many physical systems and have been explained and modeled by physicists in terms of microscopic and macroscopic relationships ever since the 19th century, when Ludwig Boltzmann created the science of statistical mechanics by conjoining the theory of molecules and classical thermodynamics. Hermann Haken (1983) developed the field in synergetics by

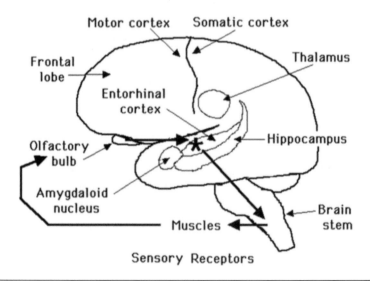

FIGURE 14.3   Pragmatists view perception as an active process.

using the state transition in lasers as his touchstone and applying the resulting theory of nonlinear dynamics and chaos to brain function.

In figure 14.3, the * marks the site of the initiation of active perception. Humans and other animals maintain a stance of attention and expectation, which embodies an expectation formed by intentional dynamics in the limbic system. This expectation is transmitted by corollary discharge to all the sensory cortices. The arrival of stimuli confirms or denies the hypothesis. The expectation is tested by state transitions giving patterns of amplitude modulation (AM) that converge into the limbic system (into the entorhinal cortex in mammals). A new expectation forms that presages one of a range of possible actions, each with its corollary discharge. The crucible of intention is in the limbic system, not in the thalamus or frontal lobe, because the hippocampus provides the neural machinery for directing intentional action through space and time. Every sensory module must be able to organize its patterns of meaning in space and time. Either it must have its own space-time register or it must share one space-time register after fusion of the multimodal patterns. The parsimonious solution of evolution does not preclude direct exchanges between sensory modules, but it indicates the unique importance of the multisensory convergence into the entorhinal cortex.

The laser was also used by Cartwright (1989) to exemplify levels of causality. She contrasted simple, direct relations of cause and effect that had no significant interactions or second-order perturbations with higher-order capacities. According to her, these capacities closely relate to Mill's (1843) tendencies, but differ by "material abstraction" (p. 226). By virtue of abstraction, the capacities have an enlarged scope of forward action but lack the circular relation between microscopic and macroscopic entities that is essential for explaining lasers—and brains. By further extrapolation, the entire intentional cycle can be seen to exemplify circular causality, because the emergence of a goal thrusts the organism's past into its future and entangles both into an intelligible whole. The action is an expression of what an animal has learned as much as of what it desires, and the perception is an actualization of patterns that were already created within the sensory areas in cooperation with the core areas.

The entanglement of time and causality becomes obvious when we take a closer look at how neurobiologists derive proof of linear causal chains by observing and measuring stimulus-response (SR) relationships in an animal. The demonstration of the invariance of the relation between cause and effect must be based on repeated trials (figure 14.4). On each trial the observers must segment the infinite time line of reality and reset the observer time to zero. Neurobiologists assume that the conditions of the experiment remain constant across trials, or they make corrections for fatigue, satiety, boredom, distractions, and cumulative learning. They collect multiple SR pairs and assemble them by aligning the zero points in a spatial display. The double dot indicates a point in real time, which irretrievably disappears from observer time.

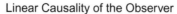

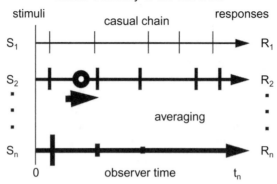

FIGURE 14.4   Linear causality.

Reprinted, by permission, from W.J. Freeman, 1999, "Reclaiming cognition," *Journal of Consciousness Studies* 6(11-12): 144-145.

Linear causality is the view that events are connected by causal chains. As seen in figure 14.4, the observer must create an artificial time, here labeled as observer time, t_n, to summarize the average of the sequence of responses to repeated stimuli over real time in which the individual events, S_1, R_1, and so on, were collected. The encircled dot represents an instant in real time. The weaknesses of this view lie in constructing explanations for assigning points in time to the beginning and end of each chain as well as to intervening events in the chain in strict order and for repeatedly observing in varying circumstances in order to connect pairs of classes of events. As Davidson (1980) remarked, events have causes; classes have relations. In the example, stimulus-dependent events such as evoked potentials are analyzed by time ensemble averaging, which degrades unsynchronized events and leads to further attempts to segment the successive peaks, thus losing sight of an event extended in time. The notion of agency is implicit in each event in the chain that acts to produce an effect that then becomes the next cause.

Some form of generalization is required over the pairs. In the example shown in figure 14.4, observers generalize by time ensemble averaging. This leads to a problem, because the response does not come with a fixed latency, and sometimes it doesn't come at all. Observers who are working in the paradigm of active perception expect this, because they see the response as self-organized, triggered sometime after the stimulus in each trial and occurring at the pleasure of the animal, but observers who are working in the paradigm of passive perception expect that each stimulus initiates a causal chain of events in each trial, such as those events indicated by the tick marks on each time segment in figure 14.4. These serial events do not reliably occur at the same latencies from the zero point, which observers typically select independently of what the animal under observation is doing. Events that are early in the chain, just after stimulus onset and therefore with short post-stimulus latencies, tend to have smaller variances in latency, so they are retained under averaging. Later events with more widely varying latencies tend to be lost. The observers attribute the variance in latency to chance or to noise, which is their rationale for averaging.

This procedure enhances the features of the response that depend on the stimulus and diminishes the contributions made by the animal, reinforcing the utility of the passive paradigm in the minds of the observers, but at the cost of an anomaly. Brains have no neural mechanisms for storing and averaging single trials in the way that observers do. On the contrary, the function of the sensory cortex, for reasons discussed, is to construct a mean-field pattern and remove the stimulus-driven activity as trash. The observers who use averaging thereby remove the self-organized constructs formed on each trial, and what they retain for analysis is brain refuse.

Circular causality is shown in figure 14.5. The encircled dot shows a point moving counterclockwise in real time on a trajectory idealized as a circle. This construction indicates that a perceptual event exists irreducibly as a state through a duration of inner time, which we can abstract and idealize as a point in real time. External stimuli from the world impinge on this state. So do internal stimuli emerging through the self-organizing dynamics within the core of the brain. Most stimuli are ineffective, but occasionally one succeeds as a hit on the brain state, and a response occurs. The impact results in a nonlinear state transition, which is followed by a change in brain structure that we identify with learning, and this change begins a new orbit. A succession of orbits can be conceived as a cylinder that has its axis in real time and extends from birth to death of an individual and its brain. Events are intrinsically not reproducible. The circular trajectories in inner time fuse the past and future into an extended present that constitutes a state that is entered and exited by state transitions.

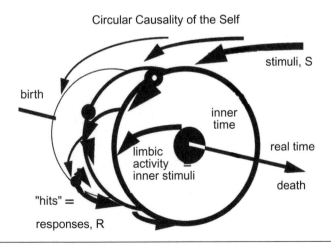

FIGURE 14.5   Circular causality.

Reprinted, by permission, from W.J. Freeman, 1999, "Reclaiming cognition," *Journal of Consciousness Studies* 6(11-12): 144-145.

In figure 14.5, circular causality expresses the interrelations among levels in the hierarchy of brain dynamics. A top-down macroscopic state simultaneously influences and constrains the microscopic particles that create and sustain the macroscopic state from the bottom up. The state exists over a span of inner time that we tend to collapse to a point in external time. Events in real time are marked by discrete transitions in the state of the system. A hit denotes the impact of an external stimulus onto a cortex prepared by preafference, so that a state transition ensues. Without such preparation, nothing happens, as is the case for the great preponderance of sensory inputs. I postulate that internal stimuli arising from self-organizing processes in the limbic system can operate in place of external stimuli in the process of imagination. The encircled dot represents the mythical moment of *now*. Circular causality is widely used in the social and physical sciences. In an example used by Haken (1983), excited atoms in a laser cause coherent light emission, and the light imposes order on the atoms. In circular causality, multiple scales of time and space are required for the different levels of brain hierarchies and the notion of an agent does not enter. A similar view was held by followers of a resilient school of philosophy, nominalism. Followers included David Hume (1739), who was led by this fundamental premise to conclude that the abstract idea of causality exists only in minds, not in the material world.

Timing in the Awareness of Action

Since we perceive action through our awareness of the intentional process, an action can be accessed in respect to either the onset of an external stimulus or an internal preafferent message presaging a goal-directed action. However, as shown in figure 14.5, there are two time lines: one linear, signifying a segment of real time, and one circular, showing perceived time. Awareness of percepts is not simultaneous with the onset of the stimulus or with the state transition that constitutes the initial planning of an act. A neural mechanism keeps perceived time sufficiently close to the flow of events in real time so that actions are effective even in exceedingly rapid external flows. This mechanism was revealed in experiments conducted by the neurophysiologist Benjamin Libet (1994), who collaborated with neurosurgeons to measure the lapse between the onset of a stimulus and awareness of the stimulus.

For diagnostic purposes, surgeons placed electrodes in the brains of patients to treat intractable epilepsy. Some patients volunteered to participate in a fundamental test, in which they remained awake and reported the effects of direct electrical stimulation of their brains after surgical exposure under local anesthesia. In some trials the surgeons stimulated a nerve in the patient's left hand, which evoked an electrical response in the right sensory cortex almost instantly by a very fast pathway to the sensory cortex. The patient reported feeling the stimulus 1/2 s later. On other trials the surgeons gave an electrical stimulus directly to the exposed left sensory cortex, which bypassed the fast pathway from the right hand and caused an immediate onset of a sensory cortical response. Again, about 1/2 s elapsed before the patient reported perceiving the stimulus, despite the very short time delay in the onset of the evoked potentials in the cortex.

Two aspects of Libet's experiment are especially important for interpretation. First, the stimulus given to the left hand could be felt no matter how brief it was, but the stimulus given directly to the left cortex had to be a pulse train lasting 1/4 to 1/2 s to achieve what Libet called "neuronal adequacy" for awareness. Briefer durations of cortical stimulation required higher stimulus intensity. Second, patients assigned awareness of the direct electrical stimulus to the left cortex to the end of the pulse train, the time required for neuronal adequacy, but backdated the awareness of the stimulus given to the left hand, which was relayed to the right cortex, to its time of occurrence. Backdating synchronizes brain function with the flow of real time, despite the obligatory delay in forming a percept. Anyone who plays on a sports team or in an orchestra knows the necessity of keeping rapid sequences of behavior in harmony with the group, despite rates of change that are too fast to allow perceptual frames in succession, yet require integration into the shared time sequences of the unfolding events.

Libet showed that the neural basis for backdating is provided by one of the two somatosensory channels, the lemniscal system. The ascending axons of the system are fast and unbranched, and the system reports to the cortex in under 30 ms exactly where and when a stimulus hits either the skin or the sensory nerves serving the cutaneous receptors. Libet found that patients could backdate if he stimulated the thalamus and included that pathway, but otherwise they could not. In contrast, axons in the other somatosensory channel, the spino-thalamic system, are slow and branch extensively into the reticular formation. The branched axons diverge the activity to many neurons, and those neurons excite each other in such a way that the cortex as the main target receives prolonged bursts known as "after-discharges" that are the basis for perceiving the stimulus 1/2 s later, but perception of the time and place of onset is based on lemniscal input. Experimental psychologists commonly use a double threshold technique to detect events in noisy time series. They use a high threshold to determine that an event with gradual onset has occurred and a low threshold to backdate the time at which it began. In constructing a mechanical model of learning, Walter (1963) used two electronic circuits, one with a step output to report that an event happened, and the other with a pulse output to report when it happened. When in other experiments, physiologists cut all spinal tracts in rats except that of the lemniscal system, and tested its function, the rats ignored all stimuli below the level of the cut (Melzack and Wall 1983), leaving the question: What does the system do? Libet's work gives an answer. It is the lemniscal system that coordinates perceived time with real time.

Although Libet's experiment has been severely criticized for its failure to develop an accurate measure of inner awareness, the facts remain that awareness is a more complex process than the induced state transitions in sensory cortices and that it requires more time. Libet and several other neurobiologists have also deduced from measurements of brain activity in human volunteers that a comparable delay exists in the onset of awareness of a self-paced action, such as when experimental subjects are asked to briefly press a switch, at their inclination, now and then over the course of an hour. In this experiment, a slow change in electric potential is recorded with scalp electrodes located between the top of the head and the base of the earlobes. This slow increase is called the readiness potential. It starts about 1 s before each self-paced movement. The change in potential is so small that it can be detected only by averaging over numerous trials, but it shows that neural activity for planning and organizing the movement precedes the awareness of an intention to act. The length of time by which awareness follows the onset of the readiness potential is comparable to the delay in the awareness of a stimulus onset. That is, when the subjects report the time they became aware of their decision to press the switch, the timing of their responses indicates that their awareness follows the onset of the readiness potential by 1/4 to 1/2 s.

The results show that both perception and action run in perceived time quite smoothly without awareness and that intention surfaces intermittently into awareness for a query or an update, filling in the gaps of awareness by remembering. This appears to be why remembered time is so much more fallible than the perceived time that precedes and underlies awareness and that continuously and effortlessly supports attempts to achieve desired goals. In accordance with this view, we perceive time through our experiences of taking action in the space around us (Rosenbaum and Collyer, 1998). Despite tours de force such as the novels of Marcel Proust (1919) and James Joyce, recall is not a reliable way to study perceptual time in reconstructing actions, owing to the sparseness with which the intentional process is monitored, sampled, and reconstructed in awareness.

Conclusion

The largest gap in our understanding of movement is in the neural dynamics by which brains predict future states, conceive these states as attainable goals, and plan elaborate sequences of actions intended to actualize those states. For many centuries, philosophers have proposed that action is prelude to perception and that movement cannot be understood except in the context of perception and what is intended by the movement. A special class of the action-perception cycle includes awareness of the self and the body in motion, which requires consideration of consciousness along with the perceptions of time and causality. Neurophysiological data indicate that perception in all modalities of sensation occurs through destabilizing areas of the cortex. Through destabilization these areas construct and transmit spatial patterns of neural activity that have been set up by limbic preafference and selected by sensory input. A useful analogy for each area of the cortex is the heart, which is bistable in having a receiving diastolic mode and a transmitting systolic mode. Each area of the heart switches back and forth, broadcasting to all other areas during systole and receiving from all other areas during diastole (Freeman, 2000c). As in the heart, the alternating jumps in the cortex are made by state transitions.

A key requirement of intentional action is embedding in space-time. Neurobiological data indicate that the requisite neural machinery is located in the medial temporal lobe, with the field of space-time located in the hippocampus. These parts of vertebrate brains have cytoarchitectures and patterns of neural activity, both mesoscopic and microscopic, that closely resemble the corresponding properties of sensory and motor cortices. The perceptions of actions and of the causal relations of actions, both antecedent and consequent, have their origins in the same intentional cycle that produces goal-directed actions accompanied by preafference, attention, and learning from the perceived consequences of acting. Therefore the main components of the limbic system are expected to have in concert similar capacities for creating spatial patterns of mesoscopic neural activity. Through preafference, these patterns set up the motor systems to initiate actions and the sensory areas to anticipate the fresh patterns of sensory input that soon will come. These anticipations are hypotheses to be tested by actions. Neural dynamics are creative by virtue of chaos, so that no repeated actions like writing a signature or catching a ball are identical. The intrinsic, individualized variance is characteristic of brain dynamics.

Chapter 15

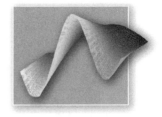

Variability of Brain Activity During Rhythmic Unimanual Finger Movements

T.D. Frank, PhD, C.E. Peper, PhD, A. Daffertshofer, PhD, and P.J. Beek, PhD

Editors' Overview

Variability is an immanent feature of the human movement system, and this chapter investigates the interplay between neural control and the behavior of movement effectors. The variability of phase differences between movement trajectories and encephalographic signals is investigated during externally paced and voluntary rhythmic finger movements. The chapter discusses previous work and two recent experiments in which the pacing frequency of finger movements was varied under different task constraints including synchronization and syncopation with a beat. Data are presented that suggest that descending neural pathways play a significant role in constraining the phase locking of brain signals and movement trajectories, leading to spatial patterns with regions of strong (low variability) and weak (high variability) couplings. These patterns seem to be invariant across task constraints (syncopation and synchronization), and they remain consistent over different participants. In a discussion of the dynamics of mutually coupled neural oscillators, readers are introduced to a stochastic model that captures the stability and variability of phase synchronization in the brain. From a dynamic systems approach, data supporting the model are presented, showing how mean-field forces emerge from the interaction of homogeneous subsystem components in the human body.

The contribution of Lieke Peper was made possible by a fellowship of the Royal Netherlands Academy of Arts and Sciences. This research was financially supported by the Netherlands Foundation for Behavioral Sciences (SGW/NWO).

In recent years, both the analysis of experimental data regarding variability and the modeling of intrinsically variable systems of motor control have become prominent research topics in human movement science. In particular, the observation of patterned yet variable brain signals and movement trajectories constitutes a fundamental challenge for understanding motor control systems as it requires the unification of two seemingly conflicting properties: coordination and variability. As we argue in the section, "Theoretical Framework," the dynamic systems approach to human movement (Beek at al., 1995; Haken, 1996; Kelso and Haken, 1995; Kelso, 1995; Tass, 1999; Uhl, 1999) allows us to address these properties within a comprehensive theoretical framework. In the section, "Coordinated Rhythmic Movements," the dynamic systems approach is worked out in more detail for rhythmic movement. The central concepts of the mean-field theory commonly used in statistical physics are introduced. Furthermore, we illustrate that measurements of variability may provide useful information about the strength and nature of couplings between constituents of motor control systems. Experimental results are reported in the section, "Experiments and Experimental Results," and discussed in view of the theoretical predictions later in this chapter.

Theoretical Framework

In the dynamic systems approach, systems for motor control are regarded as complex and dynamic, possessing a large number of subsystems that generally evolve on different characteristic timescales. In contrast to the irregular appearance of bubbles in boiling water and the random walks of atoms of dilute gases, the subsystems of motor control exhibit a coordinated and often synchronized behavior. Task- or goal-directed motor performance requires constraints that reduce the degrees of freedom of the systems of motor control (Bernstein, 1967; Turvey, 1990). In this context, we may think of control systems that, like the conductor of an orchestra, supervise human systems of motor control and ensure that the respective subsystems become active at appropriate times and in appropriate fashions. The dynamic systems approach to human movement, however, looks at the problem of the degrees of freedom from a different perspective, one in which relevant constraints are not imposed upon but are generated by the systems of motor control themselves. Like people strolling through a crowded pedestrian zone and forming a laminar biphasic flow pattern, with people on one half of the street walking in one direction and on the other half in the opposite direction, systems for motor control are believed to be able to organize themselves without the assistance of supervisory control systems. This ability is called self-organization.

Origin of Noise

To elucidate the notion of self-organization, let us consider an arbitrary task-specific system of motor control (see figure 15.1). To begin with, the system is embedded in a hosting or supporting system. In general, the supporting system includes unspecific subsystems that are unrelated to the functioning of the system of interest. Usually, they are considered to evolve much faster than the system for motor control. For example, there is thermal irregular motion in the molecules of the bone, connecting tissue, and extra- and intracellular fluids that vanishes only at 0 K, or –273 °C. Similarly, with respect to rhythmic movements performed at frequencies ranging from 2 to 3 Hz, ongoing brain

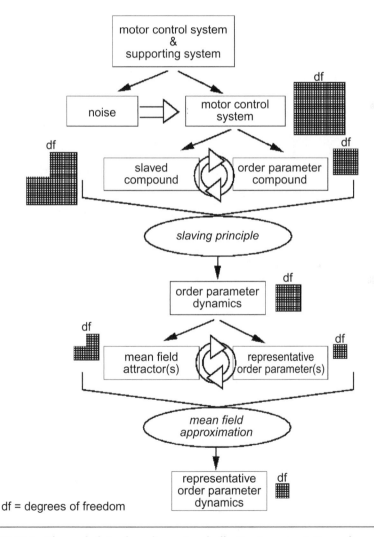

FIGURE 15.1 The underlying low-dimensional effective (representative order parameter) dynamics of a high-dimensional system for motor control embedded in a supporting structure.

activity in the range of 60 to 80 Hz can also be regarded as a fast-evolving process, and due to its phase randomness it is likely to be unspecific. When these unspecific subsystems act on task-specific systems of motor control, they manifest themselves as noise (or fluctuating forces) that permanently disturbs the functioning of the systems for motor control (Haken, 1977; Jayannavar and Mahato, 1995; Kac, 1969). Furthermore, sources of noise act in a unidirectional way, as indicated in figure 15.1.

Slaved and Order Parameter Compounds

In many cases task-specific systems of motor control can be broken into two qualitatively different compounds: slaved and order parameter. Slaved compounds contain task-specific subsystems that are fast evolving, whereas order parameter compounds consist of slowly evolving subsystems. Although in general there are mutual interactions between the two compounds, the dynamics of the slaved compounds may be expressed conveniently in terms of the evolution of the order parameter compounds as if the slaved compounds are unidirectionally driven by the order parameter compounds. The reason for this is that the slaved compounds immediately follow the variations of the order parameter compounds due to the separation in timescales (Haken, 1977). Consequently, the effect of a slaved compound on an order parameter compound can be viewed as the effect of the order parameter compound onto itself. Thus, order parameter compounds evolve as if slaved compounds are not involved in their dynamics. We may compare this situation with a conversation between two people in which one person only asks, "How so?". We can describe the dynamics of this conversation by a single speaker who is continuously explaining the meaning of her previous statement. The decomposition into slaved and order parameter compounds and the emergence of order parameter dynamics in complex systems are referred to as the slaving principle (Haken, 1977).

Mean-Field Forces

Usually there are many rapidly evolving subsystems but few slowly evolving subsystems, as is illustrated in figure 15.1. There might be a single order parameter such as the relative phase between two rhythmically moving limbs (Haken et al., 1985). But we can deal with a large set of identical order parameters, that is, with many copies of a particular subsystem. For example, cross bridges of a muscle filament (Shimizu, 1974; Shimizu and Yamada, 1972) and neural oscillators involved in rhythmic finger movements (Frank et al., 2000) have been considered as elements of an order parameter compound. Large ensembles of almost identical interacting subsystems typically produce forces that represent the averaged (or collective) effects on individual members of the ensemble. These forces are called mean-field forces, and they become particularly important in circular causality, as they are produced by ensemble members and act on these members at the same time. By virtue of the mean-field forces, order parameter compounds consisting of large sets of almost identical elements can be decomposed into mean-field forces and representative order parameters (see figure 15.1).

Mean-Field Approximation

Forces in collective ensembles (mean-field forces) can often be determined by using the so-called mean-field approximation (Desai and Zwanzig, 1978; Frank, 2001a; Frank et al., 2001a; Kuramoto, 1984; Tass, 1999). According to this approximation, the ensemble of spatially distributed order parameter subsystems (a material ensemble) can be replaced by the statistical ensemble of a single representative subsystem. For example, suppose we are interested in the statistical properties of a fully loaded hotel elevator with a maximum capacity of 20 people. To investigate the statistics of the load, we could stuff a number of different groups of 20 people into the elevator and measure the load after each filling. Alternatively, we could simplify our investigation and randomly choose 20 people, put them into the elevator, and carry out a single measurement. The first approach uses samples of material ensembles of 20 people and yields detailed information about the statistics of the load, whereas the second approach uses the statistical ensemble of a single person and provides only an estimate of the mean load. Both approaches lead to identical mean values in the absence of correlations among the elements of the material ensemble. In our example of a hotel elevator, such correlations cannot be neglected because hotels are frequently visited by tourist groups, and a group of basketball players, for example, does not usually weigh the same as a group of tourists. For large ensembles, however, such correlations can be neglected (Bonilla, 1987; Kuramoto, 1984; Neu, 1980; Tass, 1999). Consequently, in the limit of large systems, mean-field forces can be expressed by the statistical properties of representative order parameters. As a result of the mean-field approximation, the evolution of ensembles of order parameters is determined by the evolution of representative order parameters.

Solution to the Problem of Degrees of Freedom

If we measure the degrees of freedom in a system of motor control by using the number of subsystems that are sufficient for describing the system, then we realize that the slaving principle and the mean-field approximation result in the aforementioned required reduction of the degrees of freedom. This reduction is achieved by the systems of motor control themselves. Accordingly, the constraints emerging in the systems are self-inflicted and do not demand supervisory control.

Role of Transition Points

As stated earlier, the slaved compounds usually comprise the larger parts of systems for motor control. This is because the systems operate near transition points (Haken, 1996). That is, they operate in such a way that slight changes in the parameters can induce dramatic effects. For example, variations in the speed of locomotion can result in transitions between gaits and variations in perceptual key variables can initiate grasping movements. Let us now introduce the characteristic timescale. The characteristic timescale describes how fast a process relaxes from a perturbed unstable state to a stationary stable state. It can be shown that at transition points, the characteristic timescale of at least one subsystem becomes infinitely long (the critical slowing down). Consequently, compared to that particular subsystem, all other subsystems that evolve on finite timescales can be considered as rapidly evolving systems constituting the slaved compound. If there are ensembles of identical subsystems, then at a transition point the characteristic timescale of one of these ensembles tends to infinity. The corresponding ensemble can then be identified as the order parameter compound.

Affinity of Motor Control Systems to Transition Points

Why should systems of motor control operate near transition points? First, close to transition points the scope of behavioral options is enhanced, and this guarantees flexibility and adaptability in motor performance (Haken, 1996; Kelso and Haken, 1995). Second, small changes of parameters can result in large effects near transition points. In contrast, in systems far away from transition points, parameters need to be greatly varied to induce switches between characteristic patterns of behavior. Consequently, in the latter case the time required for switching is long, and the systems are in jeopardy of being destroyed before being able to adapt to changing environmental and internal demands. Third and finally, it has been suggested that when far from transition points, the slaving principle breaks down and chaos may occur (Haken, 1977). For the Lorenz attractor, this breakdown can be illustrated explicitly. Consequently, in order to avoid chaotic and unpredictable behavior, systems of motor control may primarily occupy regions in their respective parameter spaces that are close to transition points.

Lessons From Variability

From the dynamic systems approach we can draw some important conclusions regarding the couplings in subsystems of motor control (see table 15.1). In particular, the strength and nature of couplings can be assessed by measurements of variability such as variances and cross-correlations. Cross-correlations between elements of slaved compounds can be neglected in comparison to cross-correlations between slaved and order parameter compounds (Haken, 1977). Consequently, the subsystems of slaved compounds are primarily coupled indirectly via order parameter compounds. The relevant quantity for describing couplings between slaved and order parameter compounds is a conditional probability density[1] that defines the probability of finding a slaved compound

---

[1]For example, the probability that consumers buy less given that gasoline prices are rising is a conditional probability.

in a certain state given that an order parameter compound assumes a particular state (Haken, 1977). Roughly speaking, the cross-correlations between slaved and order parameter compounds provide information about the connectivity between these compounds.

If the order parameter compound consists of only a few components, the couplings between the order parameter elements of systems for motor control can be determined with various measurements of variability such as the variance and the degree of harmonicity (Amazeen et al., 1998; Peper et al., 1995; Post et al., 2000; Schöner et al., 1986; Sternad et al., 2000; Newell and Corcos, 1993). On the other hand, if the order parameter compound includes large sets of identical components, coupling strength can be expressed by the statistical deviations of the dynamics of the subsystems from respective mean-field attractors (Frank et al., 2000). Alternatively, the coupling strength can be expressed in terms of the deviations of order parameter distributions from the uniform distribution (Bhattacharya and Petsche, 2001; Gross et al., 2000; Tass et al., 1998). These analytical tools are based on a fundamental assumption that the more variable is the collective behavior of subsystems, the weaker are the couplings between them.

TABLE 15.1   Measurements of Variability for the Strength of Couplings in Structural Components of Systems for Motor Control

Couplings	Measurement
Between slaved and order parameter compounds	Conditional probability density
Within order parameter compounds	Variance, degree of harmonicity
Within ensembles of identical subsystems	Occupation probability of mean-field attractors

Coordinated Rhythmic Movements

In order to illustrate the conceptual framework laid out in the preceding sections, particularly the emergence of mean-field forces, we consider systems of motor control that (a) show transitions and (b) contain large sets of identical elements. Rhythmically coordinated movements satisfy these demands, especially if we include brain activity related to movement. For example, paced rhythmic movements exhibit involuntary transitions between intended offbeat (syncopative) patterns and unintended, simpler on-beat patterns when the pacing frequency exceeds critical threshold values (Kelso et al., 1990; Kelso, 1995).

Similarly, in bimanual polyrhythmic tapping, transitions between different poly-rhythms have been observed that were induced again by increasing the overall speed of performance (Peper et al., 1991, 1995b). During experiments such as these, brain activity can be recorded in encephalographic signals (Daffertshofer et al., 2000a,b; Fuchs et al., 1992; Kelso et al., 1992, 1998; Wallenstein et al., 1995). Taking the brain into our considerations, we are immediately confronted with an ensemble of similar subsystems in the form of populations of neurons. Movements evoke neural activity that can be measured as encephalographic signals (Creutzfeld, 1995; Shibasaki, 1982), which in turn are assumed to arise from the cooperative activity of many neurons (Nunez, 1995, 2000). In particular, oscillatory neural activity is believed to result from the interaction of large sets of almost identical neural oscillators (Ermentrout and Cowan, 1979; Gerstner and van Hemmen, 1994; Lopes da Silva et al. 1974; Schuster and Wagner, 1990; Sompolinsky et al., 1991; Wright and Liley, 1996). The notion that spatially distributed, interacting neural oscillators are the basis of neural processing is also supported by intracranial measurements (Bressler et al., 1993; Eckhorn et al., 1988; Engel et al., 1991; Gray et al., 1989; Murthy and Fetz, 1996; Salenius et al., 1997). In this context, it has been suggested that the perceptual motor system links distributed units to task-specific enti-ties (or synergies) (Singer, 1993). As stated earlier, one mechanism that can lead to cooperative behavior and synchronized ensembles is the emergence of a mean-field force. Therefore, the study of brain activity related to rhythmic coordinated movements is a favorable test bed for the applicability of the mean-field approximation in the dynamic systems approach. In what follows, we discuss some specific details of the dynamic systems approach that relate to the study of coordinated rhythmic movements.

Phase Synchronization of Neural Activity

In the case of oscillatory brain activity (as related to rhythmic movements), the cooperative behavior of neural oscillators often manifests itself as synchro-nization (Gray et al., 1989). In this context, the question arises of whether synchronization is established through coherency (Andrew and Pfurtscheller, 1996) or simply through phase synchronization (Gross et al., 2000). The latter case requires only phase locking; amplitude effects are not involved in the linking mechanism.

To quantify the phase synchronization, measurements are needed for assess-ing the variability of phase dynamics, that is, for quantifying the extent to which the phase under consideration assumes a fixed value or to which the phase is uniformly distributed. These measurements must be independent of the amplitudes of the oscillations being studied. Coherency measurements (e.g., Andrew and Pfurtscheller, 1996) capture the variability of signals but depend on oscillation amplitudes. Phase maps (Kelso et al., 1992; Silberstein, 1995) plot the mean values of the phases over recording sites. They are not confounded by amplitude effects but they cannot address issues of variability. Recently, it has been suggested to investigate the synchronization of two signals by using the distribution of differences between their time-dependent (Hilbert) phases (e.g., Tass et al., 1998). Accordingly, the absence of phase synchronization corresponds to a uniform distribution. Nonuniform distributions are interpreted as evidence for phase synchronization. Such deviations can be quantified with a scalar measurement: the difference between the entropy of the observed distribution and the (maximum) entropy of the uniform distribution. Thus, an index of relative entropy can be computed and index maps of synchronization can be plotted (see table 15.2). Phase synchronization in this statistical sense has been observed in electromyographic and magnetoencephalographic signals recorded during tremor (Tass et al., 1998) and during isometric force production (Gross et al., 2000) as well as in electroencephalographic signals recorded during the presentation of music (Bhattacharya and Petsche, 2001). In this chapter, we indicate how such statistical tools for phase synchronization can be applied to the analysis of brain activity corresponding to rhythmic movements and how the results may be interpreted. Note that the aforementioned approach to statistical phase synchronization is indifferent to mean values that may occur in the encephalographic signals. Since transitions between different modes of coordinated rhythmic movements are characterized by switches in mean values (Daffertshofer et al., 2000; Frank et al., 1999; Kelso et al., 1992; Wallenstein et al.,1995), the statistical analysis proposed by Tass et al. (1998) has recently been modified by accounting for reference phases that are defined by the attractive points of mean-field forces (Frank et al., 2000). In doing so, phase synchronization can be discussed in terms of phase synchronization variability (PSV) maps (see table 15.2) that display the probabilities of finding elements of order parameter ensembles on their corresponding mean-field attractors (occupation probabilities). This analytical tool is described in detail later in this chapter. In addition, novel findings regarding self-paced rhythmic finger movements are presented.

TABLE 15.2 Sensitivity of Analytical Methods to Variability and Amplitude Effects

Method	Sensitive to variability	Insensitive to amplitude
Coherency analysis	Yes	No
Phase maps	No	Yes
Index maps of synchronization	Yes	Yes
Phase synchronization variability (PSV) maps	Yes	Yes

Mean Values of Phase Synchronization

Having discussed the emergence of phase synchronization, the question arises of which mean phases can serve as attractors for the dynamics of neural oscillators. This empirical question requires an attempt to use neurophysiological observations to derive the attractive points of the neural mean-field forces involved in the control of rhythmic movements. To this end, we restrict our considerations to paced rhythmic movements that show characteristic unintended transitions from offbeat to on-beat patterns of movement at critical pacing frequencies. Such rhythmic movements include paced finger (Kelso et al., 1990; Kelso, 1995) and arm movements (Peper and Beek, 1998). Then we distinguish three kinds of neural activity: descending and ascending neural activities related to movement and neural activity related to the pacing signal. As we show in the following sections, these three types of neural activity can be distilled from the bulk of the brain activity by using characteristic phase relationships. To this aim, we use encephalographic data to compute the distributions of the phases of brain signals related to movement, and we plot these distributions as functions of the pacing frequency, as is illustrated schematically in figure 15.2. In general, phase distributions consist of multiple components that correspond to the aforementioned types of neural activity. These components are of particular relevance because they define the mean phases to which the dynamics of neural oscillators can be attracted.

Pacing Signals

Brain activity related to a periodic pacing signal can be distinguished from other neural activity by studying the phase locking of the observed encephalographic signals with respect to the pacing signal. This is because in the case of repetitive stimuli, one can usually observe phase locking between stimulus and brain activity (Forss et al., 1993; Silberstein, 1995). Experiments involving transitions of brain activity are particularly amenable for studies of phase locking between pacing stimulus and neural activity because neural activity (ascending and descending) related to movement may change with a transition of the manual behavior, whereas the neural activity related to the pacing signal is assumed invariant across such transitions. Consequently, neural activity related to a pacing signal gives rise to a component in the phase distribution of the bulk of the brain activity that is invariant against changes in the pacing frequency (see figure 15.2).

Ascending Neural Activity

Sensory inputs from moving or stimulated body parts can be identified by characteristic latencies. For the case of brisk, voluntary flexion and extension of the finger, several authors have suggested that ascending neural activity measured via electro- and magnetoencephalography attains its maximum value about 100 ms after the onset of the electromyographic (EMG) activity related to the finger flexion (Deecke et al., 1976; Cheyne and Weinberg, 1989; Feige et al., 1996; Kristeva et al., 1991). Delivering a vibratory stimulus to the

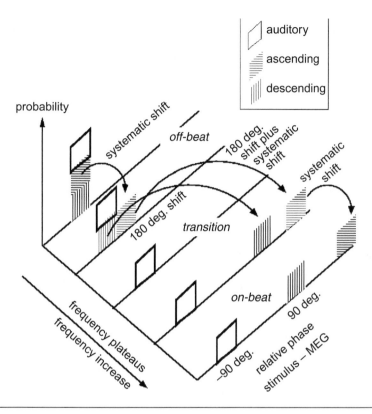

FIGURE 15.2 Components of phase distributions involving ascending and descending brain activity related to movement and to stimulus as functions of pacing frequency. The focus is on how these components evolve with changing pacing frequencies. For the sake of clarity, all components are centered at 90° in the lowest frequency plateau.

fingertips evokes neural activity that again peaks about 100 ms after stimulus onset (Hashimoto et al., 1998). Similarly, repetitive flexion and extension of the finger are accompanied by peaks occurring in encephalographic recordings of brain activity about 100 ms following the onset of EMG activity related to movement. These peaks have been interpreted to reflect peripheral sensory input (Gerloff et al., 1997, 1998). Studies on magnetic stimulation show that conduction times for descending cortical signals traveling to hand muscles are in the range of 10 to 50 ms (Gross et al. 2000 and references therein). Conversely, using phase synchronization techniques, transmission times of proprioceptive signals evoked in hand muscles during isometric contractions and terminated in cortical somatosensory regions have been estimated to range from 10 to 50 ms (Gross et al., 2000). Hence, ascending neural activity elicited in the hand is supposed to reach cortical areas after a latency of 100 ms (at most). Moreover, latencies recorded for vibratory sensory stimuli decreased only slightly with increasing stimulus frequency. Therefore, transmission delays are likely invariant against moderate changes in experimental conditions such as increasing pacing frequency. The implications of these findings for paced rhythmic movements in the range of 1 to 3 Hz (periods of 1000 to 333 ms) are at least twofold. First, in the low-frequency region (1.0 to 1.5 Hz or 1000 to 666 ms), peripheral input with latencies of 100 ms results in neural activity with a relative phase in the range of 10° to 50°.[2] Second, given the assumption that latencies do not depend on movement frequency for frequencies of 1 to 3 Hz, the relative phase between the ascending brain activity and the pacing signal changes dramatically between regions of low and high frequency. For example, a constant latency of 100 ms yields a relative phase of 10° during on-beat tapping to a rhythm of 1 Hz, but it corresponds to a relative phase of 110° during finger tapping at every 3.2 Hz. Consequently, significant contributions of ascending neural activity to the overall brain activity result in components of the phase distribution of encephalographic signals that for low frequencies, center in the 10° to 50° range, and that shift systematically as pacing frequency increases, as shown in figure 15.2 (for two frequency plateaus that precede the transition and two plateaus that follow the transition).

Descending Neural Activity

In contrast to ascending neural activity, which is characterized by particular latencies, descending neural activity related to movement is characterized by particular waveforms. For brisk, voluntary flexion and extension of the finger, brain waves measured by magnetoencephalography (MEG) typically consist of three components (see figure 15.3) (Cheyne et al., 1989; Cheyne and Weinberg, 1989; Feige et al., 1996; Kristeva et al., 1991). Immediately before the onset of EMG activity there is a rapid (accelerating) increase of MEG activity (component a). Following the EMG onset there is a time of deceleration in which MEG activity further increases and approaches a maximum (component b). Subsequently, the MEG wave drops rapidly, which leads to the aforementioned peak with a latency of about 100 ms that most probably describes the sensory input (component c).

Components a and b describe a monotonic increase of MEG activity and constitute the so-called readiness field that is believed to correspond to descending neural activity conveyed to the effector system. During paced and self-paced rhythmic flexion and extension of the finger, similar wave patterns can be observed in both electro- and magnetoencephalographic recordings (Gerloff et al., 1997, 1998). Therefore, Gerloff et al. (1998) suggested to explicitly decompose the characteristic MEG wave shown in figure 15.3 into the readiness field and the movement-evoked field and to extend the readiness field by a sinusoidal function over the whole flexion-extension cycle (see figure 15.4).

---

[2]Similarly, for latencies <100 ms we obtain relative phases <50°.

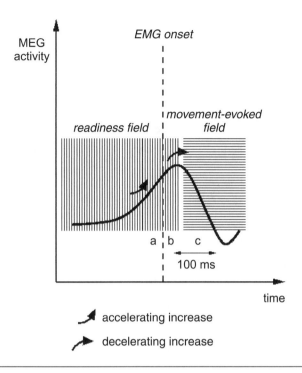

FIGURE 15.3   Schematic illustration of averaged MEG activity observed during repetitive as well as nonrepetitive flexion and extension of the finger. The EMG onset coincides with the transition from an accelerating to a decelerating change in the MEG activity.

According to this construction, the descending neural activity involved in rhythmic finger movements is shifted by about 90° with respect to the EMG onset. Because this conclusion is based on experiments involving individual voluntary as well as repetitive movements, we assume that this phase shift occurs across a wide range of movement frequencies. Consequently, descending neural activity reveals itself by relative phases of about 90° occurring between MEG signals and manual response signals. In particular, if either offbeat or on-beat patterns are performed, the corresponding descending neural activity contributes to the phase distribution of the overall brain activity with a component that is shifted by about ±90° relative to the pacing signal. Moreover, according to the model shown in figure 15.4, a transition between off- and on-beat patterns (antiphase and in-phase patterns) is accompanied by a shift of 180° in the component of descending neural activity (see figure 15.2). Whether or not these conclusions from studies on finger movements also hold for other kinds of rhythmic movements has to be sorted out in future experiments.

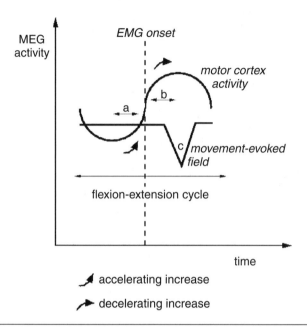

FIGURE 15.4   Decomposition of the waveform from figure 15.3 into a sinusoidal component related to motor cortex activity and a burstlike component describing feedback from the effector system.

Discriminating Ascending, Descending, and Stimulus Neural Activity

How can we discriminate among ascending, descending, and stimulus components of brain activity? The first step is to derive for each pacing frequency the probability density that describes the relative phase between the neural activity and the pacing signal. Then neural activities originating from the pacing signal make contributions to the probability densities that are independent of frequency as well as mode. In other words, the contributions are unaffected by transitions from antiphase to in-phase movements (see empty boxes in figure 15.2). Ascending neural activities characterized by constant latencies result in phase differences that depend on movement frequencies and thus yield contributions to the probability densities that shift systematically from plateau to plateau (see boxes shaded with diagonal lines in figure 15.2). Descending neural activities related to rhythmic movements are characterized by phase shifts of ±90° provided that offbeat or on-beat patterns are performed. Note that the predictions regarding ascending and descending neural activities are based on the assumption that the timing of the taps with respect to the stimuli is constant over frequency conditions.

Bipolar Neural Activity

For the sake of simplicity, the discussion so far has centered on brain activity of one kind of polarity. Usually, rhythmic movements are accompanied by bipolar patterns of brain activity (Cheyne et al., 1989; Cheyne and Weinberg, 1989, Feige et al., 1996, Gerloff et al., 1997, 1998; Kelso et al., 1998; Kristeva et al., 1991). Bipolar patterns generally imply that one also observes brain waves with a polarity opposite to that of the wave shown in figure 15.3. By analogy to the preceding discussion, these brain waves embody sinusoidal components of descending neural activity that are shifted by about $-90°$ with regard to EMG onset. Thus, brain activities related to movement that are recorded over the entire head generally yield bimodal phase distributions. Therefore, in a preparatory stage, regions of different polarity must be identified and the total recording area must be divided into two regions with signals showing a single polarity. Among other techniques, phase synchronization variability (PSV) maps can be applied for this purpose.

Experiments and Experimental Results

We report here two experiments focusing on brain activity related to paced and self-paced rhythmic finger movements. Experiment 1 involved three right-handed male drummers referred to as subjects A, B, and C (the age range was 29-34 y). They performed several tasks, as described by Daffertshofer et al. (2000b). In one task they performed a self-paced 2 or 3 Hz rhythm with their right index fingers during durations of 30 s. The subjects were first exposed to a 2 or 3 Hz stimulus signal for 30 s and instructed to tap along with this isochronous stimulus train. After this tuning, the signal was switched off and the subjects were instructed to continue tapping the required rhythm. Table 15.3 summarizes this part of the experiment.

We checked subject performance by calculating the power spectra of the manual response signals of the continuation phase obtained for each individual trial. Trials which showed a peak at a frequency differing from the required tapping frequency were excluded from the analysis, resulting in the total numbers

TABLE 15.3   Summary of a Subset of Experiment 1*

Subject	Pacing frequency	# of trials performed	# of valid trials
A	2 Hz	7	4
A	3 Hz	7	5
B	2 Hz	7	4
B	3 Hz	7	4
C	2 Hz	7	-
C	3 Hz	7	-

* Subjects were required to tap unimanually to a pacing stimulus (at 2 or 3 Hz, synchronization was 30 s) and to continue tapping at this prescribed frequency after the stimulus was switched off (continuation was 30 s).

of valid trials shown in table 15.3. The MEG signals were recorded using a full-head device with 151 channels. More details concerning the MEG device used in this study (and the study described later) can be found in Daffertshofer et al. (2000a, b). We did not evaluate MEG signals recorded from subject C because of the lack of significant peaks at the tapping frequency in the power spectra of the MEG signals.

In experiment 2, a single subject (a 22-year-old right-handed female without musical training) performed a large number of trials involving paced finger movements. We will refer to this subject as subject D. Subject D was exposed to a repetitive acoustic signal with a frequency ranging from 1 to 3.2 Hz. For 10 consecutive stimuli the stimulus frequency was fixed, and then it was increased or decreased by 0.2 Hz. In this way trials of increasing (1 to 3.2 Hz) and decreasing (3.2 to 1 Hz) frequency were conducted. Subject D was requested to tap her right index finger either in-phase (synchronization) or antiphase (syncopation) with the pacing signal. During the performance of the antiphase mode, pacing frequency was increased as in the so-called Julliard experiment (Kelso, 1995), while during the performance of the in-phase mode, pacing frequency was either increased or decreased. These experimental trials were performed in four blocks (see table 15.4). During the experiment, brain activity was recorded with the aforementioned full-head MEG device. Note that some trials were discarded because of technical problems arising during data acquisition. In addition, trials in which phase locking was lost at the high-frequency plateaus (pacing frequency $\geq$ 3 Hz) were excluded from analysis. For further experimental details see Frank et al. (2000).

TABLE 15.4 Summary of Experiment 2*

Block of trials	Task	Frequencies in Hz	# of trials performed	# of valid trials
I	Antiphase	1-3.2	20	16
II	Antiphase	1-3.2	20	17
III	In-phase	1-3.2	20	15
IV	In-phase	3.2-1	10	10

* Only one subject (D) participated. Trial duration was 65 s. Blocks I and II comprise the so-called Julliard experiment.

Temporal Analysis

In order to identify differences and similarities in paced and self-paced rhythmic finger movements, we partitioned the 30 s of self-paced tapping obtained in experiment 1 into consecutive segments, each of which consisted of 10 fictive interstimulus intervals. In doing so, for the signals recorded in experiments

1 and 2 we obtained the same segmentation in terms of 10-stimuli segments. We obtained 6 10-stimuli segments for the runs at 2 Hz and 9 for the runs at 3 Hz in the self-paced experiment, and we obtained 12 10-stimuli segments (frequency plateaus) in the paced experiment. For the self-paced conditions (2 or 3 Hz), the required tapping frequency was constant for all (6 or 9) segments. In contrast, in experiment 2, the frequency changed by 0.2 Hz from plateau to plateau (i.e., from segment to segment). For both experiments, brain activity was analyzed in regard to manual behavior. We first examined the power spectra of the tapping sequences and the MEG signals. Figure 15.5 shows power spectra averaged across 10-stimuli segments. The upper panels show the averaged power spectra obtained for subjects A and B during self-paced tapping with a frequency of 2 Hz. The lower three panels show the averaged power spectra obtained from subject D for blocks II, III, and IV. We can see from figure 15.5 that the subjects indeed tapped with the required frequency (see the small bars labeled R at the top of each panel) and that the brain activity in the range of 1 to 10 Hz was dominated by an oscillation with a frequency coinciding with that of the tapping movements. The power spectra obtained for subjects A and B under the conditions of 3 Hz (not shown here) qualitatively resembled the spectra shown in figure 15.5. However, the peaks at the tapping frequency were less pronounced, and the spectra were more diffuse. The power spectrum obtained in block I (the Julliard session) for subject D (not shown here) was both qualitatively and quantitatively similar to the spectrum shown for block II.

The peaks at the tapping frequency in the power spectra allowed us to examine the phase relationship between MEG signals and tapping behavior (see also Frank et al., 2000). To this end, Fourier phases $\Phi_i^{(\text{MEG, }l)}$ were calculated, one for each segment (frequency plateau), l, and MEG signal, $i = 1, \ldots, 151$. For experiment 2, phases of tapping sequences Φ_R (R stands for manual response) were determined on the basis of point estimates (Beek et al., 1996; Kelso et al., 1986) according to $\Phi_R^{(n, l)} := 2\pi \times \Delta t_R^{(n, l)} \times 10 / T_l$, where T_l corresponds to the total duration of the segment (frequency plateau), l. Here, $T_l / 10$ is the interstimulus interval, and $\Delta t_R^{(n, l)}$ denotes the duration between the beginning of the nth interstimulus interval and the moment when the finger hit the sensor. This assignment was also used for analyzing the self-paced finger movements performed in experiment 1. To this end, the artificially introduced stimuli segments were considered as counterparts of the frequency plateaus. Consequently, analysis could be carried out in an analogous fashion for experiments 1 and 2. For comparison with the Fourier phases, $\Phi_i^{(\text{MEG, }l)}$, we derived manual phases that can be regarded as representing a 10-stimuli segment, l. For each 10-stimuli segment, we used circular statistics to calculate the averaged phase $\Phi_R^{(l)} :< \Phi_R^{(n, l)} > cs$ from the segment phases $\Phi_R^{(1, l)}, \ldots, \Phi_R^{(10, l)}$. We obtained relative phases $\phi_i^{(\text{MEG-R, }l)} = \Phi_i^{(\text{MEG, }l)} - \Phi_R^{(l)}$ describing the phase relationship between brain activity and manual behavior. Let m denote an individual trial. Taking the number of performed trials into account, we thus obtained 151

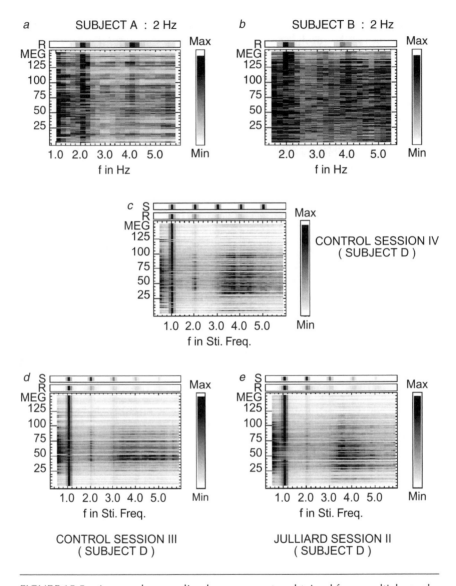

FIGURE 15.5 Averaged, normalized power spectra obtained from multichannel recordings. Power is plotted in terms of a color code (black = maximum, white = minimum). Horizontal axes show 151 MEG channels. Small bars labeled R and S give the power spectra of manual responses and stimulus signals, respectively. Power spectra for subjects A and B obtained during self-paced movements at a frequency of 2 Hz are shown in panels a and b, respectively. Power spectra for subject D are shown in panels c (block IV), d (block III), and e (block II). The vertical axes in panels c, d, and e show frequency in the units of the stimulus frequency.

$\times$ L $\times$ M values for $\phi_i^{(MEG\text{-}R, l, m)}$, where L and M are the number of segments (frequency plateaus) and valid trials, respectively. For example, $151 \times 6 \times 4$ values of $\phi_i^{(MEG\text{-}R, l, m)}$ were obtained from the 2 Hz continuation trials performed by subject A, $151 \times 9 \times 5$ values of $\phi_i^{(MEG\text{-}R, l, m)}$ were obtained from the 3 Hz continuation trials performed by subject A, $151 \times 12 \times 16$ values of $\phi_i^{(MEG\text{-}R, l, m)}$ were obtained in the paced tapping condition in block I performed by

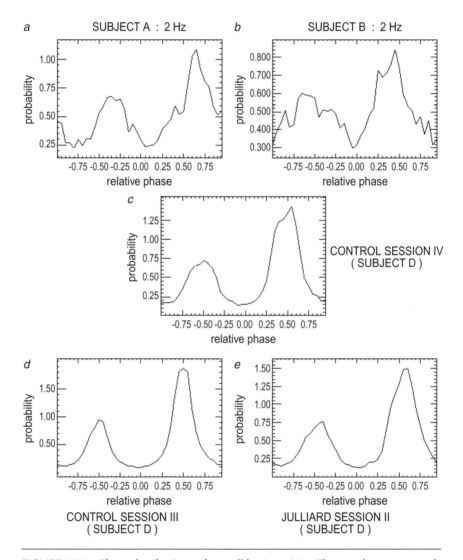

FIGURE 15.6   Phase distributions of overall brain activity. The panels are arranged as in figure 15.5.

subject D, and so on. On the basis of these large sets of values for $\phi_i^{(MEG-R, l, m)}$, we computed the distribution functions $P_{MEG-R}(\phi)$ for subjects A, B, and D and for the experiments listed in tables 15.3 and 15.4. The distribution functions $P_{MEG-R}(\phi)$ were defined by $P_{MEG-R}(\phi) \approx 1 / (151 \cdot L \cdot M) \sum_{i=1\ldots 151} \sum_{l=1\ldots L} \sum_{m=1}$ $\ldots_M \delta(\phi - \phi_i^{(MEG-R, l, m)})$, where $\delta(x)$ denotes the delta distribution. Examples of these distribution functions are shown in figure 15.6.

The phase relationship between manual response and brain activity is clearly characterized by a bimodal distribution. Bimodality seems to be independent of the subject and is observed during both self-paced (subjects A and B) and paced (subject D for both syncopation and synchronization) finger movements. Similar distributions (not shown here) were obtained for the other conditions. The maxima are separated by approximately 180°. In the case of the paced conditions (subject D), the bimodal distributions exhibit two pronounced peaks at about ±90. For subjects A and B, the maxima are slightly shifted away from ±90°. Let ϕ_{max} denote the position of the larger of the two maxima. We estimate for subject A $\phi_{max} \approx 110°$ and for subject B $\phi_{max} \approx 75°$. The two peaks in the distribution functions hint at the existence of cortical regions with different polarities (see p. 284). We therefore expect a spatial analysis to reveal two groups of MEG signals, with each group contributing to one of the two peaks.

Spatial Analysis

Our next objective is to clarify to what extent brain signals contribute to the bimodality of the relative phase distributions, $P_{MEG-R}(\phi)$, depicted in figure 15.6. There are two extreme possibilities. On the one hand, the relative phase $\phi_i(t)$ of the MEG signal, i, may perform a random walk, thereby permanently switching between the positions of the two maxima. On the other hand, $\phi_i(t)$ may be confined at all times t to positions near one of the two maxima. To assess the degree of phase synchronization, we decomposed the domain of the definition of relative phases ([0, 2π]) into two disjoint intervals of width, π, centered around the two maxima. More precisely, we introduced the intervals $I(+): = [\phi_{max} - \pi / 2, \phi_{max} + \pi / 2)$ mod 2π, (where ϕ_{max} describes the position of the larger of the two maxima as stated earlier) and $I(-): = [\phi_{max} + \pi / 2, \phi_{max} + 3\pi / 2)$ mod 2π. Next, we used the relative phases, $\phi_i^{(MEG-R, l, m)}$, with $l = 1$, . . . , L and $m = 1, \ldots , M$, to compute the probabilities $p_i(+)$ and $p_i(-)$ of finding a phase difference ϕ_i in $I(+)$ and $I(-)$, respectively. Note that by definition $p_i(+) + p_i(-) = 1$. For subject D, the result of this procedure is shown in figure 15.7, where the degree of phase synchronization expressed as $p_i(+)$ and $p_i(-)$ is plotted for each MEG signal, i.

We realize that there are two groups of MEG signals with either $p_i(+) \approx 1$ or $p_i(-) \approx 1$. When $i > 90$ the relative phases ϕ_i at all times assume phase values close to ϕ_{max} (i.e., $p_i(+) \approx 1$), whereas when $i < 30$, the relative phases are all located near the second maximum, $\phi_{max} - \pi$. For these signals there is a large probability of finding relative phases close to either ϕ_{max} or $\phi_{max} - \pi$. In this

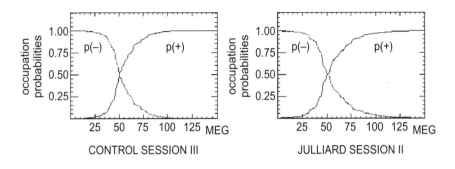

FIGURE 15.7   Occupation probabilities $p(+)$ (solid lines) and $p(-)$ (dotted lines) as functions of MEG signals computed from trials performed in the control block III (left panel) and the Julliard session II (right panel) of experiment 2.

sense, the relative phases of these MEG signals are characterized by a strong degree of phase synchronization, which implies a low variability. Cortical sites corresponding to sensor positions with $I \approx 50$ can be described by a weak degree of phase synchronization and a large variability in the corresponding phase dynamics. For subjects A and B, diagrams of phase synchronization similar to those in figure 15.7 were obtained (not shown here). In order to illustrate the spatial layout of the three types of cortical sites, $(p_i(+) \approx 1, p_i(-) \approx 1$, and $p_i(+) \approx p_i(-) \approx 0.5)$, we plotted $p_i(+)$ as a function of the recording position i (see figures 15.8 and 15.9).

The maps shown in figures 15.8 and 15.9 reveal domains of strong phase synchronization and domains lacking phase synchronization. Cortical sites with strong phase synchronization and relative phases close to ϕ_{max} and $\phi_{max} - \pi$ are displayed as white and black, respectively. Cortical sites that are indifferent in this regard (i.e., with $p_i(+) \approx p_i(-) \approx 0.5$) are gray. The patterns seem to be invariant across task conditions and subjects. On the left-hand side (contralateral to the tapping finger), a dipolar structure can be identified that might be associated with the contralateral motor cortex. In fact, in the context of rhythmic finger movements, such dipolar structures have been frequently reported in literature (e.g., Gerloff et al., 1998; Kelso et al., 1998). On the right-hand (ipsilateral) side, a band-shaped domain of strong phase synchronization with $\phi_i \approx \phi_{max}$ can be found. This observation is consistent with other studies reporting ipsilateral brain activity during unilateral limb movements (Cheyne and Weinberg, 1989; Gerloff et al., 1997, 1998; Kristeva et al., 1991, Murthy and Fetz, 1996). Finally, we would like to emphasize a slightly different interpretation of the maps in figures 15.8 and 15.9. Since $p_i(+)$ and $p_i(-)$ describe the probability of the local neural phase dynamics observed at site i to occupy an interval defined by the collective neural activity related to movement, the maps show the occupation probabilities of local neural activity being found on the attractors of collective neural activity.

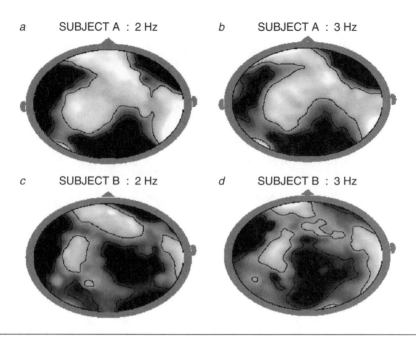

FIGURE 15.8 PSV maps obtained for subjects A (panels a and b) and B (panels c and d) when performing self-paced movements at frequencies of 2 Hz (panels a and c) and 3 Hz (panels b and d).

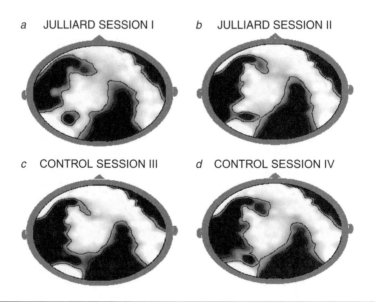

FIGURE 15.9 PSV maps obtained in experiment 2. Panels a, b, c, and d were computed from all valid trials performed in blocks I, II, III, and IV, respectively.

Spatiotemporal Analysis: Phase Synchronization Variability (PSV) Maps

As illustrated in the previous section, the maps depicted in figures 15.8 and 15.9 can describe the phenomenon of phase synchronization in an array of signals by evaluating the variability in the phase dynamics of the individual signals. Therefore, these maps are phase synchronization variability (PSV) maps. It is clear from the preceding discussion that PSV maps indeed satisfy the features listed in table 15.2, that is, the analysis of spatiotemporal signals by PSV maps is sensitive to the variability of the signals being studied and insensitive to the amplitudes of their oscillatory components. Here, we briefly summarize the construction of the PSV maps that was carried out in the preceding sections. In doing so, we demonstrate the generality of this analytical tool and relate the PSV maps to synchronization index maps (Bhattacharya and Petsche, 2001; Gross et al., 2000; Tass et al., 1998).

There are four basic steps in constructing a PSV map from a given data set (see figure 15.10). Let $q(t)$ be an N-dimensional time-dependent vector representing signals recorded at N distinct locations and at equidistant instances t_i, with $0 \leq t_i \leq T$ and $i = 1, 2, \ldots$ The first step is to determine a particular reference frequency Ω_R. To this end, we calculate the power spectra of the components of $q(t)$ and the reference signal, as shown in figure 15.10 (panel a), and then we detect the main peaks of the spectra and choose one of these peaks as the reference frequency Ω_R. This choice depends on the phenomenon of interest. In the preceding sections, the focus was on the fundamental peaks observed at the required tapping frequencies in the power spectra of the MEG signals.[3] In the second step, an appropriate reference phase Φ_{ref} is defined (earlier on p. 287, we used the phase of the manual response signal). Evaluating the Fourier transformation (FT) over the interval $[0, T]$ for the frequency Ω_R, we can assign a phase $\Phi_i^{(q)}$ and a relative phase $\Phi_i^{(q)}$ to each component q_i of q:

$$\text{FT}: \left(q_i\left(t\right), T, \Omega_R, \Phi_{ref} \right) \Rightarrow \phi_i^{(q)} := \Phi_i^{(q)} - \Phi_{ref}. \tag{15.1}$$

Consider now a set of K recordings, $\{q(t)^{(k)}\} = \{q(t)^{(1)}, \ldots, q(t)^{(K)}\}$. Each sample k yields a relative phase $\phi_i^{(q,k)}$, where $k = 1, ,K$. From the distribution of relative phases $\phi_i^{(q,k)}$ the phase distribution $P_{(q)\text{-Ref}}(\phi) \approx 1 / (N K) \Sigma_{i=1..N} \Sigma_{k=1..K} \Sigma(\phi - \phi_i^{(q,k)})$ can be calculated, where $\delta(x)$ denotes the delta-function as stated earlier. Explicitly, we obtain

$$\text{FT}: \left(q_i\left(t\right)^{(k)}, T, \Omega_R, \Phi_{ref} \right) \Rightarrow \phi_i^{(q,k)} := \Phi_i^{(q,k)} - \Phi_{ref} \Rightarrow P_{(q)\text{-Ref}}\left(\phi\right), \tag{15.2}$$

See figure 15.10 (panel b). If the signals $q_i(t)^{(k)}$ oscillate with a particular common phase difference $\phi_i^{(q)} = \phi_{max}$ with respect to Φ_{ref}, then the probability density $P_{(q)}$

---

[3]Alternatively, we could have studied phase synchronization with regard to the higher harmonics of the required movement frequencies.

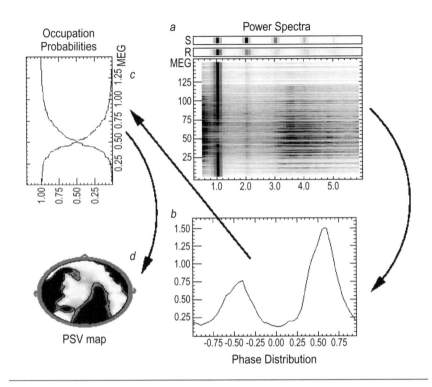

FIGURE 15.10   The four steps of constructing a PSV map.

$_{-Ref}(\phi)$ shows a pronounced maximum at this common phase difference ϕ_{max}. In general, the most probable phase difference ϕ_{max} can be defined as[4]

$$\phi_{max} : P_{(q)-Ref}\left(\phi_{max}\right) = maximal. \tag{15.3}$$

The third step in constructing a PSV map is quantifying the degree of phase synchronization in the signals $q_j(t)^{(1)}, \ldots, q_j(t)^{(K)}$. To this end, one splits the range of phase values, $[0,2\pi]$, into two separate intervals of equal width, $I(+)$: $=[\phi_{max} - \pi / 2, \phi_{max} + \pi / 2) \bmod 2\pi$ and $I(-) : = [\phi_{max} + \pi / 2, \phi_{max}+3\pi / 2)$ $\bmod 2\pi$. Subsequently, the probabilities $p_i(+)$ and $p_i(-)$ are calculated to find a phase difference ϕ in the set $\{\phi_i^{(1)}, \ldots, \phi_i^{(K)}\}$ in $I(+)$ and $I(-)$, respectively. In other words, the occupation probabilities $p_i(+)$ and $p_i(-)$ of the intervals $I(+)$ and $I(-)$ are computed for each signal i (see panel c of figure 15.10). In doing so, we obtain

$$\left(\phi_{max}, \phi_i^{(q,k)}, k = 1, \cdots, K\right) \rightarrow I\left(+\right), I\left(-\right) \rightarrow p_i\left(+\right), p_i\left(-\right). \tag{15.4}$$

---

[4]If there are multiple maxima, we have to test which of these maxima best suits our purpose. For example, on page 290, bimodal distribution functions were obtained and ϕ_{max} was assigned to the position of the larger of the two peaks.

By definition, we have $p_i(-) = 1 - p_i(+)$. The probabilities $p_i(+)$ and $p_i(-)$ can be considered as statistical measurements describing the degree of phase synchronization in a signal recorded at site i with respect to a reference signal and with respect to the intervals $I(+)$ and $I(-)$ that are defined by the collective properties of the signals recorded at all sites. The notion of this kind of phase synchronization is in line with the studies mentioned earlier (see p. 278), in which the degree of phase synchronization is described by the deviation from the uniform distribution. With the probabilities $p_i(+)$ and $p_i(-)$, we can rearrange the order of the components i of the signal vector $\boldsymbol{q}(t)$ (e.g., rearrange the labels of the MEG sensors) on the ordinate of the diagrams for the power spectra so that indices coincide with those on the abscissa of the diagrams for $p_i(+)$ and $p_i(-)$. For any signal $q_i(t)$, the power spectra and $p_i(\pm)$ diagrams together provide the essential information about its degree of phase synchronization and its spectral power (see figure 15.10, panels a and c). The fourth and final step in constructing a PSV map is the actual plotting of $p_i(+)$ and $p_i(-)$ over the locations i, which yields the phase synchronization variability maps $p(+)$ and $p(-)$, respectively (see figure 15.10, panel d). These maps provide information about the spatial distribution of the degree of phase synchronization or about the probabilistic strength of phase locking of the recorded signals as defined earlier. In particular, a uniform distribution of the phase differences $\phi i_{(q, k)}$ of a particular component i yields $p_i(+) = p_i(-) = 0.5$. Conversely, the relation of equiprobability, $p_i(+) \approx p_i(-) \approx 0.5$, hints at the absence of phase synchronization. Alternatively, PSV maps can be regarded as describing the occupation probabilities of the signals i with regard to the phase attractors defined by the intervals $I(+)$ and $I(-)$.

PSV Maps and Synchronization Index Maps

The probabilities $p_i(+)$ and $p_i(-)$ of finding a relative phase ϕ_i in one of the disjoint intervals $I(+)$ and $I(-)$ can be considered as the elements of a probability distribution $P_i^{(j)}$ defined on a binary state phase with $j = 1$ or $j = 2$. That is, for each signal i the distribution $P_i^{(j)}$ is given by $P_i^{(1)} = p_i(+)$ and $P_i^{(2)} = p_i(-)$. By exploiting the identity $p_i(-) = 1 - p_i(+)$, the Boltzmann-Gibbs-Shannon entropy, $S_i = -\sum_{j=1,2} P_i^{(j)} \ln P_i^{(j)}$, (Shannon, 1948) reads $S_i[p_i(+)] = -p_i(+) \ln p_i(+) - [1 - p_i(+)] \ln[1 - p_i(+)]$, and the maximum entropy S_{max} for the equiprobability distribution $p_i(+) = p_i(-) = 0.5$ assumes the value $S_{max} = \ln 2$. The synchronization indices ρ_i introduced in Gross et al. (2000) and Tass et al. (1998) express the deviations of the distributions $P_i^{(j)}$ from the equiprobability distribution in terms of the difference between the entropy of the distribution $P_i^{(j)}$ and the maximum entropy S_{max} as $\rho_I = (S_{max} - S_i[p_i(+)]) / S_{max}$. Consequently, we obtain

$$\rho_i \left[p_i \left(+ \right) \right] = \left(\ln 2 + p_i \left(+ \right) \ln p_i \left(+ \right) + \left[1 - p_i \left(+ \right) \right] \ln \left[1 - p_i \left(+ \right) \right] \right) / \left(\ln 2 \right). \tag{15.5}$$

Using the new variables $\Delta p_i = |p_i(+) - 0.5|$, the indices ρ_i read $\rho_i(\Delta p_i) = (\ln 2 + [0.5 - \Delta p_i] \ln[0.5 - \Delta p_i] + [0.5 + \Delta p_i] \ln[0.5 + \Delta p_i]) / \ln 2$. Then, we realize that the synchronization indices attain their minimum, $\rho_i = 0$, for the equiprobability distributions $p_i(+) = p_i(-) = 0.5 \Rightarrow \Delta p_i = 0$. Furthermore, ρ_i increases monotonically as a function of Δp_i because $d\rho_i / d\Delta p_i = -\ln[(0.5 - \Delta p_i) / (0.5 + \Delta p_i)] / \ln 2 > 0$ for $0 < \Delta p_i < 0.5$. As a result, the synchronization index maps that we obtain by plotting $\rho_i[p_i(+)]$ agree qualitatively with the PSV maps shown in figures 15.8 and 15.9. Since the indices ρ_i yield the same values for $p_i(+) = 0.5 + \epsilon$ and $p_i(+) = 0.5 - \epsilon$, however, the black domains in figures 15.8 and 15.9 appear white in the synchronization index maps. Hence, synchronization index maps merely facilitate the discrimination between white domains indicating phase synchronization and gray regions indicating a lack of phase synchronization. They cannot be used to distinguish different types of phase synchronization. In particular, they cannot be used to uncover the polarity domains described by the black and white regions in figures 15.8 and 15.9.

Spatiotemporal Analysis: Transitions

As transitions only occurred in experiment 2, the following analysis concentrates on the data obtained for subject D.

Analysis of a Single Sensor

As stated in the introduction, variations in environmental conditions can induce unintended transitions between characteristic patterns of movement. Consequently, investigating the effects of parameter variations can lead to insights into the dynamic organization of human systems for motor control. In experiment 2, parameter changes were effected by a gradual increase or decrease in the pacing frequency, as has been done in other studies on paced rhythmic finger movements and accompanying brain activity (Kelso et al., 1990, 1992; Wallenstein et al., 1995). In the case of the Julliard experiment (blocks I and II), shifts of the Fourier phases ϕ_i^{MEG} by about 180° accompanied by unintended transitions from antiphase to in-phase finger movements were observed at critical frequencies in the range of 1.6 to 2.0 Hz (Daffertshofer et al., 2000a; Frank et al., 2000). This coincidence of transitions at the behavioral and neural levels does not come as a surprise in view of the observation made in the earlier text on page 278 that phase differences calculated from brain signals and manual response signals are characterized by a large degree of phase locking irrespective of task conditions. The four panels in figure 15.11 illustrate the observed transitions at both the behavioral and neural levels. Using the horizontal midlines as reference, vertical lines pointing downward indicate acoustic stimuli whereas vertical lines pointing upward describe tapping sequences.

The upper two panels (a and b) describe control block III, in which in-phase finger movements were performed from the beginning and pacing frequency was increased. The left and right panels show low-frequency (1.2 Hz) and high-frequency (3.0 Hz) plateaus, respectively. Obviously, the task requirements are met, as the tapping sequence coincides with the stimulus trains. The lower two panels (c and d) are drawn from data of the Julliard block II, when antiphase movements were performed while the pacing frequency was increased. Left

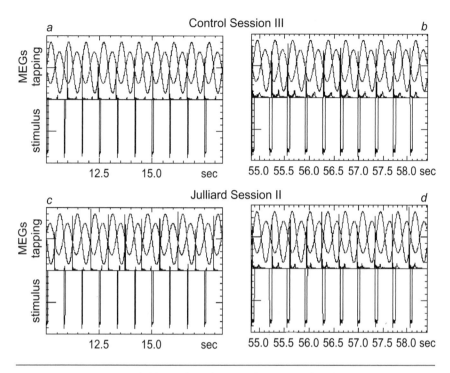

FIGURE 15.11   Sinusoidal lines describe neural activity related to movement as recorded in experiment 2 by two representative MEG sensors located in the black (solid line) and white (dotted line) polarity domains. Vertical lines represent the stimulus trains (lower halves) and tapping sequences (upper halves), with peaks indicating the moments that the switch was hit by the finger tip. Panels a and b (or c and d) show data obtained in the frequency plateaus 2 and 10 in one representative trial of the control session performed in block III (or Julliard session II).

and right panels again show low-frequency (1.2 Hz) and high-frequency (3.0 Hz) plateaus. At low frequencies, task instructions are obeyed (the taps occur between subsequent stimuli), but at high pacing frequencies task requirements are violated and in-phase movements are performed. The transitions of the Fourier phases ϕ_i^{MEG} describing oscillatory brain activity from ϕ_i^{MEG} to $\phi_i^{MEG} + \pi$ is illustrated by the sinusoidal lines in the upper halves of the panels. The oscillations with the smaller and larger amplitudes describe the oscillatory component relating to movement in the representative MEG signals of the white and black polarity domains, respectively. The oscillations are 180° out of phase and are locked with the tapping sequence (see panels c and d). Consequently, there is a change in the phases of the neural oscillations that have strong phase synchronization (corresponding to the white and black domains in figures 15.8 and 15.9) by about 180° (when compared to the stimulus) that coincides with the transition from antiphase to in-phase finger movements.

Analysis of Polarity Domains

In addition to analyzing a single sensor, we were interested in studying the overall behavior of the brain activity recorded over the two polarity domains. Relative phases were computed from MEG signals and the acoustic stimulus because the phase of the acoustic stimulus ϕ_{stim} had been fixed due to the experimental setup (see also figure 15.10). Phases of MEG signals were again expressed in terms of the Fourier phases associated with the respective tapping frequencies. For subject D, tapping frequencies coincided with the pacing frequencies (see figure 15.3). Since the issue was how phase distributions change due to variations of pacing frequency, we could not simply collapse data from different frequency plateaus, as doing so decreases the number of available data points. In order to compensate for this loss of data points, time-dependent Fourier analysis was employed instead of the time-independent Fourier analysis used in the preceding investigations. More precisely, a moving window Fourier analysis (Fuchs et al., 1992; Feige et al., 1996; Gross et al., 2000; Leocani et al., 1997; Newell et al., 1997) was applied to each MEG signal i. The basic idea of a moving window Fourier analysis is to carry out a conventional Fourier analysis on a piece of the complete time series. This piece is defined by the length and position of a window function. The window is shifted continuously along the time series, and at each new position a Fourier analysis is performed. For our purposes, a window length of two interstimulus intervals was used. Let ISI denote the length of an interstimulus interval. For frequency plateaus with N data points composed of interstimulus intervals with $ISI = N / 10$ data points, $N{-}2 \times ISI$ time-dependent Fourier phases $\phi_i^{MEG, window}$ and relative phases $\phi_i^{MEG\text{-}S, window} = \phi_i^{MEG, window} - \phi_{stim}$ were derived for all valid trials M and each session s.

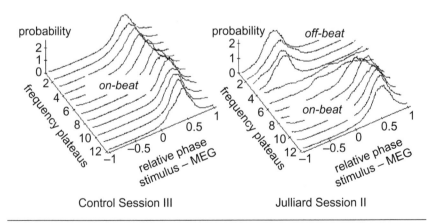

Control Session III   Julliard Session II

FIGURE 15.12   Phase distributions obtained in blocks II (right panel) and III (left panel) of experiment 2 as functions of pacing frequency (frequency plateaus).

Reprinted from *Physica D*, vol. 144, T.D. Frank, A. Daffertshofer, C.E. Peper, P.J. Beek, and H. Haken, Towards a comprehensive theory of brain activity: coupled oscillator systems under external forces, pgs. 62-86, Copyright 2000, with permission from Elsevier.

The relative phases $\phi_i^{MEG-S, window}$ of the cortical sites i belonging to either of the two domains of strong phase synchronization were pooled into two data sets. Using these data sets, probability densities $P_{MEG-S, window}(\phi)$ were computed for each plateau m (and session s) and for both polarity domains that describe the probability of finding a relative phase $\phi_{MEG-S, window}$. Figure 15.12 depicts these probability densities $P_{MEG-S, window}(\phi)$ related to the brain activity recorded over the white domains. The probability densities are shown in figure 15.7 for the control experiment III (in-phase tapping and frequency increase) and the Julliard session II (intended antiphase tapping and frequency increase).

Similar diagrams can be obtained for the probability densities $P_{MEG-S, window}$ describing brain activity recorded over the black domains in figure 15.9 (Frank et al., 2000).

Dominance of Descending Neural Activity

We discussed characteristic features of brain activity related to a pacing signal and descending and ascending brain activity related to movement (see p. 280 ; these characteristics were summarized in figure 15.2). Comparing figure 15.2 with the experimental findings depicted in figure 15.12, we can determine functional properties of the neural activities recorded in our experiments. If brain activity were dominated by contributions of the auditory system, the evolution of the probability densities obtained for the Julliard experiments would not exhibit a shift by 180° in the transition region. From figure 15.12 we can appreciate that there is indeed a shift of brain activity by about 180°. It can be shown that this shift corresponds to an unintended switch from antiphase to in-phase patterns of movement (Daffertshofer et al., 2000a; Frank et al.; 2000). Therefore, we are inclined to say that there is at most a minor contribution of the brain activity related to the stimulus to the measured brain activity. This conclusion is in line with the previous observation (see figures 15.4 and 15.5) that neural activity is first and foremost phase locked with the manual behavior. Significant contributions of ascending neural activity to the overall observed brain activity would result in systematic shifts of the probability densities from frequency plateau to frequency plateau as illustrated schematically in figure 15.2. In addition, in the low-frequency region, relative phases of ascending neural activity related to movement would be centered in the range of 10° to 50°. The phase distributions obtained in our experiment for the low-frequency regime, however, do not show peaks between 10° and 50°, and they do not show unidirectional trends as movement frequency is scaled from 1 to 3.2 Hz. Therefore, we are also inclined to say that ascending neural activity provides a minor contribution to the overall brain activity observed in our experiments. The evolution of the phase distributions shown in figure 15.12 qualitatively resembles the evolution of the phase distributions related to descending neural activity (see figure 15.2). In addition, the most probable values are found at phase differences of about ±90°, just as descending neural activity is assumed to be shifted by about ±90°

with respect to the pacing signal in the case of in- and antiphase movements (provided that the timing of the actual taps is adequate) (see also figure 15.1 in Frank et al., 2000). In recognition of these findings, we propose that the brain activity recorded for subject D during paced finger movements primarily reflects descending neural activity. Moreover, since the phase distributions (describing the relationship between the MEG and the taps) obtained in experiment 1 for self-paced movements display peaks at about ±90°, and the PSV maps reveal similar characteristic structures for paced and self-paced movements (see figures 15.8 and 15.9), we propose that the brain signals recorded from subjects A and B primarily reflect descending neural activity as well.

Phase Synchronization and Mean-Field Forces

The phase distributions of the overall brain activity related to movement shown in figure 15.5 differ from uniform distributions and reveal coherent regions of low and high probability. In line with the dynamic systems approach discussed in the introduction, the emergence of regions of high probability suggests that there is phase synchronization of the neural activity involved in performing the rhythmic finger movements. Using PSV maps, we explained the bimodality of the phase distributions in terms of the bipolarity of neural activity and identified domains of unique polarity (see figures 15.8 and 15.9). Within each polarity domain, neural activity seems to be phase synchronized with unique attractors (see figures 15.7 and 15.10) defined by relative phases between manual response and neural activity of either +90° or −90°. According to the mean-field theory, these attractors are self-organized and result from the collective interaction of their constituents. Consequently, we propose that the phase synchronization observed during rhythmic movements is due to the interaction of distributed neural activity and, in particular, to the emergence of mean-field forces entraining local oscillatory neural subsystems. Whereas in a previous study (Frank et al., 2000) this suggestion was formulated for paced movements, the findings reported here suggest that neural mean-field forces are also involved in the control of self-paced movements.

Connectivity Maps

The relevance of the maps depicted in figures 15.8 and 15.9 for our understanding of systems for human motor control is at least twofold. First, they provide an analytical tool for investigating the phase synchronization of global neural activity related to rhythmic coordinated movements. This tool is based on the variability in the relative phase dynamics of local neural activity. Second, these maps may be interpreted as layouts of cortical circuitry. According to the mean-field theory, the domains of phase synchronization observed in the experiments reported here result from couplings within and between polarity domains. Phase synchronization within a polarity domain is assumed to result from attractive couplings between cortical sites of that domain. In contrast, the observation of two clusters of phase synchronization oscillating 180° out of phase suggests that there are repulsive couplings between cortical sites belonging to different polarity domains. Furthermore, in line with our earlier suggestion that in our experiments the measured neural activity is dominated by descending cortical activity, the maps shown in figures 15.8 and 15.9 may be interpreted as task-specific connectivity maps of the efferent neural system of motor control. That is, they putatively describe for the efferent system the positions of terminals of neural pathways as well as the strength ($|p_i(+) - 0.5|$) and character (attractive or repulsive) of the effect of these terminals.

Mean-Field Haken-Kelso-Bunz Model

A stochastic theory of rhythmic finger movements is directed at understanding the variability of performance and neural activity observed during the movements. In the context of the Julliard experiment, such a theory has been developed by Schöner et al. (1986) and has been extended in several studies (Daffertshofer et al., 1999; Frank et al., 1999; Fuchs and Jirsa, 2000). These works employ stochastic descriptions in terms of Langevin equations and Fokker-Planck equations. Langevin equations can be regarded as ordinary differential equations supplemented with an element of randomness: a fluctuation, or Langevin force. In contrast, Fokker-Planck equations are diffusion equations that describe the evolution of probability densities. To model the phase synchronization in the assumed ensembles of neural oscillators in the polarity domains shown in figures 15.8 and 15.9, the stochastic model by Schöner et al. (1986) has been extended by a mean-field force (Frank et al., 2000, 2001b). Let us consider an ensemble of neural oscillators described by the phases $\phi_j(t)$ with $j = 1, \ldots, N$ in the limit of a large system size (i.e., for $N \to \infty$). Then, the phase dynamics of a representative member of the ensemble, say the neural oscillator i, is given by

$$d\phi_i(t) / dt = -dV_{\text{HKB,a,b}}(\phi_i) / d\phi_i - dV_{\text{MF,K}}(\phi_i) / d\phi_i + \Gamma(t), \tag{15.6}$$

where $\Gamma(t)$ corresponds to a delta-correlated fluctuation force with $< \Gamma(t)\,\Gamma(t') > = Q\,\delta(t - t')$ (Risken, 1989), and $Q > 0$ denotes the strength of that fluctuation force. The potential $V_{\text{HKB, a, b}}$ is the Haken-Kelso-Bunz (HKB) potential (Haken et al., 1985) involving the parameters $a \geq 0$ and $b \geq 0$ and inducing the force $h_{\text{HKB, a, b}} = -dV_{\text{HKB, a, b}} / d\phi_i$ that acts on the oscillator i.. The potential $V_{\text{MF,K}}$ describes the collective impact of the oscillator ensemble on the oscillator i and is defined by $V_{\text{MF,K}} = -N^{-1} K \Sigma_{i=1, ,N} \Sigma_{j=1, ,N} \cos(\phi_i - \phi_j)$, where $K \geq 0$ is a measure for the strength of the couplings between the oscillators. Obviously, this potential attains its minimum for the complete synchronization of the ensemble, that is, for $\phi_j = \phi^*$ with $j=1, ,N$. Therefore, the potential $V_{\text{MF,K}}$

supports a synchronization of coupled oscillator ensembles and is assumed to play an essential role in the theory of phase synchronization (Gerstner and van Hemmen, 1994; Kuramoto, 1984, 1997; Strogatz and Stewart, 1993; Strogatz, 2000; Tass, 1999, 2000)., In particular, $V_{MF,K}$ defines the coupling force $h_{MF,K}$=-$dV_{MF,K} / d\phi_i = -N^{-1} K \Sigma_{j=1, ,N} \sin(\phi_i - \phi_j)$, proposed by (Kuramoto, 1975, 1981, 1984), which is a typical example of a mean-field force that can emerge in an ensemble of interacting subsystems (see page 274). As stated earlier, mean-field forces can be determined in the limit of large system sizes (i.e., for $N \rightarrow \infty$) by means of the mean field approximation. Accordingly, the material ensemble of oscillators $j=1,. . .,N$ is replaced by a statistical ensemble of a representative oscillator ϕ leading to the mean field force $h_{MF,K}(\phi) \rightarrow h_{MF,K}(\phi)=-K < \sin(\phi - x)$ $>x$ (where the average $<. . .>$ is computed with respect to the variable x) and the stochastic phase dynamics.

$$d\phi(t) / dt = h_{HKB,a,b}(\phi) + h_{MF,K}(\phi) + \Gamma(t). \tag{15.7}$$

The evolution equation (15.7) has been studied through the corresponding Fokker-Planck equation (Frank et al., 2000, 2001b; Frank, 2001b). It has been shown that the mean-field force $h_{MF, K}(\phi)$ indeed results in the kind of phase synchronization observed in our experiments. In particular, the 3-D parameter space spanned by the appropriately rescaled parameters a', e, and K' (where $a' = a / Q$, $e = 4b / a$, and $K' = K / Q$) can be divided into two subspaces (see the upper panel of figure 15.13). For parameter values chosen from one of these subspaces, the model exhibits two stationary probability densities that correspond to the phase distributions in the low-frequency regime (plateaus 1 to 3) related to the in-phase (on-beat) and antiphase (offbeat) movements shown in the left and right panels of figure 15.12. For parameter values in the other subspace, the model admits only one stationary phase distribution. This distribution corresponds to the phase distributions observed in the high-frequency regime (plateaus 7 to 12 of figure 15.12) of the Julliard experiment. Consequently, the characteristic 180° shift of phase distribution that is observed in the Julliard experiment (shown in the right panel of figure 15.12) can be modeled as a nonequilibrium phase transition of the mean-field HKB model. This nonequilibrium phase transition is induced by a change of the model parameters such that they pass the surface separating the monostable and bistable subspaces shown in the upper panel of figure 15.13. The result of a simulation of the mean-field HKB model is shown in the lower panel of figure 15.13. The parameter e was gradually decreased, whereas the parameters a' and K' were fixed. The fixed parameters a' and K' and the initial value of e were chosen so that by decreasing e, the threshold surface was traversed from the bistable to the monostable subspace. The statistical ensemble for ϕ was initially distributed according to a noisy bell-shaped distribution centered at 180° (see *initial* in the lower panel of figure 15.13). That is, the system was initially prepared close to that stochastic state which exists only in the bistable regime and describes neural activity related to offbeat finger movements.

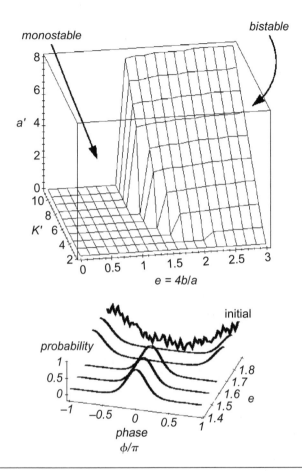

FIGURE 15.13   In the upper panel, the 3-D parameter space of the mean-field HKB model given by equation 15.6 is composed of two subspaces that describe a model with one (monostable) and two (bistable) stationary phase distributions. The lower panel shows a simulation of the model that mimics the transition observed in experiment 2 (see the right panel of figure 15.12).

Reprinted from *Physica D*, vol. 144, T.D. Frank, A. Daffertshofer, C.E. Peper, P.J. Beek, and H. Haken, Towards a comprehensive theory of brain activity: coupled oscillator systems under external forces, pgs. 62-86, Copyright 2000, with permission from Elsevier.

Implications for the Dynamic Systems Approach

In large systems subjected to noise and composed of many similar constituents, mean-field forces can emerge due to self-organization. The emergence of such a collective force in a system implies that (a) the degrees of freedom of that system are considerably reduced and (b) the variability of the system (accuracy) can be reduced (increased) without an external force. Consequently, experimental studies on the variability in distributed systems of motor control will certainly provide further hints for the presence of mean-field forces and may reveal structural organization principles. In theoretical studies, one should consider that mean-field forces can account for the reduced degrees of freedom of a large complex system with homogeneous characteristic timescales just as order parameters can account for the reduced degrees of freedom of a highly dimensional complex system with inhomogeneous characteristic timescales. While in the first case, the degrees of freedom are reduced to those of a single representative system described by a mean-field model, in the second case, the degrees of freedom are reduced to those of a low-dimensional system describing the dynamics of a few order parameters.

Outlook

It has been argued that the brain activity recorded in our experiments primarily reflects descending neural activity of the neural efferent system for motor control involved in rhythmic finger movements. Therefore, the next step is to investigate other kinds of neural activity in more detail and, in particular, to study neural activity related to stimulus and ascending neural activity related to movement. To study the neural activity related to the pacing signal, encephalographic recordings from both paced and self-paced rhythmic movements have been compared (Gerloff et al., 1997, 1998). In line with such studies, future research may compare synchronization and continuation as performed in experiment 1. Experiments in which subjects listen to the acoustic pacing signal without moving (not reported here) can provide information about the phase relationship between the stimulus and the brain activity related to the stimulus. For example, ascending neural activity originating from the proprioceptive system and the tactile sensory system can be examined in the context of paced finger movements when pacing frequency is varied (see figure 15.2). The fact that in our case study (experiment 2) ascending neural activity could not be extracted from the phase distributions describing the overall measured brain activity may not generalize to other subjects. Therefore, similar experiments involving more subjects have to be carried out and analyzed. However, ascending neural activity can also be analyzed when corresponding components in phase distributions of neural activity related to movement cannot be observed. One may evaluate the averaged waveforms of encephalographic data as discussed earlier on page 282 (see also figure 15.3).

Phase synchronization has been interpreted as an indicator of mean-field forces. Apparently, there are alternative mechanisms leading to phase synchronization in encephalographic signals. For example, long-distance fields (far fields) of dipole sources and long-distance effects of subcortical structures can result in the phase synchronization of encephalographic signals. However, in view of several studies involving intracranial measurements in which synchronization among distal cortical sites was observed (see page 278) , the dipole hypothesis is less likely to account for the synchronization observed in our experiments. The possibility of long-distance effects of subcortical structures, in contrast, cannot be ruled out on the basis of the analysis presented in this chapter. Therefore, future investigations might test the mean-field hypothesis against the hypothesis that subcortical oscillators drive neocortical areas. In particular, spatially distributed cortical structures driven by a single subcortical oscillator should reveal common random temporal patterns, namely, the fluctuations to which the subcortical oscillator is subjected. In contrast, distributed neural activity that is self-organized due to the effect of mean-field forces does not necessarily exhibit such common random patterns. Further indications for the relevance of mean-field forces in human motor control may be derived by comparing predictions of mean-field models and models without mean-field forces with experimental findings (see Frank, 2000, section 6.2).

According to the mean-field HKB model presented earlier (see page 301), there are two forces involved in the transition from antiphase to in-phase movements: the drift force related to the HKB potential and the (Kuramoto) mean-field coupling force. While the HKB drift force describes the coupling of the motor control system involved in paced rhythmic movements with respect to the pacing signal, the mean-field coupling force describes the couplings between distributed cortical sites. Consequently, the model offers two opposing explanations of the basic mechanism of transition between antiphase and in-phase patterns of movement: the transition may be induced by parameter changes exclusively affecting the HKB drift force (i.e., changes of the parameters a and b) or the mean-field force (i.e., changes of the parameter K). In principle, predictions regarding these two mechanisms can be derived from the mean-field HKB model and compared with experimental findings. In doing so, the relevance of external couplings (couplings to pacing signals) and internal couplings (couplings between task-related but distributed internal subsystems) involved in paced rhythmic movements can be addressed (at least in the context of the mean-field HKB model).

Finally, we would like to return to the issue of synchronization. As stated earlier, we can distinguish between synchronization in terms of coherency and phase synchronization. The focus in this chapter was on phase synchronization. This is not to imply that the amplitude of neural activity is irrelevant for human motor control. Therefore, future research may concentrate on the role of amplitude effects for synchronized brain activity related to movement. For example, analytical tools dependent on and independent of amplitude may be applied simultaneously (see table 15.1), and conclusions may be drawn by comparing the results thus obtained.

References

Abernethy, B. (1987). Selective attention in fast ball sports II: Expert-novice differences. *Australian Journal of Science and Medicine in Sport, 19*, 7-16.

Abernethy, B. (1990). Anticipation in squash: Differences in advance cue utilization between expert and novice players. *Journal of Sports Sciences, 8*, 17-34.

Abernethy, B. (1991). Visual search strategies and decision-making in sport. *International Journal of Sport Psychology, 22*, 189-210.

Abernethy, B., and Russell, D.G. (1984). Advance cue utilisation by skilled cricket batsmen. *Australian Journal of Science and Medicine in Sport, 16*, 2-10.

Abernethy, B., and Russell D.G. (1987). The relationship between expertise and visual search strategy in a racquet sport. *Human Movement Science, 6*, 283-319.

Adolph, K.E., Eppler, M.A., and Gibson, E.J. (1993). Development of perception of affordances. In C. Rovee-Collier and L.P. Lipsitt (Eds.), *Advances in Infancy Research* (Vol. 8, pp. 51-89). Norwood, NJ: Ablex.

Adolph, K.E., Vereijken, B., and Denny, M.A. (1998). Experience related changes in development of crawling. *Child Development, 69*, 1299-1312.

Alderson, G.J.K., Sully, D.J., and Sully, H.G. (1974). An operational analysis of a one-handed catching task using high speed photography. *Journal of Motor Behavior, 6*, 217-226.

Alexander, R.McN. (1984). Walking and running. *American Scientist, 72*, 348-354.

Alexander, R.McN. (1989). Optimization and gaits in the locomotion of vertebrates. *Physiological Reviews, 69*, 1199-1227.

Allard, F., and Starkes, J.L. (1980). Perception in sport: Volleyball. *Journal of Sport Psychology, 2*, 22-33.

Allard, P., Stokes, I.A.F., and Blanchi, J-P. (1995). *Three-dimensional analysis of human movement.* Champaign, IL: Human Kinetics.

Allum, J.H.J., Honegger, F., and Schicks, H. (1993). Vestibular and proprioceptive modulation of postural synergies in normal subjects. *Journal of Vestibular Research, 3*, 59-85.

Alvarez, R., Terrados, N., Ortolano, R., Iglesias-Cubero, G., Reguero, J.R., Batalla, A., Cortina, A., Fernandez-Garcia, B., Rodriguez, C., Braga, S., Alvarez, V. and Coto, E. (2000). Genetic variation in the renin-angiotensin system and athletic performance. *European Journal of Applied Physiology, 82*, 117-120.

Amazeen, P.G., Amazeen, E., Turvey, M.T. (1998). Dynamics of human intersegmental coordination: Theory and research. In D.A. Rosenbaum and C.E. Collyer (Eds.), *Timing of behaviour* (pp. 237-259). Cambridge, MA: MIT Press.

Amblard, B., Assaiante, C., Lekhel, H., and Marchand, A.R. (1994). A statistical approach to sensorimotor strategies: conjugate cross-correlations. *Journal of Motor Behavior, 26*, 103-112.

Anderson, D.I., and Sidaway, B. (1994). Coordination changes associated with practice of a soccer kick. *Research Quarterly for Exercise and Sport, 69*, 93-99.

Anderson, M., and Pitcairn, T. (1986). Motor control in dart throwing. *Human Movement Science, 5,* 1-18.

Andrew, C., and Pfurtscheller, G., (1996). Event-related coherence as a tool for studying dynamic interaction of brain regions. *Electroenceph. Clin. Neurophysiol. 98,* 144-148.

Arellano, R. and Pardillo, S. (1992). An evaluation of changes in the crawl-stroke technique during training periods in a swimming season. In *Biomechanics and Medicine in Swimming – Swimming Science VI* (edited by D. MacLaren, T. Reilly and A. Lees), pp. 143-149. London: EandFN Spon.

Armbruster, D.A., and Morehouse, L.M. (1950). *Swimming and diving.* St. Louis: Mosby.

Arutyunyan, G.H., Gurfinkel, V.S., and Mirskii, M.L. (1968). Investigation of aiming at a target. *Biophysics, 13,* 536-538.

Arutyunyan, G.H., Gurfinkel, V.S., and Mirskii, M.L. (1969). Organisation of movements on execution by man of exact postural task. *Biophysics, 14,* 1162-1167.

Atkinson, G., and Speirs, L. (1998). Diurnal variation in tennis service. *Perceptual and Motor Skills, 86,* 1335-1338.

Attneave, F. (1959). *Applications of information to psychology.* New York: Holt.

Bak, P. (1996). *How nature works: The science of self-organized criticality.* New York: Springer-Verlag.

Baker J. (2003). Early specialization in youth sport: A requirement for adult expertise? *High Ability Studies, 14,* 85-94.

Baker, J., Côté, J., and Abernethy, B. (2003a). Sport-specific training, deliberate practice and the development of expertise in team ball sports. *Journal of Applied Sport Psychology, 15,* 12-25.

Baker, J., Côté, J., and Abernethy, B. (2003b). Learning from the experts: Practice activities of expert decision-makers in sport. *Research Quarterly for Exercise and Sport, 74,* 342-347.

Baker, J., Deakin, J., and Côté, J. (2005). Expertise in ultra-endurance triathletes: Early sport involvement, training structure, and the theory of deliberate practice. *Journal of Applied Sport Psychology, 17,* 1-15.

Balasubramaniam, R., Riley, M.A., and Turvey, M.T. (2000). Specificity of postural sway to the demands of a precision task. *Gait Posture, 11,* 12-24.

Balasubramaniam, R., and Wing, A.M. (2002). The dynamics of standing balance. *Trends in Cognitive Science, 6,* 531-536.

Banuelos, F.S. (1976, July). Loss of precision in aim throwing due to the increase of speed of throwing. *Proceedings—International Congress on Physical Activity Sciences, Quebec City, 7,* 121-125.

Bardy, B.G. (2004). Postural coordination dynamics in standing humans. In V.K. Jirsa and J.A.S. Kelso (Eds.), *Coordination Dynamics: Issues and Trends,* Vol.1 *Applied Complex Systems* (pp. 103-121). New York: Springer Verlag.

Bardy, B.G., Faugloire, E., and Fourcade, P. (in press). Changes in postural patterns with learning and expertise. In M. Latash and F. Lestienne (Eds.), *Progress in Motor Control IV.* Springer Verlag, in press.

Bardy, B.G., and Laurent, M. (1998). How is body orientation controlled during somersaulting? *Journal of Experimental Psychology: Human Perception and Performance, 24,* 963-977.

Bardy, B.G., Marin, L., Stoffregen, T.A., and Bootsma, R.J. (1999). Postural coordination modes considered as emergent phenomena. *Journal of Experimental Psychology: Human Perception and Performance, 25,* 1284-1301.

Bardy, B.G., Oullier, O., Bootsma, R.J., and Stoffregen, T.A. (2002). Dynamics of human postural transitions. *Journal of Experimental Psychology: Human Perception and Performance, 28,* 499-514.

Bardy, B.G., Warren, W.H.J., and Kay, B.A. (1996). Motion parallax is used to control postural sway during walking. *Experimental Brain Research, 111,* 271-282.

Barnard, R.J., Edgerton, V.R., Furukava, T., and Peter, J.B., (1971). Histochemical, biochemical and contractile properties of red, white and intermediate fibers. *Am. J. Physiol., 220,* 410-414.

Barrie, J.M., Freeman, W.J., and Lenhart, M. (1996). Modulation by discriminative training of spatial patterns of gamma EEG amplitude and phase in neocortex of rabbits. *Journal of Neurophysiology, 76,* 520-539.

Barsh, G.S., Farooqi, I.S., and O'Rahilly, S. (2000). Genetics of body-weight regulation. *Nature, 404,* 644-651.

Bartlett, R.M. (1997). Current issues in the mechanics of athletic activities: a position paper. *Journal of Biomechanics, 30,* 477-486.

Bartlett, R.M. (1999). *Sports biomechanics: Reducing injury and improving performance.* London: E and FN Spon.

Basar, E. (Ed.). (1990). *Chaos in brain function.* New York: Springer-Verlag.

Bassingthwaighte, J.B., Liebovitch, L.S., West, B.J. (1994). *Fractal physiology.* Oxford, UK: Oxford University Press.

Bates, B.T. (1996). Single-subject methodology: an alternative approach. *Medicine and Science in Sports and Exercise, 28,* 631-638.

Bates, B.T., James, S.L., and Osternig, L.R. (1978). Foot function during the support phase of running. *Running, 3,* 24-29.

Bates, B.T., Zhang, S., Dufek, J.S., and Chen, F.C. (1996). The effects of sample size and variability on the correlation coefficient. *Medicine and Science in Sports and Exercise, 28,* 386-391.

Batschelet, E. (1981). *Circular statistics in biology.* London: Academic Press.

Bauer, H.U., and Schöllhorn, W. (1997). Self-organizing maps for the analysis of complex movement patterns. *Neural Processing Letters, 5,* 193-199.

Baumann, W. (1981). Application of biomechanics research to sport. In H. Matsui and K. Kobayashi (Eds.), *Biomechanics VIII-B* (pp. 722-734). Champaign, IL: Human Kinetics.

Baumann, W. (1987). Biomechanics of sports—current problems. In G. Bergmann, R. Kolbel, and A. Rohlmann (Eds.), *Biomechanics: Basic and applied research* (pp. 51-58). Lancaster, UK: Academic Publishers.

Baumann, W. (1989). Methodological approach to study of sports biomechanics. *Proceedings of the 1st IOC World Congress on Sport Sciences, Colorado Springs,* 244-248.

Baumann, W. (1992). Perspectives in methodology in biomechanics of sport. In R. Rodano, G. Ferrigno, and G. Santambrogio (Eds.), *Proceedings of the 5th Symposium of the International Society of Biomechanics in Sports* (pp. 97-104). Milan: Edi Ermes.

Bawa, P., Binder, M.D., Ruenzel, P., and Henneman, E. (1984). Recruitment order of motoneurons in stretch reflexes is highly correlated with their axonal conduction velocity. *J. Neurophysiol., 52*(3), 410-420.

Becker, W.J, Kunesch, E., and Freund, H-J. (1990). Coordination of a multi-joint movement in normal humans and in patients with cerebellar dysfunction. *Canadian Journal of Neurological Science, 17,* 264-274.

Beek, P.J., Peper, C.E., and Stegeman, D.F. (1995). Dynamical models of movement coordination. *Human Movement Science, 14,* 573-608.

Beek, P.J., Rikkert, W.E.I., and van Wieringen, P.C.W. (1996). Limit cycle properties of rhythmic forearm movements. *Journal of Experimental Psychology: Human Perception and Performance, 22,* 1077-1093.

Beek, P.J., and Van Santvoord, A.A.M. (1992). Learning the cascade juggle: a dynamical systems analysis. *Journal of Motor Behaviour, 24,* 85-94.

Belkin, D.S., and Eliot, J.F. (1997). Motor skill acquisition and the speed-accuracy trade-off in a field based task. *Journal of Sport Behavior, March,* 16-28.

Bellew, J.W. (2002). The effect of strength training on control of force in older men and women. *Aging (Milano), 14*(1), 35-41.

Beltrami, E. (1999). *What is random? Chance and order in mathematics and life.* New York: Copernicus.

Bernstein, N. (1967). *The co-ordination and regulation of movement.* Elmsford, NY: Pergamon Press.

Berthier, N.E., Rosenstein, M.T. and Barto, A.G. (2005). Approximate optimal control as a model for motor learning. *Psychological Review 112,* 329-346.

Berthoz, A. (2000). *The brain's sense of movement.* Cambridge, MA: Harvard University Press.

Beuter, A., Flashner, H. and Arabyan, A. (1986). Phase plane modeling of leg motion. *Biological Cybernetics, 53,* 273-284.

Bhattacharya, J. and Petsche, H. (2001). Enhanced phase synchrony in the electroencephalography gamma band for musicians while listening to music. *Phys. Rev. E, 64,* 012902.

Bober, T. (1981). Biomechanical aspects of sports techniques. In A. Morecki, K. Fidelus, K. Kedzior, and A. Wit (Eds.), *Biomechanics VII* (pp. 501-509). Baltimore: University Park Press.

Bonilla, L.L. (1987). Stable nonequilibrium probability densities and phase transitions for mean-field models in the thermodynamic limit. *J. Stat. Phys. 46,* 659-678.

Bonnard, M., Pailhous, J., and Danion, F. (1997). Intentional on-line adaptation of rhythmic movements during a hyper- to microgravity change. *Motor Control, 1,* 247-262.

Bottinelli, R., Betto, R., Schiaffino, S. and Reggiani, C. (1994). Unloaded shortening velocity and myosin heavy chain and alkali light chain isoform composition in rat skeletal muscle fibres. *J. Physiol. 478,* 341-349.

Bottinelli, R., Canepari, M., Pellegrino, M.A., and Reggiani, C. (1996). Force-velocity properties of human skeletal muscle fibres: Myosin heavy chain isoform and temperature dependence. *J. Physiol. (Lond.), 495,* 573-586.

Bottinelli, R., Coviello, D.A., Redwood, C.S., Pellegrino, M.A., Maron, B.J., Spirito, P., Watkins, H., and Reggiani, C. (1998). A mutant tropomyosin that causes hypertrophic cardiomyopathy is expressed in vivo and associated with an increased calcium sensitivity [see comments]. *Circ. Res., 82,* 106-115.

Bottinelli, R., and Reggiani, C. (2000). Human skeletal muscle fibres: molecular and functional diversity. *Progr. Biophys. Mol. Biol., 73,* 195-262.

Bottinelli, R., Schiaffino, S., and Reggiani, C. (1991). Force-velocity relations and myosin heavy chain isoform compositions of skinned fibres from rat skeletal muscle. *J. Physiol., 437,* 655-672.

Bouchard C., Daw E.W., Rice T., Pérusse L., Gagnon J., Province M.A., Leon A.S., Rao D.C., Skinner J.S., Wilmore J.H.. (1998). Familial resemblance for $\dot{V}O_2$ max in the sendentary state: The HERITAGE family study. *Medicine and Science in Sports and Exercise, 30,* 252-258.

Bouchard, T.J. (1997). IQ similarity in twins reared apart: Findings and responses to critics. In R.J. Sternberg and E. Grigorenko (Eds.), *Intelligence, heredity, and environment* (pp.126-162). Cambridge, MA: Cambridge University Press.

Breitbart, R.E. and Nadal-Ginard, B. (1986). Complete nucleotide sequence of the fast skeletal troponin T gene. Alternatively spliced exons exhibit unusual interspecies divergence. *J. Mol. Biol. 188*(3), 313-324.

Breitbart, R.E., and Nadal-Ginard, B. (1987). Developmentally induced, muscle-specific trans factors control the differential splicing of alternative and constitutive troponin T exons. *Cell., 49*(6), 793-803.

Bressler, S.L., Coppola, R., Nakamura, R. (1993). Episodic multiregional cortical coherence at multiple frequencies during visual task performance. *Nature, 366,* 153-156.

Bretag, A.H. (1987). Muscle chloride channels. *Physiol. Rev., 67*(2), 618-724.

Brisson, T.A., and Alain, C. (1996). Should common optimal movement patterns be identified as the criterion to be achieved? *Journal of Motor Behavior, 28,* 211-223.

Broadbent, D.E. (1958). *Perception and communication.* New York: Pergamon Press.

Brooke, M.H., and Kaiser, K.K. (1970). Muscle fiber types: How many and what kind? *Arch. Neurol., 23*(4), 369-379.

Brooks, V.B. (1986). *The neural basis of motor control.* Oxford, UK: Oxford University Press.

Brown, R.M., and Counsilman, J.E. (1971). The role of lift in propelling swimmers. In J.M. Cooper (Ed.), *Biomechanics* (pp. 179-188). Chicago, IL: The Athletic Institute.

Buchanan, J.J., and Horak, F.B. (1999). Emergence of postural patterns as a function of vision and translation frequency. *Journal of Neurophysiology, 81,* 2325-2339.

Buchanan, J.J., and Horak, F.B. (2001). Transitions in a postural task: Do the recruitment and suppression of degrees of freedom stabilize posture? *Experimental Brain Research, 139,* 482-494.

Bunn, J.W. (1972). *Scientific principles of coaching* (2nd Ed.). Englewood Cliffs, NJ: Prentice Hall.

Burgess-Limerick, R., Abernethy, B., and Neal, R.J. (1991). Note: A statistical problem in testing invariance of movement using the phase plane model. *Journal of Motor Behavior, 23,* 301-303.

Burke, R.E., Levine, D.N., Tsairis, P., and Zajac, F.E. (1973). Physiological types and histochemical profiles in motor units of the cat gastrocnemius. *J. Physiol., 234,* 723-748.

Burke, R.E., Levine, D.N., and Zajac, F.E., (1971). Mammalian motor units: Physiological-histochemical correlation in three types in cat gastrocnemius. *Science, 174,* 709-712.

Burnett, R.A., Laidlaw, D.H., and Enoka, R.M. (2000). Coactivation of the antagonist muscle does not covary with steadiness in old adults. *Journal of Applied Physiology, 89*(1), 61-71.

Burton, A.W., and Davis, W.E. (1996). Ecological task analysis: Utilising intrinsic measures in research and practice. *Human Movement Science, 15,* 285-314.

Button, C. (2002). The effect of removing auditory information of ball projection on the coordination of one-handed ball catching. In K. Davids, G. Savelsbergh, S. Bennett, and J. van der Kamp (Eds.), *Interception actions in sport: Information and movement* (pp. 184-194). London: Taylor and Francis.

Button, C., Bennett, S.J., and Davids, K. (1998). Coordination dynamics of rhythmical and discrete prehension: Implications for the scanning procedure and individual differences. *Human Movement Science, 17*(6), 801-820.

Button, C., Macleod, M., Coleman, S., and Sanders, R. (2003). Examining movement variability in the throwing action at different skill levels. *Research Quarterly in Exercise and Sport.*

Calancie, B., and Bawa, P. (1990). Motor unit recruitment in humans. In M.D. Binder and L.M. Mendell (Eds.), *The segmental motor system* (pp. 75-95). New York: Oxford University Press.

Caldwell, J.H., Campbell, D.T., and Beam, K.G. (1986). Na channel distribution in vertebrate skeletal muscle. *J. Gen. Physiol., 87*(6), 907-932.

Calvin, W.H. (1983). A stone's throw and its launch window: Timing precision and its implication for language and hominid brains. *Journal of Theoretical Biology, 104,* 121-135.

Card, S.K., English, W.K., and Burr, B.J. (1978). Evaluation of mouse, rate-controlled isometric joystick, step keys, and text keys for text selection on CRT. *Ergonomics, 21,* 601-613.

Carlton, L.G., Kim K-H., Liu, Y-T., and Newell, K.M. (1993). Impulse variability in isometric tasks. *Journal of Motor Behavior, 25,* 33-43.

Carlton, L.G., and Newell, K.M. (1993). Force variability and characteristics of force production. In K.M. Newell and D.M. Corcos (Eds.), *Variability and motor control* (pp. 15-36). Champaign, IL: Human Kinetics.

Cartwright, N. (1989). *Nature's capacities and their measurement.* Oxford, UK: Clarendon Press.

Cauraugh, J.H., Gabert, T.E., and White, J.J. (1990). Tennis serving velocity and accuracy. *Perceptual and Motor Skills, 70,* 719-722.

Cavanagh, P.R. (1987). The biomechanics of lower extremity action in distance running. *Foot and Ankle, 7,* 197-217.

Cavanagh, P.R. (1989). Biomechanical studies of elite distance runners: Directions for future research. In J.S. Skinner, C.B. Corbin, D.M. Landers, P.E. Martin, and C.L. Wells (Eds.), *Future directions in exercise and sport science research* (pp. 163-179). Champaign, IL: Human Kinetics.

Cavanagh, P.R. (1990). Biomechanics: A bridge builder among the sport sciences. *Medicine and Science in Sports and Exercise, 22,* 546-557.

Cavanagh, P.R., and Hinrichs, R. (1981). Biomechanics of sport: The state of the art. In G.A. Brooks (Ed.), *Perspectives of the academic discipline of physical education* (pp. 137-157). Champaign, IL: Human Kinetics.

Chamberlin, C., and Lee, T. (1993). Arranging practice conditions and designing instruction. In R.N. Singer, M. Murphy, and L.K. Tennant (Eds.), *Handbook of research on sport psychology* (pp.213-241). New York: Macmillan.

Chanaud, C.M., Pratt, C.A., and Loeb, G.E. (1991). Functionally complex muscles of the cat hindlimb. V. The roles of histochemical fiber-type regionalization and mechanical heterogeneity in differential muscle activation. *Exp. Brain. Res., 85,* 300-313.

Charness, N., Krampe, R., and Myr, U. (1996). The role of practice and coaching in entrepreneurial skill domains: An international comparison of life-span chess skill acquisition. In K.A. Ericsson (Ed.), *The road to excellence: The acquisition of expert performance in the arts and sciences, sports and games* (pp. 51-80). Mahwah, NJ: Erlbaum.

Charteris, J. (1982). Human gait cyclograms: Conventions, speed relationships and clinical applications. *Journal of Rehabilitation Research, 5,* 507-518.

Chase, W.G., and Simon, H.A. (1973). Perception in chess. *Cognitive Psychology, 4,* 55-81.

Chatfield, C. (1984). *The analysis of time series* (3rd ed.). London: Chapman and Hall.

Chen, Y., Ding, M., and Kelso, J.A.S. (2001). Origins of timing errors in human sensorimotor coordination. *Journal of Motor Behavior, 33,* 3-8.

Cheyne, D., and Weinberg, H. (1989). Neuromagnetic fields accompanying unilateral finger movements: Pre-movement and movement-evoked fields. *Exp. Brain Res., 78,* 604-612.

Cheyne, D., Kristeva, R., Lang, W., Lindinger, G., and Deecke, L. (1989). Neuromagnetic localisation of sensorimotor cortex sources associated with voluntary movements in humans. In S.J. Williamson, M. Hoke, G. Stroink, and M. Kotani (Eds.), *Advances in biomagnetism* (pp. 177-180). New York: Plenum Press.

Chollet, D., Chalies, S. and Chatard, J.C. (2000). A new index of coordination for the crawl: description and usefulness. *International Journal of Sports Medicine, 21,* 54-59.

Chow, J.W., Carlton, L.G., Lim, Y-T., Chae W-S., Shim, J-H., Kuenster, A.F., and Kokubun, K. (in press). Comparing the pre-and post-impact ball and racquet kinematics of elite tennis players' first and second serves—A preliminary study. *Journal of Sport Sciences*.

Christou, E.A., and Carlton, L.G. (2001). Old adults exhibit greater motor output variability than young adults only during rapid discrete isometric contractions. *Journal of Gerontology A: Biol. Sci. Med. Sci., 56*(12), B524-532.

Christou, E.A., and Carlton, L.G. (2002). Age and contraction type influence motor output variability in rapid discrete tasks. *Journal of Applied Physiology, 93,* 489-499.

Christou, E.A., Grossman, M., and Carlton, L.G. (2002). Modeling variability of force during isometric contractions of the quadriceps femoris. *Journal of Motor Behavior, 34*(1), 67-81.

Christou, E.A., Shinohara, M., and Enoka, R.M. (2001, August). *The changes in EMG and steadiness with variation in movement speed differ for concentric and eccentric contractions.* Paper presented at the meeting of the Proceedings of the 25th Annual Meeting of the American Society of Biomechanics, San Diego, CA.

Christou, E.A., Shinohara, M. and Enoka, R.M. (2003). Force fluctuations impair accuracy during anisometric contractions performed by young and old adults. *Journal of Applied Physiology,* 95, 373-384.

Christou, E.A., Tracy, B.L., and Enoka, R.M. (2002). The steadiness of lengthening contractions. In M.L. Latash (Ed.), *Progress in motor control II* (pp. 195-207). Champaign, IL: Human Kinetics.

Christou, E.A., Yang, Y. and Rosengren, K. (2003). Taiji training improves knee extensor strength and force control in older adults. *Journal of Gerontology Series A: Biological Sciences and Medical Sciences 58,* 763-766.

Christova, P., and Kossev, A. (2000). Human motor unit activity during concentric and eccentric movements. *Electromyography and Clinical Neurophysiology, 40*(6), 331-338.

Clark, J.E. (1995). On becoming skillful: Patterns and constraints. *Research Quarterly for Exercise and Sport, 66,* 173-183.

Clark, J.E., and Phillips, S.J. (1993). A longitudinal study of intra-limb coordination in the first year of independent walking: A dynamical systems analysis. *Child Development, 64,* 1143-1157.

Clarke, T.E., Frederick, E.C., and Hamill, C. (1984). The study of rearfoot movement in running. In E.C. Frederick (Ed.), *Sports shoes and playing surfaces* (pp. 166-189). Champaign, IL: Human Kinetics.

Cole, K.J., and Beck, C.L. (1994). The stability of precision grip force in older adults. *Journal of Motor Behavior, 26,* 171-177.

Cole, K.J., Rotella, D.L., and Harper, J.G. (1999). Mechanisms for age-related changes of fingertip forces during precision gripping and lifting in adults. *Journal of Neuroscience, 19*(8), 3238-3247.

Coleman, S. (2002). Biomechanics and its application to coaching practice. In N. Cross and J. Lyle (Eds.), *The coaching process: Principles and practice for sport* (pp. 130-151). Oxford, UK: Butterworth-Heinemann.

Collins, J.J., Imhoff, T.T., and Grigg, P. (1996). Noise-enhanced tactile sensation. *Nature, 383,* 770.

Cooper, J.M., and Glassow, R.B. (1976). *Kinesiology* (4th ed.). St. Louis: Mosby.

Cope, T.C., and Pinter, M.J. (1995). The size principle: Still working after all these years. *NIPS, 10,* 281-286.

Corbetta, D., and Thelen, E. (1996). The developmental origins of bimanual coordination: A dynamic perspective. *Journal of Experimental Psychology: Human Perception and Performance, 22,* 502-522.

Corbetta, D., and Veriejken, B. (1999). Understanding development and learning of motor coordination in sport: The contribution of dynamic systems theory. *International Journal of Sport Psychology, 30*(44), 507-530.

Cordo, P., Carlton, L., Bevan, L., Carlton, M., and Kerr, G.K. (1994). Proprioceptive coordination of movement sequences: Role of velocity and position information. *Journal of Neurophysiology, 71*(5), 1848-1861.

Cordo, P., Inlgis, J.T., Verschueren, S., Collins, J.J., Merfeld, D.M., Rosenblum, S., Buckley, S., Moss, F. (1996). Noise in human muscle spindles. *Nature, 383,* 769-770.

Corna, S., Tarantola, J., Nardone, A., Giordano, A., and Schieppati, M. (1999). Standing on a continuously moving platform: Is body intertia counteracted or exploited? *Experimental Brain Research, 124,* 331-341.

Côté, J. (1999). The influence of the family in the development of talent in sports. *The Sports Psychologist, 13,* 395-417.

Côté, J., and Hay, J. (2002). Children's involvement in sport: A developmental perspective. In J.M. Silva and D. Stevens (Eds.), *Psychological foundations of sport* (2nd ed.). Boston: Merrill.

Counsilman, J.E. (1968). *The science of swimming.* Englewood Cliffs, NJ: Prentice Hall.

Counsilman, J.E. (1969). The role of sculling movements in the arm pull. *Swimming World, 10,* 6-7.

Counsilman, J.E. (1971). The application of Bernoulli's principle to human propulsion in water. In L. Lewillie and J.P. Clarys (Eds.), *Swimming I* (pp. 59-71). Brussels: Université Libre de Bruxelles.

Cox, J.S. (1985). Patellofemoral problems in runners. *Clinics in Sports Medicine, 4,* 699-707.

Craig, A.B. and Pendergast, D.R. (1979). Relationships of stroke rate, distance per stroke and velocity in competitive swimming. *Medicine and Science in Sport,* 11, 278-283.

Creath, R., Kiemel, T., Horak, F., Peterka, R., and Jeka, J. (2005). A unified view of quiet and per-turbed stance: simultaneous co-existing excitable modes. *Neuroscience Letters, 377,* 75-80.

Creutzfeld, O.D. (1995). *Cortex cerebri.* Oxford, UK: Oxford University Press.

Crossman, E.R.F.W. (1959). A theory of the acquisition of speed-skill. *Ergonomics, 2,* 153-166.

Crossman, E.R.F.W., and Szafran, J. (1956). Changes with age in the speed of information intake and discrimination. *Exerientia Supplementum IV, Symposium on Experimental Gerontology, 4,* 128-135.

Cureton, T.K. (1930). Mechanics and kinesiology of swimming. *Research Quarterly, 1,* 87-121.

Daffertshofer, A., Peper, C.E., and Beek, P.J. (2000). Spectral analyses of event-related encepha-lographic signals. *Phys. Lett. A, 266,* 290-302.

Daffertshofer, A., Peper, C.E., Frank, T.D., and Beek, P.J. (2000). Spatio-temporal patterns of encephalographic signals during polyrhythmic tapping. *Hum. Movement Sci., 19,* 475-498.

Daffertshofer, A., van den Berg, C., Beek, P.J. (1999). A dynamical model for mirror movements. *Physica D, 132,* 243-266.

Danieli Betto, D., Betto, R., and Midrio, M. (1990). Calcium sensitivity and myofibrillar protein isoforms of rat skinned skeletal muscle fibres. *Pflugers Arch., 417,* 303-308.

Danion, F., Duarte, M., and Grosjean, M. (1999). Fitts' law in human standing: The effect of scaling. *Neurosciences Letters, 277,* 131-133.

d'Aquino, T. (1952). ("Aquinas") The summa theologica. In Fathers of the English Dominican Province (Trans.) and D.J. Sullivan (Ed.), *Great Books Series* (Vol. 19). Chicago: Encyclopedia Britannica. (Original work published in 1272).

Darling, W.G., Cooke, J.D., and Brown, S.H. (1989). Control of simple arm movements in elderly humans. *Neurobiology of Aging, 10*(2), 149-157.

Darrah, J., Redfern, L., Maguite, T.O., Beaulne, P., and Watt, J. (1998). Intra-individual stability of rate of gross motor development in full-term infants._Early Human Development, 52, 169-179.

Darwin, C. (1877). Biographical sketch of an infant. *Mind, 2,* 285-294.

Davids, K., Bennett, S.J., Handford, C., and Jones, B. (1999). Acquiring coordination in self-paced extrinsic timing tasks: A constraints led perspective. *International Journal of Sport Psychology, 30,* 437-61.

Davids, K., Button, C. and Bennett, S.J. (in press). *Acquiring movement skill: A constraints-led perspective.* Champaign, Ill.: Human Kinetics.

Davids, K., Glazier, P.S., Araújo, D., and Bartlett, R.M. (2003). Movement systems as dynamical systems: The role of functional variability and its implications for sports medicine. *Sports Medicine, 33,* 245-260.

Davids, K., Handford, C.H., and Williams, A.M. (1994). The natural physical alternative to cognitive theories of motor behaviour: An invitation for interdisciplinary research in sports science? *Journal of Sports Sciences, 12,* 495-528.

Davids, K., Kingsbury, D., Bennett, S.J., and Handford, C. (2001). Information-movement coupling: Implications for the organisation of research and practice during acquisition of self-paced extrinsic timing skills. *Journal of Sports Sciences, 19,* 117-27.

Davids, K., Shuttleworth, R. Button, C., Renshaw, I. and Glazier, P. (2004). "Essential noise" - enhancing variability of informational constraints benefits movement control: A comment on Waddington and Adams (2003). *British Journal of Sports Medicine* 38, 601-605.

Davidson, D. (1980). Actions, reasons, and causes. In D.Davidson (Ed.), *Essays on actions and events* (pp. 3-19). Oxford, UK: Clarendon Press.

Davis, W.E., and Burton, A.W. (1991). Ecological task analysis: Translating movement behaviour theory into practice. *Applied Physical Activity Quarterly, 8,* 154-77.

de Guzman, G.C., Kelso, J.A.S., and Buchanan, J.J. (1997). Self-organization of trajectory formation. II. Theoretical model. *Biological Cybernetics, 76,* 275-284.

De Luca, C.J. (1988). The common drive of motor units. In W. Wallings, H.B.K. Boom, and J. de Vries (Eds.), *Electrophysiological kinesiology* (pp. 35-38). Amsterdam: Elsevier Science.

De Luca, C.J., Foley, P.J., and Erim, Z. (1996). Motor unit control properties in constant force isometric contractions. *Journal of Neurophysiology, 76,* 1503-1516.

De Luca, C.J., Le Fever, R.S., McCue, M.P., and Xenakis, A.P. (1982). Control scheme governing concurrently active human motor units during voluntary contractions. *Journal of Physiology, 329,* 129-142.

de Rugy, A., Taga, G., Montagne, G., Buekers, M.J., and Laurent, M. (2002). Perception-action coupling model for human locomotor pointing. *Biological Cybernetics, 87,* 141-150.

Deecke, L., Grozinger, B., Kornhuber, H.H. (1976). Voluntary finger movement in man: Cerebral potentials and theory. *Biological Cybernetics, 23,* 99-119.

Delbono, O., O'Rourke, K.S., and Ettinger, W.H. (1995). Excitation-calcium release uncoupling in aged single human skeletal muscle fibers. *J. Membr. Biol., 148*(3), 211-222.

DeLeo, A., Dierks, T.A., Ferber, R. and Davis, I.S. (2004). Lower extremity joint coupling during running: a current update. *Clinical Biomechanics, 19,* 983-991,

Dennis, C. (2005). Rugby team converts give gene tests a try. *Nature, 434,* 260.

Desai, R.C., and Zwanzig, R. (1978). Statistical mechanics of a nonlinear stochastic model. *J. Stat. Phys., 19,* 1-24.

Desmedt, J.E., and Godaux, E. (1977). Fast motor units are not preferentially activated in rapid voluntary contractions in man. *Nature, 267,* 717-719.

Deutsch, K.M., and Newell, K.M. (2001). Age differences in noise and variability of isometric force production. *Journal of Experimental Child Psychology, 80,* 392-408.

Deutsch, K.M., and Newell, K.M. (2002). Children's coordination of force output in a pinch grip task. *Developmental Psychobiology, 41,* 253-264.

Deutsch, K.M., and Newell, K.M. (2003). *Noise, variability, and the development of children's perceptual-motor skills.* Manuscript submitted for publication.

Deutsch, K.M., and Newell, K.M. (in press). Deterministic and stochastic processes in children's isometric force variability. *Developmental Psychobiology.*

Diedrich, F.J., and Warren Jr., W.H. (1995). Why change gaits? Dynamics of the walk-run transition. *Journal of Experimental Psychology: Human Perception and Performance, 21,* 183-202.

Diedrich, F.J., and Warren, W.H. (1998). The dynamics of gait transitions: Effects of grade and load. *Journal of Motor Behavior, 30,* 60-78.

Dijkstra, T.M., Schöner, G., Giese, M.A., and Gielen, C.C. (1994). Frequency dependence of the action-perception cycle for postural control in a moving visual environment: relative phase dynamics. *Biological Cybernetics, 71,* 489-501.

Dijkstra, T.M.H., Gielen, C.C.A.M., and Melis, B.J.M. (1992). Postural responses to stationary and moving scenes as a function of distance to the scene. *Human Movement Science, 11,* 195-203.

Dillman, C.J. (1989). Improving elite performance through precise biomechanical measures. In J.S. Skinner, C.B. Corbin, D.M. Landers, P.E. Martin, and C.L. Wells (Eds.), *Future directions in exercise and sport science research* (pp. 91-95). Champaign, IL: Human Kinetics.

Dingwell, J.B., Cusumano, J.P., Cavanagh, P.R., Sternad, D. (2001). Local dynamic stability versus kinematic variability of continuous overground and treadmill walking. *Journal of Biomechanical Engineering, 123,* 27-32.

Dixon, S.J., and Kerwin, D.G. (1998). The influence of heel lift manipulation on Achilles tendon loading in running. *Journal of Applied Biomechanics, 14,* 374-389.

Draeger, A., Weeds, A.G., and Fitzsimons, R.B. (1987). Primary, secondary and tertiary myotubes in developing skeletal muscle: A new approach to the analysis of human myogenesis. *J. Neurol. Sci., 81*(1), 19-43.

Drucker, E.G. (1996). The use of gait transition speed in comparative studies of fish locomotion. *American Zoologist, 36,* 555-556.

Duarte, M., and Zatsiorsky, V.M. (2000). On the fractal properties of natural human standing. *Neuroscience Letters, 283,* 173-176.

Dufek, J.S., Bates, B.T., and Davis, H.P. (1995). The effect of trial size and variability on statistical power. *Medicine and Science in Sports and Exercise, 27,* 288-295.

Dufek, J.S., Bates, B.T., Stergiou, N., and James, C.R. (1995). Interactive effects between group and single-subject patterns. *Human Movement Science, 14,* 301-323.

Duffey, M., Martin, D., Cannon, DW, Craven, T., and Messier, S.P. (2000). Etiologic factors associated with anterior knee pain in runners. *Medicine and Science in Sports and Exercise, 32,* 1825-1832.

Dupuy, M.A., Mottet, S., and Ripoll, H. (2000). The regulation of release parameters in underarm precision throwing. *Journal of Sport Sciences, 18,* 375-382.

Eckhorn, R., Bauer, R., Jordan, W., Brosch, M., Kurse, W., Munk, M., Reitboeck, H.J. (1988). Coherent oscillations: A mechanism of feature linking in the visual cortex? *Biol. Cybern., 60,* 121-130.

Edman, K.A. (1979). The velocity of unloaded shortening and its relation to sarcomere length and isometric force in vertebrate muscle fibres. *J. Physiol. (Lond.), 291,* 143-159.

Edman K.A.P., and Reggiani C. (1987). The sarcomere length-tension relation determined in short segments of intact muscle fibres of the frog. *J. Physiol., 385,* 709-732.

Eisen, A., Entezari-Taher, M., and Stewart, H. (1996). Cortical projections to spinal motoneurons: Changes with aging and amyotrophic lateral sclerosis. *Neurology, 46,* 1396-1404.

Elble, R.J., and Koller, W.C. (1990). *Tremor.* Baltimore: Johns Hopkins University Press.

Elliott, B.C. (1997). Causal mechanisms for improved performance or injury reduction: An essential part of sports biomechanics research. In J. Wilkerson, K. Ludwig, and W. Zimmermann (Eds.), *Proceedings of the 15th Symposium on Biomechanics in Sports* (pp. 45-49). Denton, TX: Texas Woman's University.

Elliott, B.C. (1999). Biomechanics: An integral part of sport science and sport medicine. *Journal of Science and Medicine in Sport, 2,* 299-310.

Elliott, B.C. (2002). Biomechanics of injury: Its role in prevention, rehabilitation and orthopaedic outcomes. In Y. Hong (Ed.), *International research in sports biomechanics* (pp. 109-115). London: Taylor and Francis.

Elliott, B.C., Hardcastle, P.H., Burnett, A.F., and Foster, D.H. (1992). The influence of fast bowling and physical factors on radiological features in high performance young fast bowlers. *Sports Medicine, Training and Rehabilitation, 3,* 113-130.

Elliott, D., Helsen, W.F., and Chua, R. (2001). A century later: Woodworth's (1899) two-component model of goal-directed aiming. *Psychological Bulletin, 127,* 342-357.

Engel, A.K., König, P., Kreiter, A.K., Singer, W. (1991). Interhemispheric synchronization of oscillatory neuronal responses in cat visual cortex. *Science, 252,* 1177-1179.

Engelhorn, R. (1997). Speed and accuracy in the learning of a complex motor skill. *Perceptual and Motor Skills, 85,* 1011-1017.

Enoka, R.M. (1997). Neural strategies in the control of muscle force. *Muscle and Nerve, 5*(9) (Suppl.), S66-69.

Enoka, R.M. (2004). Biomechanics and neuroscience: a failure to communicate. *Exercise and Sports Sciences Reviews, 32,* 1-3.

Enoka, R.M., and Fuglevand, A.J. (2001). Motor unit physiology: Some unresolved issues. *Muscle and Nerve, 24*(1), 4-17.

Ericsson, K.A. (Ed.). (1996). *The road to excellence: The acquisition of expert performance in the arts and sciences, sports and games.* Mahwah, NJ: Erlbaum.

Ericsson, K.A. and Charness, N. (1994). Expert performance: Its structure and acquisition. *American Psychologist, 49,* 725-747.

Ericsson, K.A., Krampe, R.T., and Tesch-Römer, C. (1993). The role of deliberate practice in the acquisition of expert performance. *Psychological Review, 100*(3), 363-406.

Ericsson, K.A., and Lehmann, A.C. (1996). Expert and exceptional performance: Evidence of maximal adaptation and task constraints. *Annual Review of Psychology, 47,* 273-305.

Erim, Z., Beg, M.F., Burke D.T., and De Luca C.J. (1999). Effects of aging on motor-unit control properties. *Journal of Neurophysiology, 82,* 2081-2091.

Ermentrout, G.B., and Cowan, J.D. (1979). A mathematical theory of visual hallucination patterns. *Biol. Cybern., 34,* 137-150.

Essen, B., Jansson, E., Henriksson, J., Taylor, A.W., and Saltin, B. (1975). Metabolic characteristics of fibre types in human skeletal muscle. *Acta Physiol. Scand., 95,* 153-165.

Essen-Gustavsson, B., and Henriksson, J. (1984). Enzyme levels in pools of microdissected human muscle fibres of identified type. Adaptive response to exercise. *Acta Physiol. Scand., 120,* 505-515.

Etnyre, B.R. (1998). Accuracy characteristics of throwing as a result of maximum force effort. *Perceptual and Motor Skills, 86*, 1211-1217.

Eubank, S.G., and Farmer, J.D. (1997). Probability, random processes, and the statistical description of dynamics. In L. Lam (Ed.), *Introduction to nonlinear physics* (pp. 106-178). New York: Springer-Verlag.

Eusebi, F., Miledi, R., and Takahashi, T. (1980). Calcium transients in mammalian muscles. *Nature, 284*(5756), 560-561.

Evarts, E.V., Wise, S.A.P., and Bousfield, D. (Eds.). (1985). *The motor system in neurobiology.* Amsterdam: Elsevier Science.

Everitt, B.S., Landau, S., and Leese, M. (2000). *Cluster analysis* (4th ed.). London: Arnold.

Everts, M.E., Andersen, J.P., Clausen, T., and Hansen, O. (1989). Quantitative determination of Ca2+-dependent Mg2+-ATPase from sarcoplasmic reticulum in muscle biopsies. *Biochem. J., 260*(2), 443-448.

Faugloire, E., Bardy, B.G., Merhi, O., and Stoffregen, T.A. (2005). Exploring coordination dynamics of the postural system with real-time visual feedback. *Neuroscience Letters, 374*, 136-141.

Faugloire, E., Bardy, B.G., and Stoffregen, T.A. (submitted). *The dynamics of learning new postural patterns.*

Feige, B., Kristeva-Feige, R., Rossi, S., Pizzella, V., Rossini, P-M. (1996). Neuromagnetic study of movement-related changes in rhythmic brain activity. *Brain Res., 734*, 252-260.

Feitosa M.F., Gaskill S.E., Rice T., Rankinen T., Bouchard C., Rao D.C., Wilmore J.H., Skinner J.S. and Leon A.S.. (2002). Major gene effects on exercise ventilatory threshold: The HERITAGE Family Study. *Journal of Applied Physiology, 93*, 1000-1006.

Field-Fote, E.C., and Tepavac, D. (2002). Improved intralimb coordination in people with incomplete spinal cord injury following training with body weight support and electrical stimulation. *Physical Therapy, 82*, 707-715.

Fink, R.H., Stephenson, D.G., and Williams, D.A. (1990). Physiological properties of skinned fibres from normal and dystrophic (Duchenne) human muscle activated by Ca2+ and Sr2+. *J. Physiol. (Lond.), 420*, 337-353.

Fitts, P.M. (1951). Engineering psychology and equipment design. In S.S. Stevens (Ed.), *Handbook of experimental psychology* (pp. 1287-1340). New York: Wiley.

Fitts, P.M. (1954). The information capacity of the human motor system in controlling the amplitude of movement. *Journal of Experimental Psychology, 47*, 381-391.

Fitts, P.M., and Peterson, J.R. (1964). Information capacity of discrete motor responses. *Journal of Experimental Psychology, 67*, 103-112.

Fitts, P.M., and Posner, M.I. (1967). *Human performance.* Belmont, CA: Brooks/Cole.

Folland, J., Leach, B., Little, T., Hawker, K., Myerson, S., Montgomery, H. and Jones, D. (2000). Angiotensin-converting enzyme genotype affects the response of human skeletal muscle to functional overload. *Experimental Physiology, 85*, 575-579.

Forss, N., Mäkelä, J.P., McEvoy, L., and Hari, R. (1993). Temporal integration and oscillatory responses of the human auditory cortex revealed by evoked magnetic fields to click trains. *Hearing Res., 68*, 89-96.

Foster, D.H., John, D., Elliott, B., Ackland, T., and Fitch, K. (1989). Back injuries to fast bowlers in cricket: A prospective study. *British Journal of Sports Medicine, 23*, 150-154.

Fourcade, P., Bardy, B.G., and Bonnet, C. (2003). Modeling human postural transitions. In S. Rogers and J. Effken (Eds.), *Studies in perception and action VII.* Hillsdale, NJ: Erlbaum.

Fox, P.W., Hershberger, S.L., and Bouchard, T.J. (1996). Genetic and environmental contributions to the acquisition of a motor skill. *Nature, 384*, 356-358.

Frank, T.D. (2000). *Stochastic properties of human motor control: Nonlinear Fokker-Planck equations.* PhD Thesis, Vrije Universiteit, Amsterdam, the Netherlands. Amstelveen.

Frank, T.D. (2001a). H-theorem for Fokker-Planck equations with drifts depending on process mean values. *Phys. Lett. A, 280,* 91-96.

Frank, T.D. (2001b). A Langevin approach for the microscopic dynamics of nonlinear Fokker-Planck equations. *Physica A, 301,* 52-62.

Frank, T.D., Daffertshofer, A., Beek, P.J. (2001). Multivariate Ornstein-Uhlenbeck processes with mean field dependent coefficients—Application to postural sway. *Phys. Rev. E, 63,* 011905.

Frank, T.D., Daffertshofer, A., Beek, P.J., Haken, H. (1999). Impacts of noise on a field theoretical model of the human brain. *Physica D, 127,* 233-249.

Frank, T.D., Daffertshofer, A., Peper, C.E., Beek, P.J., Haken, H. (2000). Towards a comprehensive theory of brain activity: Coupled oscillator systems under external forces. *Physica D, 144,* 62-86.

Frank, T.D., Daffertshofer, A., Peper, C.E., Beek, P.J., Haken, H. (2001). H-theorem for a mean field model describing coupled oscillator systems under external forces. *Physica D, 150,* 219-236.

Frederiksen, H. and Christensen, K. (2003). The influence of genetic factors on physical functioning and exercise in second half of life. *Scandinavian Journal of Medicine and Science in Sports 13,* 9-18.

Freeman, H. (1961). A technique for the classification and recognition of geometric patterns. In *Proceedings of the 3rd International Congress on Cybernetics,* pp. 348-368,. Namur, Belgium: ICC.

Freeman, W.J. (1975). *Mass action in the nervous system.* New York: Academic Press.

Freeman, W.J. (1991). The physiology of perception. *Scientific American, 264,* 78-85.

Freeman, W.J. (1992) Tutorial in neurobiology: From single neurons to brain chaos. *International Journal of Bifurcation and Chaos 2:* 451-482.

Freeman, W.J. (1995). *Societies of brains. A study in the neuroscience of love and hate.* Mahwah, NJ: Erlbaum.

Freeman, W.J. (2000a). *Neurodynamics. An exploration in mesoscopic brain dynamics.* London: Springer-Verlag.

Freeman, W.J. (2000b). Perception of time and causation through the kinesthesia of intentional action. *Cognitive Processing, 1,* 18-34.

Freeman, W.J. (2000c) Mesoscopic neurodynamics. From neuron to brain. *Journal of Physiology (Paris), 94,* 303-322.

Freeman, W.J. (2001). The olfactory system: Odor detection and classification. In *Frontiers in biology, Vol. 3. Intelligent systems. Part II brain components as elements of intelligent function* (pp. 509-526). New York: Academic Press.

Freeman, W.J., and Barrie, J.M. (1994). Chaotic oscillations and the genesis of meaning in cerebral cortex. In G. Buzsáki, R. Llinás, W. Singer, A. Berthoz, and Y. Christen (Eds.), *Temporal coding in the brain* (pp. 13-37). Berlin: Springer-Verlag.

Fryer, M.W., and Neering, I.R. (1989). Actions of caffeine on fast- and slow-twitch muscles of the rat. *J. Physiol., 416,* 435-454.

Fuchs, A., Jirsa, V.K. (2000). The HKB model revisited: How varying the degree of symmetry controls dynamics. *Hum. Movement Sci., 19,* 425-449.

Fuchs, A., and Kelso, J.A.S. (1994). A theoretical note on models of interlimb coordination. *Journal of Experimental Psychology: Human Perception and Performance, 20,* 1088-1097.

Fuchs, A., Kelso, J.A.S., and Haken, H. (1992). Phase transitions in the human brain: Spatial mode dynamics. *Int. J. Bif. and Chaos, 2*, 917-939.

Fuglevand, A.J., Winter, D.A., and Patla, A.E. (1993). Models of recruitment and rate coding organization in motor-unit pools. *Journal of Neurophysiology, 70*(6), 2470-2488.

Fullerton, G.S., and Cattell, J.M. (1892). *On the perception of small differences. (Philosophical Monograph Series No. 2).* Philadelphia: University of Pennsylvania Press.

Gabell, A., and Nayak, U.S.L. (1984). The effect of age on variability in gait. *Journal of Gerontology, 39*, 662-666.

Galganski, M.E., Fuglevand, A.J., and Enoka, R.M. (1993). Reduced control of motor output in a human hand muscle of elderly subjects during submaximal contractions. *Journal of Neurophysiology, 69*(6), 2108-2115.

Gardner, C.W. (1983). *Handbook of stochastic methods.* Berlin: Springer-Verlag.

Gasteiger, E.L., and Brust-Carmona, H. (1964). On the relation of spinal reflex variability to internal noise. *Transactions of the New York Academy of Sciences, 26*, 688-696.

Gayagay, G., Yu, B., Hambly, B., Boston, T., Hahn, A., Celermajer, D.S. and Trent R.J. (1998). Elite endurance athletes and the ACE I allele—The role of genes in athletic performance. *Human Genetics, 103*, 48-50.

George, K.P., Wolfe, L.A., and Burggraf, G.W. (1991). The "Athletic Heart Syndrome:" A critical review. *Sports Medicine, 11*, 300-331.

Gerloff, C., Toro, C., Uenishi, N., Cohen, L.G., Leocani, L., and Hallett, M. (1997). Steady-state movement-related cortical potentials: A new approach to assessing cortical activity associated with fast repetitive finger movements. *Electroenceph. Clin. Neurophysiol., 102*, 106-113.

Gerloff, C., Uenishi, N., Nagamine, T., T. Kunieda, M.H., and Shibasaki, H. (1998). Cortical activation during fast repetitive finger movements in humans: Steady-state movement-related magnetic fields and their cortical generators. *Electroenceph. Clin. Neurophysiol., 109*, 444-453.

Gerstner, W., and van Hemmen, J.L. (1994). Coding and information processing in neural networks. In E. Domany, J.L. van Hemmen, and K. Schulten (Eds.), *Models of neural networks II: Temporal aspects of coding and information processing in biological systems* (pp. 1-93). Berlin: Springer-Verlag.

Gesell, A. (1929). Maturation and infant behavior pattern. *Psychological Review, 36*, 307-319.

Gesell, A. (1946). The ontogenesis of infant behavior. In L. Carmichael (Ed.), *Manual of child psychology* (pp. 295-331). New York: Wiley.

Ghez, C., and Sainberg, R. (1995). Proprioceptive control of interjoint coordination. *Canadian Journal of Physiology and Pharmacology, 73*, 273-284.

Gibson, E.J. (1988). Exploratory behavior in the development of perceiving, acting, and the acquiring of knowledge. *Annual Review of Psychology, 39*, 1-41.

Gibson, J.J. (1979). *The ecological approach to visual perception.* Boston: Houghton Mifflin.

Gilden, D.L., Thornton, T., and Mallon, M.W. (1995). 1/f noise in human cognition. *Science, 267*, 1837-1839.

Gitter, J.A. and Czerniecki, M.J. (1995). Fractal analysis of the electromyographic interference pattern. *Journal of Neuroscience Methods, 58*, 103-108.

Glass, L., and Mackey, M.C. (1988). *From clocks to chaos: The rhythms of life.* Princeton, NJ: Princeton University Press.

Glazier, P.S., Davids, K., and Bartlett, R.M. (2003). Dynamical systems theory: A relevant framework for performance-oriented sports biomechanics research? *Sportscience* [Online], 7. Available: www.sportsci.org/jour/03/psg.htm.

Goldfield, E.C., Kay, B.A., and Warren, W.H. (1993). Infant bouncing: The assembly and tuning of action systems. *Child Development, 64,* 1128-1142.

Goodman, D., and Kelso, J.A.S. (1980). Are movements prepared in parts? Not under compatible (naturalized) conditions. *Journal of Experimental Psychology: General, 109,* 475-95.

Gordon A.M., Huxley, A.F., and Julian, F. (1966). The variation in isometric tension with sarcomere length in vertebrate muscle fibres. *J. Physiol., 184,* 170-192.

Grabiner, P.C., Biswas, S.T., and Grabiner, M.D. (2001). Age-related changes in spatial and temporal gait variables. *Archives of Physical Medicine and Rehabilitation, 82*(1), 31-35.

Graves, A.E., Kornatz, K.W., and Enoka, R.M. (2000). Older adults use a unique strategy to lift inertial loads with the elbow flexor muscles. *Journal of Neurophysiology, 83,* 2030-2039.

Gray, C.M., König, P., Engel, A.K., and Singer, W. (1989). Oscillatory responses in cat visual cortex exhibit inter-columnar synchronization which reflects global stimulus properties. *Nature, 338,* 334-337.

Green, D.M., and Swets, J.A. (1966). *Signal detection theory and psychophysics.* New York: Wiley.

Greenhaff, P.L., Soderlund, K., Ren, J-M., and Hultman, E. (1993). Energy metabolism in single human muscle fibres during intermittent contraction with occluded circulation. *J. Physiol., 460,* 443-453.

Gregor, R.J. (1989). Locomotion: A commentary. In J.S. Skinner, C.B. Corbin, D.M. Landers, P.E. Martin, and C.L. Wells (Eds.), *Future directions in exercise and sport science research* (pp. 195-199). Champaign, IL: Human Kinetics.

Gregor, R.J., Broker, J.P., and Ryan, M.M. (1992). Performance feedback and new advances in biomechanics. In R.W. Christina and H.M. Eckert (Eds.), *Enhancing human performance in sport: New concepts and developments* (pp. 19-32). Champaign, IL: Human Kinetics.

Gregory, R.L. (1974). *Concepts and mechanisms of perception.* New York: Scribner's.

Grieve, D.W. (1968). Gait patterns and the speed of walking. *Biomedical Engineering, 3,* 119-122.

Grieve, D.W. (1969). The assessment of gait. *Physiotherapy, 55,* 452-460.

Grillner, S., Halbertsma, J., Nilsson, J. and Thorstensson, A. (1979). The adaptation to speed in human locomotion. *Brain Research, 165,* 177-182.

Grimston, S.K. and Hay, J.G. (1986). Relationships among anthropometric and stroking characteristics of college swimmers. *Medicine and Science in Sports and Exercise, 18,* 60-68.

Groppel, J.L. (1984). *Tennis for advanced players and those who would like to be.* Champaign, IL: Human Kinetics.

Gross, J., Tass, P.A., Salenius, S., Hari, R., Freund, H., and Schnitzler, A. (2000). Cortico-muscular synchronization during isometric muscle contraction in humans as revealed by magnetoencephalography. *J. Physiology, 527,* 623-631.

Gross, J.B., and Gill, D. (1982). Competition and instructional set effects on the speed and accuracy of a throwing task. *Research Quarterly for Exercise and Sport, 53,* 125-132.

Guiard, Y. (1997). Fitts' law in the discrete vs. cyclical paradigm. *Human Movement Science, 16,* 97-131.

Gurfinkel, E.V. (1973). Physical foundations of stabilography. *Agressologie, 14,* 9-13.

Gustin, W.C. (1985). The development of exceptional research mathematicians. In B.S. Bloom (Ed.), *Developing talent in young people* (pp. 139-192). New York: Ballantine.

Guth, L., and Samaha, F.J. (1969). Qualitative differences between actomyosin ATPase of slow and fast mammalian muscle. *Exp. Neurol., 25*(1), 138-152.

Guthrie, E.R. (1935). *The psychology of learning.* New York: Harper and Row.

Hagberg, J.M., Ferrell, R.E., McCole, S.D., Wilund, K.R., and Moore, G.E. (1998). VO$_2$max is associated with ACE genotype in postmenopausal women. *Journal of Applied Physiology, 85,* 1842-1846.

Haken, H. (1977). *Synergetics: An introduction: Nonequilibrium phase transitions and self-organization in physics, chemistry, and biology.* Berlin: Springer-Verlag.

Haken, H. (1983). *Synergetics—An Introduction.* Berlin: Springer-Verlag.

Haken, H. (1996). *Principles of brain functioning.* Berlin: Springer-Verlag.

Haken, H., Kelso, J.A.S., and Bunz, H. (1985). A theoretical model of phase transitions in human hand movements. *Biological Cybernetics, 51,* 347-356.

Halliday, D.M., Conway, B.A., Farmer, S.F., and Rosenberg, J.R. (1999). Load-independent contributions from motor-unit synchronization to human physiological tremor. *Journal of Neurophysiology, 82,* 664-75.

Hamill, J., Haddad, J.M., and McDermott, W.J. (2000). Issues in quantifying variability from a dynamical systems perspective. *Journal of Applied Biomechanics, 16,* 407-418.

Hamill, J., Van Emmerik, R.E.A., Heiderscheit, B.C., and Li, L. (1999). A dynamical systems approach to lower extremity running injuries. *Clinical Biomechanics, 14,* 297-308.

Hancock, P.A., and Newell, K.M. (1985). The movement speed-accuracy relationship in space-time. In H. Heuer, U. Kleinbeck, and K.H. Schmidt (Eds.), *Motor behavior: Programming, control and acquisition* (pp. 153-188). Berlin: Springer-Verlag.

Handford, C., Davids, K., Bennett, S., and Button, C. (1997). Skill acquisition in sport: Some applications of an evolving practice ecology. *Journal of Sports Sciences, 15,* 621-40.

Harris, C.M., and Wolpert, D.M. (1998). Signal-dependent noise determines motor planning. *Nature, 394,* 780-784.

Hartmann, W.M. (1997). *Signals, sound, and sensation.* Woodbury, NY: American Institute of Physics.

Hashimoto, I., Mashiko, T., Kimura, T., and Imada, T. (1998). Human somatosensory evoked magnetic fields to vibratory stimulation of the index finger: Is there frequency organization in SI? *Electroenceph. Clin. Neurophysiol., 109,* 454-461.

Hatze, H. (1998). Biomechanics of sports: Selected examples of successful applications and future perspectives. In H. Riehle and M. Vieten (Eds.), *Proceedings of the 16th International Symposium on Biomechanics in Sports* (pp. 2-22). Germany: University of Konstanz.

Hausdorff, J.M., Cudkowicz, M.E., Firtion, R., Wei, Y.G., and Goldberger, A.L. (1998). Gait variability and basal ganglia disorders: Stride-to-stride variations of gait cycle timing in Parkinson's disease and Huntingdon's disease. *Movement Disorders, 13,* 428-437.

Hausdorff, J.M., Edelberg, H.K., Mitchell, S.L., Goldberger, A.L., Wei, J.Y. (1997). Increased gait unsteadiness in community-dwelling elderly fallers. *Archives of Physical Medicine and Rehabilitation, 78,* 278-283.

Hausdorff, J.M., Purdon, L., Peng, C-K., Ladin, Z., Wei, J.Y., Goldberger, A.L. (1996). Fractal dynamics of human gait: Stability of long-range correlations in stride interval fluctuations. *Journal of Applied Physiology, 80,* 1448-1457.

Hay, J.G. (1973). *The biomechanics of sports techniques.* Englewood Cliffs, NJ: Prentice Hall.

Hay, J.G. (1983). Biomechanics of sport: An overview. In G.A. Wood (Ed.), *Collected papers on sports biomechanics* (pp. 1-21). Nedlands, WA: University of Western Australia Press.

Hay, J.G. (1985). Issues in sports biomechanics. In *Biomechanics: Current Interdisciplinary Research* (edited by S.M. Perren and E. Schneider), pp. 49-60. Dordrecht: Martinus Nijhoff.

Hay, J.G. and Guimaraes, A.C. (1983). A quantitative look at swimming biomechanics. *Swimming Technique, 20* (2), 11-17.

Hay, J.G., Liu, Q., and Andrews, J.G. (1993). Body role and hand path in freestyle swimming: A computer simulation. *Journal of Applied Biomechanics, 9*, 227-237.

Hay, J.G., and Reid, J.G. (1988). *Anatomy, mechanics and human motion.* Englewood Cliffs, NJ: Prentice Hall.

Hay, J.G., Vaughan, C.L., and Woodworth, G.G. (1981). Technique and performance: Identifying the limiting factors. In A. Morecki, K. Fidelus, and A. Wit (Eds.), *Biomechanics VII-B* (pp. 511-520). Baltimore: University Park Press.

Hayes, J.R. (1981). *The complete problem solver.* Philadelphia: Franklin Institute Press.

He, Z-H., Bottinelli, R., Pellegrino, M.A., Ferenczi, M.A., and Reggiani, C. (2000). ATP consumption and efficiency of human single muscle fibers with different myosin isoform composition. *Biophys. J., 79*, 945-961.

Heene, R. (1975). *Experimental myopathies and muscular dystrophy.* Berlin: Springer-Verlag.

Heiderscheit, B.C. (2000a). *Locomotion variability and joint pain.* Unpublished doctoral dissertation, University of Massachusetts, Amherst.

Heiderscheit, B.C. (2000b). Movement variability as a clinical measure for locomotion. *Journal of Applied Biomechanics, 16*, 419-427.

Heiderscheit, B.C., Hamill, J., and Van Emmerik, R.E.A. (1999). Q-angle influences on the variability of lower extremity coordination during running. *Medicine and Science in Sports and Exercise, 31*, 1313-1319.

Heiderscheit, B.C., Hamill, J., and Van Emmerik, R.E.A. (2002). Variability of stride characteristics and joint coordination among individuals with unilateral patellofemoral pain. *Journal of Applied Biomechanics, 18*, 110-121.

Helsen, W.F., Starkes, J.L., and Hodges, N.J. (1998). Team sports and the theory of deliberate practice. *Journal of Sport and Exercise Psychology, 20*, 12-34.

Henderson, G., Tomlinson, B.E., and Gibson, P.H. (1980). Cell counts in human cerebral cortex in normal adults throughout life using an image analysing computer. *Journal of Neurological Science, 46*, 113-136.

Hendriks-Jansen, H. (1996). *Catching ourselves in the act: Situated activity, interactive emergence, evolution, and human thought.* Cambridge, MA: MIT Press.

Henneman, E., Clamann, H.P., Gillies, J.D., and Skinner, R.D. (1974). Rank order of motoneurons within a pool: Law of combination. *J. Neurophysiol., 37*(6), 1338-1349.

Hennig, R., and Lomo, T. (1985). Firing patterns of motor units in normal rats. *Nature, 314*(6007), 164-166.

Herrick, C.J. (1948). *The brain of the tiger salamander.* Chicago: University of Chicago Press.

Hershler, C., and Milner, M. (1980). Angle-angle diagrams in the assessment of locomotion. *American Journal of Physical Medicine, 59*, 109-125.

Higgins, J.R. (1977). *Human movement: An integrated approach.* St. Louis: Mosby.

Hintermann, B., and Nigg, B.M. (1998). Pronation in runners: Implications for injuries. *Sports Medicine, 26*, 169-176.

Hobbes, T. (1904). *Leviathan; or, The matter, forme and power of commonwealth, ecclesiasticall and civill.* (A.R. Waller, Ed.). Cambridge, UK: Cambridge University Press. (Original work published 1651).

Hochmuth, G. (1984). *Biomechanics of athletic movement.* Berlin: Sportverlag.

Hodge, T., and Deakin, J. (1998). Deliberate practice and expertise in the martial arts: The role of context in motor recall. *The Journal of Sport and Exercise Psychology, 20*, 260-279.

Hodges, N.J., Kerr, T., Starkes, J.L., Weir, P.L., and Nananidou, A. (2004). Predicting performance from deliberate practice hours for the multi-sport athlete: Issues of transfer, circumventing constraints and defining practice. *Journal of Experimental Psychology: Applied, 10,* 219-237.

Hodges, N.J., and Starkes, J.L. (1996). Wrestling with the nature of expertise: A sport-specific test of Ericsson, Krampe and Tesch-Römer's (1993) theory of "deliberate practice." *International Journal of Sport Psychology, 27,* 400-424.

Hogan, N. (1985). The mechanics of multi-joint posture and movement control. *Biological Cybernetics, 52*(5), 315-331.

Holt, K.G., Jeng, S.F., Ratcliffe, R., and Hamill, J. (1995). Energetic cost and stability during human walking at the preferred stride frequency. *Journal of Motor Behavior, 27,* 164-178.

Hopkins, W.G. (2001). Genes and training for athletic performance. *Sportscience* 5(1) [Online]: Available sportsci.org/jour/0101/wghgene.htm.

Horak, F.B., and MacPherson J.M. (1996). Postural orientation and equilibrium. In L.B. Rowell and J.T. Sheperd (Eds.), *Handbook of physiology: A critical, comprehensive presentation of physiological knowledge and concepts* (pp. 256-292). New York: Oxford University Press.

Horak, F.B., and Nashner, L.M. (1986). Central programming of postural movements: Adaptation to altered support-surface configurations. *Journal of Neurophysiology, 55,* 1369-1381.

Horak, F.B., Nashner, L.M., and Diener, H.C. (1990). Postural strategies associated with somatosensory and vestibular loss. *Experimental Brain Research, 82,* 167-77.

Hore, J., Watts, S., Martin, J., and Miller, B. (1995). Timing of finger opening and ball release in fast and accurate overarm throws. *Experimental Brain Research, 103,* 277-286.

Hore, J., Watts, S., and Tweed, D. (1996). Errors in the control of joint rotations associated with inaccuracies in overarm throws. *Journal of Physiology, 75,* 1013-1025.

Horstmann, G.A., and Dietz, V. (1988). The contribution of vestibular input to the stabilization of human posture: A new experimental approach. *Neuroscience Letters, 95,* 179-184.

Hortobagyi, T., and DeVita, P. (1999). Altered movement strategy increases lower extremity stiffness during stepping down in the aged. *Journal of Gerontology A Biological Science Medical Science, 54*(2), B63-70.

Hortobagyi, T., Tunnel, D., Moody, J., Beam, S., and DeVita, P. (2001). Low- or high-intensity strength training partially restores impaired quadriceps force accuracy and steadiness in aged adults. *Journal of Gerontology A Biological Science Medical Science, 56*(1), B38-47.

Hoyt, D.F., and Taylor, C.R. (1981). Gait and energetics of locomotion in horses. *Nature, 292,* 239-240.

Hreljac, A. (1995). Determinants of the gait transition speed during human locomotion: kinematic factors. *Journal of Biomechanics, 28,* 669-677.

Hume, D. (1739). *Treatise on human nature.* London: J Noon.

Indermill, C., and Husak, W.S. (1984). Relationship between speed and accuracy in an over-arm throw. *Perceptual and Motor Skills, 59,* 219-222.

James, C.R., and Bates, B.T. (1997). Experimental and statistical design issues in human movement research. *Measurement in Physical Education and Exercise Science, 1,* 55-69.

James, S.L., and Jones, D.C. (1990). Biomechanical aspects of distance running injuries. In P.R. Cavanagh (Ed.), *Biomechanics of distance running* (pp. 249-270). Champaign, IL: Human Kinetics.

Jantzen, K.J., Steinberg, F.L., and Kelso, J.A.S. (2004). Brain networks underlying human timing behavior are influenced by prior context. *Proceedings of the National Academy of ScienceUSA,* 101, 6815-6820.

Jayannavar, A.M., and Mahato, M.C. (1995). Macroscopic equation of motion in inhomogeneous media: A microscopic treatment. *Pramana—Journal of Physics, 45,* 369-376.

Jeng, S., Holt, K.G., Fetters, L., and Certo, C. (1996). Self-optimization of walking in nondisabled children and children with spastic hemiplegic cerebral palsy. *Journal of Motor Behavior, 28*, 15-27.

Johnson, J. (1957). Tennis serve of advanced women players. *Research Quarterly, 28*, 123-131.

Johnston, T.D., and Edwards, L. (2002). Genes, interactions and the development of behaviour. *Psychological Review, 109*, 26-34.

Jones, A., Montgomery, H.E., and Woods, D.R. (2002). Human performance: A role for the ACE genotype? *Exercise and Sport Sciences Reviews, 30*, 184-190.

Jones, K., Hamilton, A., and Wolpert, D.M. (2002). The sources of signal dependent noise during isometric force production. *Journal of Neurophysiology, 88*, 1533-1544.

Jones, K.E., de C. Hamilton, A.F., and Wolpert, D.M. (2001). Sources of signal-dependent noise during isometric force production. *Journal of Neurophysiology, 88*, 1533-1544.

Jones, R.S. (1999). *Almost like a whale: The origin of the species updated.* London: Anchor Press.

Joseph, J. (2001). Separated twins and the genetics of personality differences: A critique. *American Journal of Psychology, 114*(1), 1-30.

Joseph, J.A. (Ed.). (1988). Central determinants of age-related declines in motor function. *Annals of the New York Academy of Sciences* (Vol. 515). New York: The New York Academy of Sciences.

Kac, M. (1969). The physical background of Langevin equations. In Aziz, A.K. (Ed.), *Lectures in differential equations. Vol. II* (pp. 147-166). New York: Van Nostrand Reinhold.

Kail, R. (1997). The neural noise hypothesis: Evidence from processing speed in adults with multiple sclerosis. *Aging, Neuropsychology, and Cognition, 4*, 157-165.

Kalinowski, A.G. (1985). The development of Olympic swimmers. In B.S. Bloom (Ed.), *Developing talent in young people* (pp. 139-192). New York: Ballantine.

Kamm, K., Thelen, E., and Jensen, J.L. (1990). A dynamical systems approach to motor development. *Physical Therapy, 70*, 763-775.

Kanda, K., Burke, R.E., and Walmsley, B. (1977). Differential control of fast and slow twitch motor units in the decerebrate cat. *Exp. Brain Res., 29*, 57-74.

Kant, I. (1974). *Kritik der reinen vernunft* [Critique of Pure Reason]. (W. von Weischedel, Ed.). Frankfurt, Germany: Suhrkamp-Verlag. (Original work published 1781).

Kantowitz, B.H. (Ed.). (1974). *Human information processing: Tutorials in performance and cognition.* Hillsdale, NJ: Erlbaum.

Kantz, H., and Schreiber, T. (1997). *Nonlinear time series analysis.* Cambridge: Cambridge University Press.

Kaplan, D., and Glass, L. (1995). *Understanding nonlinear dynamics.* New York: Springer-Verlag.

Karst, G.M., and Hasan, Z. (1987). Antagonist muscle activity during human forearm movements under varying kinematic and loading conditions. *Experimental Brain Research, 67*(2), 391-401.

Kawai, M., Savelsbergh, G.J.P., and Wimmers, R.H. (1999). Newborns spontaneous arm movements are influenced by the environment. *Early Human Development, 54*, 15-27.

Kay, B.A. (1988). The dimensionality of movement trajectories and the degrees of freedom problem: A tutorial. *Human Movement Science, 7*, 343-364.

Kay, L.M., and Freeman W.J. (1998). Bidirectional processing in the olfactory-limbic axis during olfactory behavior. *Behavioral Neuroscience, 112*, 541-553.

Keele, S.W. (1968). Movement control in skilled motor performance. *Psychological Bulletin, 70*, 387-403.

Keen, D.A., Yue, G.H., and Enoka, R.M. (1994). Training-related enhancement in the control of motor output in elderly humans. *Journal of Applied Physiology, 77*(6), 2648-2658.

Kelso, J.A.S. (1981). On the oscillatory basis of movement. *Bulletin of Psychonomic Society, 18,* 63.

Kelso, J.A.S. (1984). Phase transitions and critical behavior in human bimanual coordination. *American Journal of Physiology: Regulatory, Integrative and Comparative Physiology, 15,* R1000-R1004.

Kelso, J.A.S. (1991). Anticipatory dynamical systems, intrinsic pattern dynamics and skill learning. *Human Movement Science, 10,* 93-111.

Kelso, J.A.S. (1995). *Dynamic patterns: The self-organization of brain and behavior.* Cambridge, MA: MIT Press.

Kelso, J.A.S. (1997). Relative timing in brain and behavior: Some observations about the generalized motor program and self-organized coordination dynamics. *Human Movement Science, 16,* 453-460.

Kelso, J.A.S., Bressler, S.L., Buchannan, S., DeGuzman, G.C., Ding, M., Fuchs, A., and Holroyd, T. (1992). A phase transition in human brain and behavior. *Phys. Lett. A, 169,* 134-144.

Kelso, J.A.S., Buchanan, J.J., and Wallace, S.A. (1991). Order parameters for the neural organization of single, multijoint limb movement patterns. *Experimental Brain Research, 85,* 432-444.

Kelso, J.A.S., DelColle, J.D., and Schöner, G. (1990). Action-perception as a pattern formation process. In M. Jeannerod (Ed.), *Attention and performance XIII* (pp. 139-169). Hillsdale, NJ: Erlbaum.

Kelso, J.A.S., and Ding, M. (1993). Fluctuations, intermittency, and controllable chaos in biological coordination. In K.M. Newell and D.M. Corcos (Eds.), *Variability and motor control* (pp. 292-316). Champaign, IL: Human Kinetics.

Kelso, J.A.S., Ding, M., and Schöner, G. (1992). Dynamic pattern formation: A primer. In A. Baskin and J. Mittenthal (Eds.), *Principles of organization in organisms* (pp. 397-439). Santa Fe, NM: Addison-Wesley.

Kelso, J.A.S., Fink, P.W., DeLaplain, C.R., and Carson, R.G. (2001). Haptic information stabilizes and destabilizes coordination dynamics. *Proceedings of the Royal Society of London Series B-Biological Sciences, 268,* 1207-1213.

Kelso, J.A.S., Fuchs, A., Lancaster, R.T., Holroyd, D.C., and Weinberg, H. (1998). Dynamic cortical activity in the human brain reveals motor equivalence. *Nature, 392,* 814-818.

Kelso, J.A.S., and Haken, H. (1995). New laws to be expected in the organism: Synergetics of brain and behaviour. In M.P. Murphy and L.A.J. O'Neill, (Eds.), *What is life? The next fifty years* (pp. 137-160). Cambridge, MA: Cambridge University Press.

Kelso, J.A.S., Holt, K.G., Rubin, P. and Kugler, P.N. (1981). Patterns of human interlimb coordination from the properties of non-linear, limit cycle oscillatory processes: theory and data. *Journal of Motor Behavior, 13,* 226-261.

Kelso, J.A.S. and Jeka, J.J. (1992). Symmetry breaking dynamics of human multilimb coordination. *Journal of Experimental Psychology: Human Perception and Performance, 18,* 654-668.

Kelso, J.A.S., Scholz, J.P., and Schöner, G. (1986). Nonequilibrium phase-transitions in coordinated biological motion—Critical fluctuations. *Physics Letters A, 118,* 279-284.

Kelso, J.A.S., Scholz, J.P., and Schöner, G. (1988). Dynamics govern switching among patterns of coordination. *Physics Letters A, 134,* 8-12.

Kelso, J.A.S., and Schöner, G. (1988). Self-organization of coordinative movement patterns. *Human Movement Science, 7,* 27-46.

Kelso, J.A.S., Schöner, G., Scholz, J.P., and Haken, H. (1987). Phase-locked modes, phase transitions and component oscillators in biological motion. *Physica Scripta, 35,* 79-87.

Kelso, J.A.S., Southard, D.L., and Goodman, D. (1979). On the coordination of two-handed movements. *Journal of Experimental Psychology: Human Perception and Performance, 5,* 229-238.

Kelso, J.A.S., and Zanone, P.G. (2002). Coordination dynamics of learning and transfer across different effector systems. *Journal of Experimental Psychology: Human Perception and Performance, 28,* 776-797.

Keogh, J., and Sugden, D. (1985). *Movement skill development.* New York: Macmillian.

Keskinen, K.L. (1993). *Stroking characteristics of front crawl swimming.* Unpublished doctoral dissertation, University of Jyväskylä, Finland.

Keskinen, K.L., Tilli, L.J. and Komi, P.V. (1989). Maximum velocity swimming: interrelationships of stroking characteristics, force production and anthropometric variables. *Scandinavian Journal of Sports Science,* 11, 87-92.

Kevles, D.J., and Hood, L. (1992). *The code of codes: Scientific and social issues in the human genome project.* Boston: Harvard University Press.

Kiemel, T., Oie, K.S., and Jeka, J.J. (2002). Multisensory fusion and the stochastic structure of postural sway. *Biological Cybernetics, 87,* 262-277.

Kim, S., Carlton, L.G., Liu, Y.T., and Newell, K.M. (1999). Impulse and movement space-time variability. *Journal of Motor Behavior, 31,* 341-357.

Kiphut, R.J.H. (1942). *Swimming.* New York: Barnes.

Ko, Y.G., Challis, J.H., and Newell, K.M. (2001). Postural coordination patterns as a function of dynamics of the support surface. *Human Movement Science, 20,* 737-764.

Ko, Y.G., Challis, J.H., and Newell, K.M. (2003). Learning to coordinate redundant degrees of freedom in a dynamic balance task. *Human Movement Science, 22,* 47-66.

Kobayahi, M., and Musha, T. (1982). 1/f fluctuations of heartbeat period. *IEEE Transactions in Biomedical Engineering, 29,* 456-457.

Kohonen, T. (1995). Self-organizing maps. In T.S. Huang, T. Kohonen, and M.R.Schroeder (Eds.) *Springer Series in Information Science* (Vol. 30). Berlin: Springer-Verlag.

Kolers, P.A. (1975). Memorial consequences of automatized encoding. *Journal of Experimental Psychology: Human Learning and Memory, 1,* 689-701.

Konczak, J. (1990). Toward an ecological theory of motor development: The relevance of the Gibsonian approach to vision for motor development research. In J. Clark and J. Humphrey (Eds.), *Advances in motor development research 3* (pp.201-224). New York: AMS Press.

Konczak, J., Borutta, M., Topka, H., and Dichgans, Y. (1995). The development of goal-directed reaching in infants: Hand trajectory formation and joint torque control. *Experimental Brain Research, 106,* 156-168.

Kornatz, K.W., Christou, E.A., and Enoka, R.M. (2002). *Steadiness training reduces the variability of motor unit discharge rate in isometric and anisometric contractions performed by old adults.* Paper presented at Motoneurones and Muscles: The Output Machinery, Groningen, Holland.

Kornatz, K.W., Christou, E.A., and Enoka, R.M. (2005). Practice reduces motor unit discharge variability in a hand muscle and improves manual dexterity in old adults. *Journal of Applied Physiology* 98(6), 2072-2080.

Kossev, A., and Christova, P. (1998). Discharge pattern of human motor units during dynamic concentric and eccentric contractions. *Electroencephalography in Clinical Neurophysiology,* 109(3), 245-255.

Kristeva, R., Cheyne, D., and Deecke, L. (1991). Neuromagnetic fields accompanying unilateral and bilateral voluntary movements: Topography and analysis of cortical sources. *Electroenceph. Clin. Neurophysiol., 81,* 284-298.

Krizkova, M., Hlavacka F., and Gatev, P. (1993). Visual control of human stance on a narrow and soft support surface. *Physiological Research, 42,* 267-272.

Kugelberg, E. (1973). Histochemical composition, contraction speed and fatiguability of rat soleus motor units. *J. Neurol. Sci., 20,* 177-198.

Kugelberg, E., and Lindgren, B. (1979). Transmission and contraction fatigue of rat motor units in relation to succinate dehydrogenase activity of motor unit fibres. *J. Physiol., 288,* 285-300.

Kugelberg, E., and Thornell, L.E. (1983). Contraction time, histochemical type, and terminal cisternae volume of rat motor units. *Muscle Nerve, 6*(2), 149-153.

Kugler, P.N. (1986). A morphological perspective on the origin and evolution of movements patterns. In M.G. Wade, and H.T.A. Whiting (Eds.), *Motor development in children: Aspects of coordination and control* (pp. 459-858). Boston: Martinus Nijhoff.

Kugler, P.N., Kelso, J.A.S., and Turvey, M.T. (1980). On the concept of coordinative structures as dissipative structures: I. Theoretical lines of convergence. In G.E. Stelmach and J. Requin (Eds.), *Tutorials in motor behavior* (pp. 3-48). Amsterdam: North-Holland.

Kugler, P.N., Kelso, J.A.S., and Turvey, M.T. (1982). On the control and coordination of naturally developing systems. In J.A.S. Kelso and J.E. Clark (Eds.), *The development of movement control and coordination* (pp. 5-78). New York: Wiley.

Kugler, P.N., and Turvey, M.T. (1987). *Information, natural law, and the self-assembly of rhythmic movements.* Hillsdale, NJ: Erlbaum.

Kuo, A.D. (1995). An optimal control model for analyzing human postural balance. *IEEE Transcripts of Biomedical Engineering, 42,* 87-101.

Kuo, A.D., Speers, R.A., Peterka, R.J., and Horak, F.B. (1998). Effect of altered sensory conditions on multivariate descriptors of human postural sway. *Experimental Brain Research, 122,* 185-195.

Kuramoto, Y. (1975). Self-entrainment of a population of coupled nonlinear oscillators. In H. Araki (Ed.), *Int. symposium on mathematical problems in theoretical physics* (pp. 420-422). Berlin: Springer-Verlag.

Kuramoto, Y. (1981). Rhythms and turbulence in populations of chemical oscillators. *Physica A, 106,* 128-143.

Kuramoto, Y. (1984). *Chemical oscillations, waves, and turbulence.* Berlin: Springer-Verlag.

Kuramoto, Y. (1997). Phase- and center-manifold reductions for large populations of coupled oscillators with application to non-locally coupled systems. *Int. J. Bif. and Chaos, 7,* 789-805.

Kurz, M.J., and Stergiou, N. (2002). Effect of normalization and phase angle calculations on continuous relative phase. *Journal of Biomechanics, 35,* 369-374.

Kvålseth, T.O. (1980). An alternative to Fitts' law. *Bulletin of the Psychonomic Society, 16,* 371-373.

LaFiandra, M., Wagenaar, R.C., Holt, K.G., and Obusek, J.P. (2003). How do load carriage and walking speed influence trunk coordination and stride parameters? *Journal of Biomechanics, 36,* 87-95.

Lafortune, M.A., Cavanagh, P.R., Sommer, H.J., and Kalenak, A. (1994). Foot inversion-eversion and knee kinematics during walking. *Journal of Orthopaedic Research, 12,* 412-420.

Lagarde J.F., and Kelso, J.A.S. (2004). Multimodal coordination dynamics: The binding of movement, sound, and touch. *Journal of Sport and Exercise Psychology, 26,* S12-S12.

Laidlaw, D.H., Bilodeau, M., and Enoka, R.M. (2000). Steadiness is reduced and motor unit discharge is more variable in old adults. *Muscle and Nerve, 23,* 600-612.

Laidlaw, D.H., Kornatz, K.W., Keen, D.A., Suzuki, S., and Enoka, R.M. (1999). Strength training improves the steadiness of slow lengthening contractions performed by old adults. *Journal of Applied Physiology, 87*(5), 1786-1795.

Lamoth, C.J.C., Beek, P.J., and Meijer, O.G. (2002). Pelvis-thorax coordination in the transverse plane during gait. *Gait and Posture, 16,* 101-114.

Langolf, G.D., Chaffin, D.B., and Foulke, J.A. (1976). An investigation of Fitts' law using a wide range of movement amplitudes. *Journal of Motor Behavior, 8,* 113-128.

Lankford, E.B., Epstein, N.D., Fananapazir, L., and Sweeney, H.L. (1995). Abnormal contractile properties of muscle fibers expressing beta-myosin heavy chain gene mutations in patients with hypertrophic cardiomyopathy. *J. Clin. Invest., 95,* 1409-1414.

Largo, R.H., Molinari, L., Wber, M., Comenale Pinto, L., and Duc, G. (1985). Early development of locomotion: Significance of prematurity, cerebral palsy and sex. *Developmental Medicine and Child Neurology, 27,* 183-191.

Larsson, L. (1992). Is the motor unit uniform? *Acta Physiol. Scand., 144,* 143-154.

Larsson, L., Li, X., Berg, H.E., and Frontera, W.R. (1996). Effects of removal of weight-bearing function on contractility and myosin isoform composition in single human skeletal muscle cells. *Pflugers Arch., 432,* 320-328.

Larsson, L., Li, X., and Frontera, W.R. (1997). Effects of aging on shortening velocity and myosin isoform composition in single human skeletal muscle cells. *Am. J. Physiol., 272,* C638-649.

Larsson, L., and Moss, R.L. (1993). Maximum velocity of shortening in relation to myosin isoform composition in single fibres from human skeletal muscles. *Journal of Physiology, 472,* 595-614.

Latash, M.L. (1996). The Bernstein problem: How does the central nervous system make its choices? In M.L. Latash and M.T. Turvey, (Eds.), *Dexterity and its development* (pp. 277-304). Mahwah, NJ: Erlbaum.

Latash, M.L. (1998). *Neurophysiological basis of movement.* Champaign, IL: Human Kinetics.

Latash, M.L., Scholz, J.P., and Schoner, G. (2002). Motor control strategies revealed in the structure of motor variability. *Exercise and Sport Sciences Reviews, 30,* 26-31.

Ledebt, A. (2000). Changes in arm posture during the early acquisition of walking. *Infant Behavior and Development, 23,* 79-89

Lee, D.N., and Lishman, R. (1975). Visual proprioceptive control of stance. *Journal of Human Movement Studies, 1,* 87-95.

Lees, A. (1992). Biomechanics in teaching and coaching—Systematic approaches to the identification of mechanisms in performance and injury. In R. Rodano, G. Ferrigno, and G. Santambrogio (Eds.), *Proceedings of the Xth Symposium of the International Society of Biomechanics in Sports* (pp. 171-177). Milan: Edi Ermes.

Lees, A. (1999). Biomechanical assessment of individual sports for improved performance. *Sports Medicine, 28,* 299-305.

Lees, A. (2002). Technique analysis in sports: A critical review. *Journal of Sports Sciences, 20,* 813-828.

Leocani, L., Toro, C., Manganotti, P., and Hallett, M. (1997). Event-related coherence and event-related desynchronization/sychronization in the 10 Hz and 20 Hz EEG during self-paced movements. *Electroenceph. Clin. Neurophysiol., 104,* 199-206.

Lestienne, F., Soechting, J., and Berthoz, A. (1977). Postural readjustments induced by linear motion of visual scenes. *Experimental Brain Research, 28,* 363-384.

Lewontin, R. (2000). *It ain't necessarily so: The dream of the human genome and other illusions.* London: Granta Books.

Li, L., van den Bogert, E.C.H., Caldwell, G.E., Van Emmerik, R.E.A., and Hamill, J. (1999). Coordination patterns of walking and running at a similar speed and stride frequency. *Human Movement Science, 18,* 67-85.

Libet, B. (1994). *Neurophysiology of consciousness: Selected papers and new essays.* Boston: Birkhauser.

Liebovitch, L.S. (1998). *Fractals and chaos: Simplified for the life sciences.* New York: Oxford University Press.

Lintem, G. (1991). Instructional strategies. In J.E. Morrison (Ed.), *Training for performance: Principles of applied human learning,* pp.167-191. Chichester, England: Wiley.

Lipsitz, L.A. (2002). Dynamics of stability: The physiologic basis of functional health and frailty. *Journal of Gerontology A Biological Science Medical Science, 57,* B115-125.

Lipsitz, L.A., and Goldberger, A.L. (1992). Loss of "complexity" and aging. *Journal of the American Medical Association, 267,* 1806-1809.

Liu, Q., Hay, J.G., and Andrews, J.G. (1993). Body role and hand path in freestyle swimming: An experimental study. *Journal of Applied Biomechanics, 9,* 238-253.

Liu, Y-T., Mayer-Kress, G., and Newell, K.M. (1999). A piecewise linear map model for the sequential trial strategy of discrete timing tasks. *Acta Psychologica, 103,* 207-228.

Logan, G.D. (1988). Towards an instance theory of automisation. *Psychological Review, 95,* 492-527.

Lopes da Silva, F.H., Hoeks, A., Smits, H., and Zetterberg, L.H. (1974). Model of brain rhythmic activity. *Kybernetik, 15,* 27-37.

Lowry, C.V., Kimmey, J.S., Felder, S., Chi, M.M.Y., Kaiser, K.K., Passoneau, P.N., Kirk, K.A., and Lowry, O.H. (1978). Enzyme patterns in single human muscle fibres. *J. Biol. Chem., 253,* 8269-8277.

Lytton, J., Westlin, M., Burk, S.E., Shull, G.E., and MacLennan, D.H. (1992). Functional comparisons between isoforms of the sarcoplasmic or endoplasmic reticulum family of calcium pumps. *J. Biol. Chem., 267*(20), 14483-14489.

Magill, R. (1998). *Motor learning: Concepts and applications* (5th ed.). New York: McGraw-Hill.

Mah, C.D., Hulliger, M., Lee, R.G., and O'Callaghan, I.S. (1994). Quantitative analysis of human movement synergies: Constructive pattern analysis for gait. *Journal of Motor Behavior, 26*(2), 83-102.

Maki, B. (1997). Gait changes in older adults: Predictors of falls or indicators of fear? *Journal of American Geriatric Society, 45,* 313-320.

Mandelbrot, B. (1983). *The fractal geometry of nature.* New York: Freeman.

Mardia, K.V. (1971). *Statistics of directional data.* London: Academic Press.

Marin, L. (1997). Biomechanics as a (limited) constraint on postural coordination. In M.A. Schmuckler and J.M. Kennedy (Eds.), *Studies in Perception and Action III* (pp. 167-170). Hillsdale, NJ: Erlbaum.

Marin, L., Bardy, B.G., Baumberger, B., Flückiger, M., and Stoffregen, T.A. (1999). Interaction between task demands and surface properties in the control of goal-oriented stance. *Human Movement Science, 18,* 31-47.

Marin, L., Bardy, B.G., and Bootsma, R.J. (1999). Level of gymnastic skill as an intrinsic constraint on postural coordination. *Journal of Sport Sciences, 17,* 615-626.

Marin, L., and Oullier, O. (2001). When robots fail: The complex processes of learning and development. *Behavioral and Brain Sciences, 24,* 1067-1068.

Marisi, D.Q. (1977). Genetic and extragenetic variance in motor performance. *Acta Genetica Medica, 26,* 3-4.

Marteniuk, R.G. (1976). *Information processing in motor skills.* New York: Holt, Rinehart and Winston.

Masakado, Y., Noda, Y., Nagata, M., Kimura, A., Chino, N., and Akaboshi, K. (1994). Macro-EMG and motor unit recruitment threshold: Differences between the young and the aged. *Neuroscience Letters, 179,* 1-4.

Matthews, P.B.C. (1972). *Mammalian muscle receptors and their central actions.* London: Arnold.

Mayer-Kress, G., Deutsch, K.M., and Newell, K.M. (2002). Modeling the control of isometric force production with piece-wise linear, stochastic maps of multiple time-scales. *Fluctuations and Noise Letters, 3,* L23-30.

Mayer-Kress, G., and Holzfuss, J. (1987). Analysis of the human electroencephalogram with methods from nonlinear dynamics. In L. Rensing, van der Heyden, and M.C. Mackey (Eds.), *Proceedings of temporal disorder in human oscillatory systems, Springer Series in Synergetics* (Vol. 36, pp. 57-68). Berlin: Springer-Verlag.

Mayer-Kress, G., and Newell, K.M. (2003). Stochastic iterative maps with multiple time-scales for modeling human motor behavior. *Nonlinear Phenomena in Complex Systems, 4,* 1-8.

Mayer-Kress, G., Yates, F.E, Benton, L., Keidel, M., Tirsch, W., Poppl, S., and Geist, K. (1988). Dimensional analysis of nonlinear oscillations in brain, heart and muscle. *Mathematical Biosciences, 90,* 155-182.

McArdle, D. and Reilly, T. (1992). Consequences of altering stroke parameters in front crawl swimming and its simulation. In *Biomechanics and Medicine in Swimming – Swimming Science VI* (edited by D. MacLaren, T. Reilly and A. Lees), pp. 125-130. London: E and FN Spon.

McAuley, J.H., and Marsden, C.D. (2000). Physiological and pathological tremors and rhythmic central motor control. *Brain, 123*(8), 1545-1567.

McClay, I., and Manal, K. (1997). Coupling parameters in runners with normal and excessive pronation. *Journal of Applied Biomechanics, 13,* 109-124.

McClay, I.S. (2000). The evolution of the study of running mechanics: relationships to injury. *Journal of the American Podiatric Society,* 90,133-148.

McCloskey, D.I. (1978). Kinesthetic sensibility. *Physiology Review, 58,* 763-820.

McCollum, G., and Leen, T.K. (1989). Form and exploration of mechanical stability limits in erect stance. *Journal of Motor Behavior, 21,* 225-244.

McDonald, P.V., Van Emmerik, R.E.A., and Newell, K.M. (1989). The effects of practice on limb kinematics in a throwing task. *Journal of Motor Behavior, 21,* 245-264.

McGehee, R. (1997). The virtual wall: A key to learning the basic tennis serve. *Journal of Physical Recreation and Dance, 68,* 10-12.

McGinnis, P.M., and Newell, K.M. (1982). Topological dynamics: A framework for describing movement and its constraints. *Human Movement Science, 1,* 289-305.

McGraw, M. (1935). *Growth: A study of Johnny and Jimmy.* New York: Appleton-Century-Crofts.

McIntyre, D.R., and Pfautsch, E.W. (1982). A kinematic analysis of the baseball batting swing involved in opposite-field and same-field hitting. *Research Quarterly for Exercise and Sport, 53,* 206-213.

McPherson, S.L. (1993). Knowledge representation and decision-making in sport. In J.L. Starkes and F. Allard (Eds.), *Cognitive issues in motor expertise* (pp. 159-188). Amsterdam: North-Holland.

McPherson, S.L. and French, K. E. (1991). Changes in cognitive strategies and motor skills in tennis. *Journal of Sport and Exercise Psychology, 25,* 249-265.

Mégrot, F., Bardy, B.G., and Dietrich, G. (2002). Dimensionality and the dynamics of human unstable equilibrium. *Journal of Motor Behavior, 34,* 323-328.

Melzack, R., and Wall, P.D. (1983). *Textbook of Pain.* New York: Churchill Livingstone.

Mendoza, L., and Schöllhorn, W.I. (1990). Technical training in the field of high performance athletes with a biomechanical feedback system. In G.P. Brüggemann and J.K. Rühl (Eds.), *Techniques in athletics—The first international conference, Cologne, 7-9 June 1990* (pp. 412-419). Köln: Strauss.

Merleau-Ponty, M. (1962). *Phenomenology of perception.* (C. Smith, Trans.). New York: Humanities Press. (Original work published 1945).

Messier, S.P., Davis, S.E., Curl, W.W., Lowery, R.B., and Pack, R.J. (1991). Etiologic factors associated with patellofemoral pain in runners. *Medicine and Science in Sports and Exercise, 23,* 1008-1015.

Messier, S.P., and Pittala, K.A. (1988). Etiologic factors associated with selected running injuries. *Medicine and Science in Sports and Exercise, 20,* 501-505.

Metzger, W. (1975). *Gesetze des sehens [Laws of vision].* Frankfurt, Germay: Kramer.

Meyer, D.E., Abrams, R.A., Kornblum, S., Wright, C.E., and Smith, J.E.K. (1988). Optimality in human motor performance: Ideal control of rapid aimed movements. *Psychological Review, 95,* 340-370.

Michaels, C.F., and Carello, C. (1981). *Direct perception.* Englewood Cliffs, NJ: Prentice Hall.

Mill, J.S. (1843/1965). *Of liberty and necessity, Ch. II, Book VI, A system of logic* (18th ed.). London: Longman.

Miller, D.I. (1981). Biomechanical considerations in lower extremity amputee running and sports performance. *Australian Journal of Sports Medicine, 13,* 55-67.

Minetti, A.E. (1994). Contraction dynamics in antagonist muscles. *J. Theoret. Biol., 169*(3), 295-304.

Minetti, A.E., Ardigò, L.P., Susta, D., and Cotelli, F. (1998). Using leg muscles as shock absorbers: Theoretical predictions and experimental results of human drop landing. *Ergonomics, 41*(12): 1771-1791

Monno, A., Chardenon, A., Temprado, J.J., Zanone, P.G., and Laurent, M. (2000). Effects of attention on phase transitions between bimanual coordination patterns: A behavioral and cost analysis in humans. *Neuroscience Letters, 283,* 93-96.

Monsaas, J.A. (1985). Learning to be a world-class tennis player. In B.S. Bloom (Ed.), *Developing talent in young people* (pp. 211-269). New York: Ballantine.

Monster, A.W., Chan, H., and O'Connor, D. (1978). Activity patterns of human skeletal muscles: Relation to muscle fiber type composition. *Science, 200*(4339), 314-317.

Montgomery, H.E., Clarkson, P., Barnard, M., Bell, J.D., Brynes, A.E., Dollery, C.M., Hajnal, J., Hemingway, H., Mercer, D., Jarman, P., Marshall, R., Prasad, K., Rayson, M., Saeed, N., Talmud, P., Thomas, L., Jubb, M., World, M., and Humphries, S. (1999). Angiotensin-converting enzyme gene insertion/deletion polymorphism and response to physical training. *Lancet, 353,* 541-545.

Montgomery, H.E., Marshall R., Hemingway H., Myerson S., Clarkson P., Dollery C., Hayward M., Holliman D.E., Jubb M., World M., Thomas E.L., Brynes A.E., Saeed N., Barnard M., Bell J.D., Prasad K., Rayson M., Talmud P.J. and Humphries S.E. (1998). Human gene for physical performance. *Nature, 393,* 221-222.

Montgomery, H.E. and Payne, J. (2004). Angiotensin-converting enzyme and human physical performance. *Equine and Comparative Exercise Physiology 4,* 255-260.

Morange, F., and Bloch, H. (1996). Laterlization of the approach movement and the prehension movement in infants from 4 to 7 months. *Early Development and Parenting, 5,* 81-92.

Morrison, S., and Newell, K.M. (1996). Inter- and intra-limb coordination in a postural pointing task. *Experimental Brain Research, 110,* 455-464.

Morriss, C.J. (1998). Coordination patterns in the performance of an elite javelin-thrower. *Journal of Sports Sciences, 16,* 12-13.

Müller, H., and Loosch, E. (1999). Functional variability and an equifinal path of movement during targeted throwing. *Journal of Human Movement Studies, 36,* 103-126.

Müller, H., Reiser, M., and Daugs, R. (1998). Performance strategies for achieving high result consistencies in aimed throwing tasks. In P. Blaser (Ed.), *Sport kinetics '97* (pp. 105-109). Hamburg: Czwalina.

Müller, H., and Sternad, D. (2004). Decomposition of variability in the execution of goal-oriented tasks: Three components of skill improvement. *Journal of Experimental Psychology: Human Perception and Performance 30,* 212-233.

Mullineaux, D.R., Bartlett, R.M., and Bennett, S. (2001). Research design and statistics in biomechanics and motor control. *Journal of Sports Sciences, 19,* 739-760.

Mullineaux, D.R., and Wheat, J.S. (2002). Quantifying coordination in kinematic data: A running example. In K.E. Gianikellis (Ed.), *Scientific Proceedings of the XXth International Symposium on Biomechanics in Sports* (pp. 515-518). Caceres, Spain: Universidad de Extremadura.

Murthy, V.N., and Fetz, E.E. (1996). Oscillatory activity in sensorimotor cortex of awake monkeys: Synchronization of local field potentials and relation to behavior. *J. Neurophysiology, 76,* 3949-3967.

Musha, T. (1981). 1/f fluctuations in biological systems. In P.H.E. Meijer, R.D. Mountain, and R.J. Soulen, Jr. (Eds.), *Sixth International Conference On Noise in Physical Systems* (pp. 143-146). Washington, DC: U.S. Department of Commerce and National Bureau of Standards.

Myerson, S., Hemingway, H., Budget, R., Martin, J., Humphries, S.E., and Montgomery, H.E. (1999). Human angiotensin I-converting enzyme gene and endurance performance. *Journal of Applied Physiology, 87,* 1313-1316.

Nakamura, T., Meguro, K. and Sasaki, H. (1996). Relationship between falls and stride length variability in senile dementia of the Alzheimer type. *Gerontology, 42,* 108-113.

Nardone, A., Romano, C., and Schieppati, M. (1989). Selective recruitment of high-threshold human motor units during voluntary isotonic lengthening of active muscles. *J. Physiol. (Lond.), 409,* 451-471.

Nashner, L.M., and McCollum, G. (1985). The organization of postural movements: A formal basis and experimental synthesis. *Behavioral and Brain Sciences, 26,* 135-172.

Nashner, L.M., Shupert, C.L., Horak, F.B., and Black, F.O. (1989). Organization of posture controls: An analysis of sensory and mechanical constraints. *Progress in Brain Research, 80,* 411-418.

Nawoczenski, D.A., Saltzman, C.L., and Cook, T.M. (1998). The effect of foot structure on the three-dimensional kinematic coupling behavior of the leg and rear foot. *Physical Therapy, 78,* 404-416.

Nazarov, I.B., Woods, D.R., Montgomery, H.E., Shneider, O.V., Kazakov, V.I., Tomilin, N.V., and Rogozkin, V.A. (2001). The angiotensin converting enzyme I/D polymorphism in Russian athletes. *European Journal of Human Genetics, 9,* 797-801.

Nelson, R.C. (1971). Biomechanics of sport: an overview. In *Biomechanics* (edited by J.M. Cooper), pp. 31-37. Chicago, IL: The Athletic Institute.

Nelson, R.C. (1989). Biomechanics for better performance and protection from injury. In *Future directions in exercise and sport science research,* ed. J.S. Skinner, C.B. Corbin, D.M. Landers, P.E. Martin, and C.L. Wells, 5-12. Champaign, IL: Human Kinetics.

Nemeth, P., Pette, D., and Vrbova, G. (1981). Comparison of enzyme activities among single muscle fibres within defined motor units. *J. Physiol., 311,* 489-495.

Neu, J.C. (1980). Large populations of coupled chemical oscillators. SIAM *Journal on Applied Mathematics, 38,* 305-316. (SIAM stands for Society for Industrial and Applied Mathematics)

Neville, W. (1994). *Serve it up: Volleyball for life.* San Francisco: Mayfield.

Newell, A., and Rosenbloom, P.S. (1981). Mechanisms of skill acquisition and the law of practice. In J.R. Anderson (Ed.), *Cognitive skills and their acquisition* (pp. 1-55). Hillsdale, NJ: Erlbaum.

Newell, K.M. (1981). Skill learning. In D. Holding (Ed.), *Human skills* (pp. 203-226). Chichester, England: Wiley.

Newell, K.M. (1985). Coordination, control and skill. In *Differing Perspectives in Motor Learning, Memory, and Control,* ed. D. Goodman, R.B. Wilberg, and I.M. Franks, 295-317. Amsterdam: Elsevier Science.

Newell, K.M. (1986). Constraints on the development of coordination. In M.G. Wade and H.T.A. Whiting (Eds.), *Motor development in children: Aspects of coordination and control* (pp. 341-360). Boston: Martinus Nijhoff.

Newell, K.M. (1998). Degrees of freedom and the development of postural center of pressure profiles. In K.M. Newell and P.C.M. Molenaar (Eds.), *Applications of nonlinear dynamics to developmental process modeling* (pp. 63-84). Hillsdale, NJ: Erlbaum.

Newell, K.M., Broderick, M.P., Deutsch, K.M., and Slifkin, A.B. (2003). Task constraints and change in degrees of freedom with motor learning. *Journal of Experimental Psychology: Human Perception and Performance, 29,* 379-387.

Newell, K.M., Carlton, L.G., and Kim, S. (1994). Time and space-time movement accuracy. *Human Performance, 7,* 1-21.

Newell, K.M., Carlton, L.G., Carlton, M.J., and Halbert, J.A. (1980). Velocity as a factor in movement timing accuracy. *Journal of Motor Behavior, 12,* 47-56.

Newell, K.M., Challis, S., and Morrison, S. (2000). Dimensional constraints on limb movements. *Human Movement Science, 19,* 175-201.

Newell, K.M., and Corcos, D.M. (Eds.). (1993). *Variability and motor control.* Champaign, IL: Human Kinetics.

Newell, K.M., Deutsch, K., and Morrison, S. (2000). On learning to move randomly. *Journal of Motor Behavior, 32,* 314-320.

Newell, K.M., Hoshizaki, L.E.F., Carlton, M.J., and Halbert, J.A. (1979). Movement time and velocity as determinants of movement timing accuracy. *Journal of Motor Behavior, 11,* 49-58.

Newell, K.M., Liu, Y.T., and Mayer-Kress, G. (1997). The sequential structure of movement outcome in learning a discrete timing task. *Journal of Motor Behavior, 29,* 366-382.

Newell, K.M., Liu, Y-T., and Mayer-Kress, G. (2001). Time scales in motor learning and development. *Psychological Review, 108,* 57-82.

Newell, K.M., and McDonald, P.V. (1991). Practice: A search for task solutions. In R. Christina and H.M. Eckert (Eds.), *American Academy of Physical Education Papers: Enhancing human performance in sport: New concepts and developments* (pp. 51-60). Champaign, IL: Human Kinetics.

Newell, K.M., and Molenaar, P.M.C. (Eds.). (1998). *Applications of nonlinear dynamics to developmental process modeling.* Hillsdale, NJ: Erlbaum.

Newell, K.M., Scully, D., McDonald, P.V., and Baillargeon, R. (1989). Body scale and the development of prehension. *Developmental Psychobiology, 22,* 1-13

Newell, K.M., and Slifkin, A.B. (1998). The nature of movement variability. In J.P. Piek (Ed.), *Motor behavior and human skill: A multidisciplinary perspective* (pp. 143-160). Champaign, IL: Human Kinetics.

Newell, K.M., Slobounov, S.M., Slobounova, E., and Molenaar, P.C.M. (1997a). Deterministic and stochastic processes in center of pressure profiles. *Experimental Brain Research, 113,* 158-164.

Newell, K.M., Slobounov, S.M., Slobounova, E., and Molenaar, P.M.C. (1997b). Short-term non stationarity and the development of postural control. *Gait and Posture, 6,* 56-62.

Newell, K.M., and Vaillancourt, D.E. (2001). Dimensional change in motor learning. *Human Movement Science, 20,* 695-715.

Newell, K.M., and Van Emmerik, R.E.A. (1989). The acquisition of coordination: Preliminary analysis of learning to write. *Human Movement Science, 8,* 17-32.

Newell, K.M., Van Emmerik, R.E.A., Lee, D., and Sprague, R.L. (1993). On postural variability and stability. *Gait and Posture, 4,* 225-230.

Nigg, B.M. (1985). Biomechanics, load analysis and sports injuries in the lower extremities. *Sports Medicine, 2,* 367-379.

Nigg, B.M. (1993). Sports science in the twenty-first century. *Journal of Sports Sciences, 11,* 343-347.

Nigg, B.M. (1998). Biomechanics as applied to sports. In M. Harries, C. Williams, W.D. Stanish, and L.J. Micheli (Eds.), *Oxford textbook of sports medicine* (pp. 153-171). Oxford, UK: Oxford University Press.

Nigg, B.M., and Bobbert, M. (1990). On the potential of various approaches in load analysis to reduce the frequency of sports injuries. *Journal of Biomechanics, 23,* 3-12.

Norman, R.W. (1985). Biomechanics: Are there substantive issues? *International Society of Biomechanics Newsletter, 18,* 2-4.

Norman, R.W. (1989). A barrier to understanding human motion mechanisms: A commentary. In J.S. Skinner, C.B. Corbin, D.M. Landers, P.E. Martin, and C.L. Wells (Eds.), *Future directions in exercise and sport science research* (pp. 151-161). Champaign, IL: Human Kinetics.

Norrie, M.L. (1967). Effects of practice on true score and intra-individual variability for reaction and movement times for simple and complex movements. *Research Quarterly, 38,* 457-467.

Novacheck, T.F. (1998). The biomechanics of running. *Gait and Posture, 7,* 77-95.

Nunez, P.L. (1995). *Neocortical dynamics and human EEG rhythms.* New York: Oxford University Press.

Nunez, P.L. (2000). Towards a quantitative description of large scale neocortical dynamic function and EEG. *Behav. Brain Sci., 23,* 371-398.

Ogata, T., and Mori, M. (1964). Histochemical studies of oxidative enzymes in vertebrate muscles. *J. Histochem. Cytochem., 12,* 171-182.

Ohl, F.W., Scheich, H., and Freeman, W.J. (2001). Change in pattern of ongoing cortical activity with auditory category learning. *Nature, 412,* 733-736.

O'Keefe, J., and Nadel, L. (1978). *The hippocampus as a cognitive map.* Oxford, UK: Clarendon Press.

Olree, K.S., and Vaughan, C.L. (1995). Fundamental pattern of bilateral muscle activity in human locomotion. *Biological Cybernetics, 73,* 409-414.

Oullier, O., Bardy, B.G., and Bootsma, R.J. (2001). Intrinsic and informational coupling in stance. In G. Burton and R.C. Schmidt (Eds.), *Studies in perception and action VI* (pp. 169-172). Mawah, N.J.: Erlbaum.

Oullier, O., Bardy, B.G., Bootsma, R.J., and Stoffregen, T.A. (1999). On the dynamical nature of human postural transitions. In M.A. Grealy and J.A. Thomson (Eds.), *Studies in perception and action V* (pp. 330-333). Mawah, N.J.: Erlbaum.

Oullier, O., Bardy, B.G., Stoffregen, T.A., and Bootsma, R.J. (2002). Postural coordination in looking and tracking tasks. *Human Movement Science, 21,* 147-167.

Oullier, O., Bardy, B.G., Stoffregen, T.A., and Bootsma, R.J. (2004). Task-specific stabilization of postural coordination during stance on a beam. *Motor Control, 8,* 174-87.

Oullier, O., de Guzman G. C., Jantzen, K. J., and Kelso, J.A.S. (2003). On context dependence of behavioral variability in inter-personal coordination. *International Journal of Computer Science in Sport, 2,* 126-128.

Oullier, O., de Guzman, G.C., Jantzen, K.J., and Kelso, J.A.S. (2003). The role of spatial configuration and homologous muscle activation in coordination between two individuals. *Journal of Sport and Exercise Psychology, 25, S104-S105.*

Oullier, O., Jantzen, K. J., Steinberg, F. L., and Kelso, J.A.S. (2005). Neural substrates of real and imagined sensorimotor coordination. *Cerebral Cortex, 15,* 975-985.

Out, L., Savelsbergh, G.J.P., and van Soest, A. (2001). Interceptive timing in early infancy. *Journal of Human Movement Studies, 40,* 185-206

Out, L., Savelsbergh, G.J.P., van Soets, A.J., and Hopkins, B. (1997). Influence of mechanical factors on movement units in infant reaching. *Human Movement Science,16,* 733-748.

Out, L., van Soest, J., Savelsbergh, G.J.P., and Hopkins, B. (1998). The effect of posture on early reaching movements. *Journal of Motor Behaviour, 30,* 260-272.

Oyama, S. (2000). *The ontogeny of information: Developmental systems and evolution* (2nd ed.). Durham, NC: Duke University Press.

Padykula, H.A., and Gauthier, G.F. (1967). Morphological and cytochemical characteristics of fiber types in normal mammalian skeletal muscle. In A.T. Milhorat (Ed.), *Exploratory concepts in muscle dystrophy and related disorders* (pp. 117-131). New York: Excerpta Medica.

Pai, Y-C., and Patton, J.L. (1997). Center of mass velocity-position predictions for balance control. *Journal of Biomechanics, 30,* 347-354.

Pardhan, S., Gilchrist, J., Elliott, D.B., and Beh, G.K. (1996). A comparison of sampling efficiency and internal noise level in young and old subjects. *Vision Research, 36,* 1641-1648.

Peper, C.E., and Beek, P.J. (1998). Are frequency-induced transitions in rhythmic coordination mediated by a drop in amplitude? *Biol. Cybern., 79,* 291-300.

Peper, C.E., Beek, P.J., and van Wieringen, P.C.W. (1991). Bifurcations in bimanual tapping: In search of Farey principles. In J. Requin and G.E. Stelmach (Eds.), *Tutorials in motor neuroscience* (pp. 413-431). Dordrecht, the Netherlands: Kluwer Academic Publisher.

Peper, C.E., Beek, P.J., and van Wieringen, P.C.W. (1995a). Coupling strength in tapping a 2:3 polyrhythm. *Hum. Movement Sci., 14,* 217-245.

Peper, C.E., Beek, P.J., and van Wieringen, P.C.W. (1995b). Frequency-induced transitions in bimanual tapping. *Biol. Cybern., 73,* 301-309.

Person, R.S., and Kudina, L.P. (1972). Discharge frequency and discharge pattern of human motor units during voluntary contraction of muscle. *Electroencephalography and Clinical Neurophysiology, 32*(5), 471-483.

Peter, J.B., Barnard, R.J., Edgerton, V.R., Gillespie, C.A., and Stempel, K.E. (1972). Metabolic profiles of three fiber types of skeletal muscle in guinea pig and rabbit. *Biochemistry, 11,* 2627-2633.

Peters, B.T., Haddad, J.M., Heiderscheit, B.C., Van Emmerik, R.E.A., and Hamill, J. (2003). Limitations in the use and interpretation of continuous relative phase. *Journal of Biomechanics, 36,* 271-274.

Petlichkoff, L.M. (1993). Coaching children: Understanding the motivational process. *Sport Science Review, 2,* 49-61.

Pette, D., and Staron, R.S. (1997). Mammalian skeletal muscle fiber type transitions. *Int. Rev. Cytol., 170,* 143-223.

Pette, D., Wimmer, M., and Nemeth, P. (1981). Do enzyme activities vary along muscle fibres? *Histochemistry, 67,* 225-231.

Pew, R.W. (1969). The speed-accuracy operating characteristic. *Acta Psychologica, 30,* 16-26.

Piaget, J. (1930). *The child's conception of physical causality.* New York: Harcourt Brace Jovanovich, Inc.

Pick, H. (2003). Development and learning: An historical perspective on acquisition of motor control. *Infant Behavior and Development, 26,* 441-448.

Piek, J.P. (2002). The role of variability in early motor development. *Infant Behavior and Development,* 25, 252-265.

Pierce, J.R. (1963). *An introduction to information theory: Symbols, signals and noise* (2nd ed.). New York: Dover.

Pincus, S.M. (1991). Approximate entropy as a measure of system complexity. *Proceedings of the National Academy of Sciences, 88,* 2297-2301.

Piotrkiewicz, M. (1999). An influence of after hyperpolarization on the pattern of motorneuronal rhythmic activity. *Journal of Physiology (Paris), 93,* 125-133.

Pollard, C. (2002). *Potential mechanisms of ACL injury: The gender bias.* Unpublished doctoral dissertation, University of Massachusetts, Amherst.

Port, N.L., Lee, D., Dassonville, P., and Georgopoulos, P. (1997). Manual interception of moving targets. I. Performance and movement initiation. *Experimental Brain Research, 116,* 406-420.

Post, A.A., Daffertshofer, A., and Beek, P.J. (2000). Principle components in three-ball cascade juggling. *Biological Cybernetics, 82,* 143-152.

Post, A.A., Peper, C.E., Daffertshofer, A., and Beek, P.J. (2000). Relative phase dynamics in perturbed interlimb coordination: Stability and stochasticity. *Biol. Cybern., 83,* 443-459.

Prechtl, H.F.R. (1970). Discussion. In K.J. Connolly (Ed.), *Mechanisms of motor skill development* (pp. 190). London: Academic Press.

Preyer, W. (1888). *The mind of the child: Part I. The senses and the will* (N.W. Brown, Trans.). New York: Appleton. (Original work published 1880).

Priplata, A., Niemi, J., Salen, M., Harry, J., Lipsitz, L.A., and Collins, J.J. (2002). Noise-enhanced human balance control. *Physical Review Letters, 89,* 238101-4.

Pritchard, W.S. (1992). The brain in fractal time: 1/f-like power spectrum scaling of the human electroencephalogram. *International Journal of Neuroscience, 66,* 119-129.

Proust, M. (1919). *A la recherche du temps perdu.* [Remembrance of Time Past]. Paris: Gallimard.

Provine, R.R., and Westerman, J.A. (1979). Crossing the midline: Limits of early eye-hand behavior. *Child Development, 50,* 437-441.

Pufall, P.B., and Dunbar, C. (1992). Perceiving whether or not the world affords stepping onto and over: A developmental study. *Ecological Psychology, 4,* 17-38.

Pusch, M., and Jentsch, T.J. (1994). Molecular physiology of voltage-gated chloride channels. *Physiol. Rev., 74*(4), 813-827.

Ranganathan, V.K., Siemionow, V., Sahgal, V., Liu, J.Z., and Yue, G.H. (2001). Skilled finger movement exercise improves hand function. *Journal of Gerontology A Biological Science Medical Science, 56*(8), M518-522.

Rankinen, T., Perusse, L., Gagnon, J., Chagnon, Y.C., Leon, A.S., Skinner, J.S., Wilmore, J.H., Rao, D.C., and Bouchard, C. (2000). Angiotensin-converting enzyme ID polymorphism and fitness phenotype in the HERITAGE Family Study. *Journal of Applied Physiology, 88,* 1029-1035.

Regan, T. (1998). On the web, speed instead of accuracy. *Nieman Reports, 52*(1), 81.

Reichmann, H., and Pette, D., 1982. A comparative microphotometric study of succinate dehydrogenase activity levels in type I, IIA and IIB fibres of mammalian and human muscles. *Histochemistry, 74,* 27-41.

Reisman, D.S., Scholz, J.P., and Schoner, G. (2002). Coordination underlying the control of whole body momentum during sit-to-stand. *Gait and Posture, 15,* 45-55.

Riccio, G.E. (1993). Information in movement variability about the qualitative dynamics of posture and orientation. In K.M. Newell and D.M. Corcos (Eds.), *Variability and motor control* (pp. 317-357). Champaign, IL: Human Kinetics.

Riccio,G.E., and McDonald,V.P. (1998). *Multimodal perception and multicriterion control of nested systems: I. Coordination of postural control and vehicular control* (NASA Technical Rep. No. TP 3703) Houston, Tx.: NASA.

Riccio, G.E., and Stoffregen, T.A. (1988). Affordances as constraints on the control of stance. *Human Movement Science, 7*, 265-300.

Richardson, M. J., Marsh, K. L., and Schmidt, R. C. (2005). Effects of visual and verbal interaction on unintentional interpersonal coordination. *Journal of Experimental Psychology: Human Perception and Performance, 31*, 62-79.

Richman, J.S., and Moorman, J.R. (1999). Physiological time-series analysis using approximate entropy and sample entropy. *American Journal of Physiology: Heart and Circulation Physiology, 278*, H2039-2049.

Riley, M.A., and Turvey, M. (2002). Variability and determinism in motor behavior. *Journal of Motor Behavior, 34*, 99-125.

Ringer, L.B. and Adrian, M.J. (1969). An electrogoniometric study of the wrist and elbow in the crawl arm stroke. *The Research Quarterly, 40*, 353-363.

Risken, H. (1989). *The Fokker-Planck equation—Methods of solution and applications.* Berlin: Springer-Verlag.

Ritter, H., Martinetz, T., and Schulten, K. (1992). *Neural computation and self-organizing maps.* Reading, MA: Addison-Wesley.

Rochat, P. (1992). Self-sitting and reaching in 5- to 8- month old infants: The impact of posture and its development on early eye-hand coordination. *Journal of Motor Behavior, 24*, 210-220.

Roos, M.R., Rice, C.L., and Vandervoort, A.A. (1997). Age-related changes in motor unit function. *Muscle and Nerve, 20*(6), 679-690.

Rosen, R. (1970). *Dynamical systems theory in biology: Stability theory and its application.* New York: Wiley.

Rosen, R. (1983). Role of similarity principles in data extrapolation. *American Journal of Physiology, 244*, R591-599.

Rosenbaum, D.A., and Collyer, C.E. (1998). *Timing of behavior. Neural, psychological, and computational perspectives.* Cambridge, MA: MIT Press.

Rosengren, K.S., and Savelsbergh, G.J.P. (2003). Development and learning: A TASC-based perspective on the acquisition of perceptual motor behaviors. *Infant Behavior and Development, 26*, 473-494.

Rosenberg, S., Weber, N., Crocq, M-A., Duval, F., and Macher, J-P. (1990). Random number generation by normal, alcoholic and schizophrenic participants. *Psychological Medicine, 20*, 953-960.

Rosengren, K.S., Pick, H.L., and von Hofsten, C. (1988). Role of visual information in ball catching. *Journal of Motor Behavior, 20*, 150-164.

Rosengren, K.S., Savelsbergh, G.J.P. and Van der Kamp, J. (2003). Development and learning: A TASC-based perspective on the acquisition of perceptual motor behaviors. *Infant Behavior and Development, 26*, 473-494.

Rosenstein, M.T., Collins, J.J., and De Luca, C.J. (1993). A practical method for calculating largest Lyapunov exponents from small data sets. *Physica D, 65*, 117-134.

Rosser, B.W.C., and Hochamba, P.W. (1993). Metabolic capacity of muscle fibers from high altitude natives. *Eur. J. Appl. Physiol., 67*, 513-517.

Rothwell, J. (1994). *Control of human voluntary movement* (2nd Ed.). London: Chapman and Hall.

Ruelle, D. (1991). *Chance and chaos*. Princeton, NJ: Princeton University Press.

Ruff, R.L. (1996). Sodium channel slow inactivation and the distribution of sodium channels on skeletal muscle fibres enable the performance properties of different skeletal muscle fibre types. *Acta. Physiol. Scand., 156*(3), 159-168.

Ruff, R.L., and Whittlesey, D. (1992). Na+ current densities and voltage dependence in human intercostal muscle fibres. *J. Physiol., 458,* 85-97.

Ruff, R.L., and Whittlesey, D. (1993a). Comparison of Na+ currents from type IIa and IIb human intercostal muscle fibers. *Am. J. Physiol., 265,* C171-177.

Ruff, R.L., and Whittlesey, D. (1993b). Na+ currents near and away from endplates on human fast and slow twitch muscle fibers. *Muscle Nerve, 16*(9), 922-929.

Sahlin, K., Tonkonogi, M., and Soderlund, K. (1998). Energy supply and muscle fatigue in humans. *Acta Physiol. Scand., 162,* 261-266.

Salenius, S., Portin, K., Kajola, M., Salmelin, R., Hari, R. (1997). Cortical control of human motoneuron firing during isometric contraction. *J. Neurophysiology, 77,* 3401-3405.

Salesse, R., Oullier, O., and Temprado, J.J. (in press). Plane of motion mediates the coalition of constraints in rhythmic bimanual coordination. *Journal of Motor Behavior*, in press.

Saltzman, E.L., and Kelso, J.A.S. (1985). Synergies: Stabilities, instabilities and modes. *Behavioral and Brain Sciences, 8,* 161-163.

Salviati, G., Betto, R., Danieli Betto, D., and Zeviani, M. (1984). Myofibrillar-protein isoforms and sarcoplasmic-reticulum Ca2+-transport activity of single human muscle fibres. *Biochem. J.* 224(1), 215-225.

Sanders, R.H. (1998). Lifting performance in aquatic sports. In H.J. Riehle and M.M. Vieten (Eds.), *Proceedings of the XVIth International Symposium on Biomechanics in Sports* (pp. pp.25-39). Germany: University of Konstanz.

Sanders, R.H. (1999). Hydrodynamic characteristics of a swimmers hand. *Journal of Applied Biomechanics,15,* 3-36.

Savelsbergh, G.J.P. (1993). *The development of coordination in infancy*. North Holland, Netherlands: Elsevier Science.

Savelsbergh, G.J.P., and Van der Kamp, J. (1994). The effect of body orientation to gravity on early infant reaching. *Journal of Experimental Child Psychology, 58,* 510-528.

Savelsbergh, G.J.P., and Van der Kamp, J. (2000). Information in learning to coordinate and control movements: Is there a need for specificity of practise? *International Journal of Sport Psychology, 31,* 476-484

Savelsbergh, G.J.P., Van der Maas, H., and Van Geert, P. (1999). *Non-linear developmental processes*. Amsterdam: Elsevier Science.

Savelsbergh, G.J.P., von Hofsten, C., and Jonsson, B. (1997). The coupling of head, reach and grasp component in nine month old infant prehension. *Scandinavian Journal of Psychology, 38,* 325-333.

Savelsbergh, G.J.P., Whiting, H.T.A., and Bootsma, R.J. (1991). "Grasping" tau. *Journal of Experimental Psychology: Human Perception and Performance, 19,* 315-322.

Savelsbergh, G.J.P., Whiting, H.T.A., Pijpers, J.R., and van Santvoord, A.A.M. (1993). The visual guidance of catching. *Experimental Brain Research, 93,* 146-156.

Scanlan, T.K., Carpenter, P.J., Schmidt, G.W., Simons, J.P., and Keeler, B. (1993). An introduction to the sport commitment model. *Journal of Sport and Exercise Psychology, 15,* 1-15.

Schachat, F.H., Bronson, D.D., and McDonald, O.B. (1985). Heterogeneity of contractile proteins. A continuum of troponin-tropomyosin expression in mammalian skeletal muscle. *J. Biol. Chem., 260,* 1108-1113.

Schiffman, J.M., and Luchies, C.W. (2001). The effects of motion on force control abilities. *Clinical Biomechanics (Bristol, Avon), 16*(6), 505-513.

Schleihauf, R.E. (1974). A biomechanical analysis of freestyle. *Swimming Technique, 11,* 89-95.

Schleihauf, R.E. (1979). A hydrodynamic analysis of swimming propulsion. In J. Terauds and E.W. Bedingsfield (Eds.), *Swimming III* (pp. 70-109). Baltimore: University Park Press.

Schleihauf, R.E.,Gray, L., and DeRose, J. (1983). Three-dimensional analysis of swimming propulsion in the sprint front crawl stroke. In *Biomechanics and Medicine in Swimming* (edited by A.P. Hollander, P.A. Huijing and G.D. Groot). pp.173-184. Champaign, IL: Human Kinetics.

Schmidt, R.A. (1982). Generalized motor programs and schemas for movement. In J.A.S. Kelso (Ed.), *Human motor behavior: An introduction* (pp. 187-235). Hillsdale, NJ: Erlbaum.

Schmidt, R.A. (1985). The search for invariance in skilled movement behavior. The 1984 C.H. McCloy Research Lecture. *Research Quarterly for Exercise and Sport, 56,* 188-200.

Schmidt, R.A., and Lee, T.D. (1998). *Motor control and learning: A behavioral emphasis* (3rd ed.). Champaign, IL: Human Kinetics.

Schmidt, R.A., and Sherwood, D.E. (1982). An inverted-U relation between spatial error and force requirements in rapid limb movements: Further evidence for the impulse-variability model. *Journal of Experimental Psychology: Human Perception and Performance, 8,* 158-170.

Schmidt, R.A., Zelaznik, H.N., Hawkins, B., Frank, J.S., and Quinn, J.T. (1979). Motor-output variability: A theory for the accuracy of rapid motor acts. *Psychological Review, 86,* 415-441.

Schmidt, R.C., Carello, C., and Turvey, M.T. (1990). *Journal of Experimental Psychology: Human Perception and Perception, 16,* 227-247.

Schneider, K., and Zernicke, R.F. (1989). Jerk-cost modulations during the practice of rapid arm movements. *Biological Cybernetics, 60,* 221-230.

Schneider, K., and Zernicke, R.F. (1992). Mass, center of mass, and moment of inertia estimates for infant limb segment. *Journal of Biomechanics, 25,* 145-148.

Schneider, K., Zernicke, R.F., Schmidt, R.A., and Hart, T.J. (1989). Changes in limb dynamics during the practice of rapid arm movements. *Journal of Biomechanics, 22,* 805-817.

Schneider, K., Zernicke, R.F., Ulrich, B.D., Jensen, J.L., and Thelen, E. (1990). Understanding movement control in infants through the analysis of limb intersegmental dynamics. *Journal of Motor Behavior, 22,* 493-520.

Schöllhorn, W., and Bauer, H.U. (1998). Identification of individual running patterns by means of neural nets. In J. Perl and J. Mester (Eds.), *Computer science in sport* (pp. 169-176). Cologne, Germany: Sport-Buch Strauss.

Schöllhorn, W.I. (1993). Process-oriented analysis of movement patterns. In S. Bouisset (Ed.), *International Society of Biomechanics XIVth Congress Paris 4-8 July 1993* (pp. 1212-1213). Paris, France: ISB.

Schöllhorn, W.I. (1995) Time course oriented analysis of biomechanical movement patterns by means of orthogonal reference functions. In Häkkinen,K. Keskinen, K.L. Komi,P.V. Mero, A. (Eds.), *XVth Congress of the International Society of Biomechanics* (pp. 824-825). Jyväskylä, Finland: Gummerus Printing.

Schöllhorn, W.I. (1998). *System dynamische betrachtung komplexer bewegungsmuster im lernprozess* [System dynamic consideration of complex movement patterns during a learning process]. Frankfurt: Peter Lang.

Schöllhorn, W.I. (2000). Applications of systems dynamic principles to technique and strength training. *Acta Academiae Olympiquae Estoniae, 8,* 67-85.

Scholz, J.P. (1990). Dynamic pattern theory—Some implications for therapeutics. *Physical Therapy, 70,* 827-843.

Scholz, J.P. and Kelso, J.A.S. (1989). A quantitative approach to understanding the formation and change of coordinated movement patterns. *Journal of Motor Behavior, 21,* 122-144.

Scholz, J.P., and Kelso, J.A.S. (1990). Intentional switching between patterns of bimanual coordination depends on the intrinsic dynamics of the patterns. *Journal of Motor Behavior, 22,* 98-124.

Scholz, J.P., Kelso, J.A.S., and Schöner, G. (1987). Nonequilibrium phase transitions in coordinated biological motion: Critical slowing down and switching. *Physics Letters A, 123,* 390-394.

Scholz, J.P., and Schöner, G. (1999). The uncontrolled manifold concept: Identifying control variables for a functional task. *Experimental Brain Research, 126,* 289-306.

Schöner, G. (1991). Dynamic theory of action-perception patterns: The "moving room" paradigm. *Biological Cybernetics, 64,* 455-462.

Schöner, G.S., Haken, H., and Kelso, J.A.S. (1986). A stochastic theory of phase transitions in human hand movement. *Biol. Cybern., 53,* 247-257.

Schöner, G., and Kelso, J.A.S. (1988). Dynamic pattern generation in behavioral and neural systems. *Science, 239,* 1513-1520.

Schroeder, M. (1991). *Fractals, chaos, power laws: Minutes from an infinite paradise.* New York: Freeman, Cooper.

Schultz, A.B., Alexander, N.B., and Ashton-Miller, J.A. (1992). Biomechanical analyses of rising from a chair. *Journal of Biomechanics, 25*(12), 1383-1391.

Schuster, H.G., and Wagner, P. (1990). A model for neural oscillators in the visual cortex. 1. Mean-field theory and derivation of the phase equations. *Biol. Cybern., 64,* 77-82.

Seidler-Dobrin, R.D., He, J., and Stelmach, G.E. (1998). Coactivation to reduce variability in the elderly. *Motor Control, 2*(4), 314-330.

Semmler, J., Kornatz, K., Miles, T., and Enoka, R. (2002). *Low frequency (2-12 HZ) motor unit coherence differs between shortening and lengthening contractions of a hand muscle.* Paper presented at the meeting of the Society for Neuroscience Abstracts, Orlando, FL.

Semmler, J.G., Steege, J.W., Kornatz, K.W., and Enoka, R.M. (2000). Motor-unit synchronization is not responsible for larger motor-unit forces in old adults. *Journal of Neurophysiology, 84*(1), 358-366.

Shannon, C.E. (1948). A mathematical theory of communication. *Bell System Tech. J., 27,* 379-423.

Shannon, C.E., and Weaver, W. (1949). *The mathematical theory of communication.* Urbana, IL: University of Illinois Press.

Sherrington, C.S. (1906). *The integrative action of the nervous system.* New Haven, CT: Yale University Press.

Sherwood, D.E., and Schmidt, R.A. (1980). The relationship between force and force variability in minimal and near-maximal static and dynamic contractions. *Journal of Motor Behavior, 12,* 75-89.

Shibasaki, H. (1982). Movement-related cortical potentials. In A.M. Halliday (Ed.), *Evoked potentials in clinical testing* (pp. 471-482). Edinburgh: Churchill Livingstone.

Shimizu, H. (1974). Muscular contraction mechanism as a hard mode instability. *Prog. Theor. Phys., 52,* 329-330.

Shimizu, H., and Yamada, T. (1972). Phenomenological equations of motion of muscular contraction. *Prog. Theor. Phys., 47,* 350-351.

Shirley, M.M. (1931). *The first two years: A study of twenty-five babies. Vol. 1. Postural and locomotor development.* Minneapolis, MN: University of Minnesota Press.

Sidaway, B., Heise, G., and Schoenfelder-Zohdi, B. (1995). Quantifying the variability of angle-angle plots. *Journal of Human Movement Studies, 29,* 181-197.

Silberstein, R.B. (1995). Steady-state visually evoked potentials, brain resonances and cognitive processes. In P.L. Nunez (Ed.), *Neocortical dynamics and human EEG rhythms* (pp. 272-303). New York: Oxford University Press.

Simon, H.A., and Chase, W.G. (1973). Skill in chess. *American Scientist, 61,* 394-403.

Singer, R.N., and Janelle, C.M. (1999). Determining sport expertise: From genes to supremes. *International Journal of Sport Psychology, 30,* 117-150.

Singer, W. (1993). Synchronization of cortical activity and its putative role in information processing and learning. *Annu. Rev. Physiol., 55,* 349-374.

Slifkin, A.B., and Newell, K.M. (1999a). Is variability in human performance a reflection of system noise? *Current Directions in Psychological Science, 7,* 170-176.

Slifkin, A.B., and Newell, K.M. (1999b). Noise, information transmission, and force variability. *Journal of Experimental Psychology: Human Perception and Performance, 25,* 837-851.

Snedecor, G.W., and Cochran, W.G. (1989). *Statistical methods.* Ames, IA: Iowa State University Press.

Snoddy, G.S. (1926). Learning and stability. *Journal of Applied Psychology, 10,* 1-36.

Sogaard, K., Christensen, H., Jensen, B.R., Finsen, L., and Sjogaard, G. (1996). Motor control and kinetics during low level concentric and eccentric contractions in man. *Electroencephalography and Clinical Neurophysiology, 101*(5), 453-460.

Sompolinsky, H., Golomb, D., and Kleinfeld, D. (1991). Cooperative dynamics in visual processing. *Phys. Rev. A, 43,* 6990-7011.

Sonna, L.A., Sharp, M.A., Knapik, J.J., Cullivan, M., Angel, K.C., Patton, J.F. and Lilley, C.M. (2001). Angiotensin-converting enzyme genotype and physical performance during US Army basic training. *Journal of Applied Physiology, 91,* 1355-1363.

Sosniak, L.A. (1985). Learning to be a concert pianist. In B.S. Bloom (Ed.), *Developing talent in young people* (pp. 19-67). New York: Ballantine.

Southard, D. (1989). Changes in limb striking pattern: Effects of speed and accuracy. *Research Quarterly for Exercise and Sport, 60,* 348-356.

Sparrow, W.A., Donovan, E., Van Emmerik, R.E.A., and Barry, E.B. (1987). Using relative motion plots to measure changes in intra-limb and inter-limb coordination. *Journal of Motor Behavior, 19,* 115-129.

Sparrow, W.H., and Newell, K.M. (1998). Metabolic energy expenditure and the regulation of movement economy. *Psychonomic Bulletin and Review, 5,* 173-196.

Sperry, R.W. (1950). Neural basis of the spontaneous optokinetic response. *Journal of Comparative Physiology, 43,* 482-489.

Spiegel, K.M., Stratton, J., Burke, J.R., Glendinning, D.S., and Enoka, R.M. (1996). The influence of age on the assessment of motor unit activation in a human hand muscle. *Experimental Physiology, 81*(5), 805-819.

Spray, J.A., and Newell, K.M. (1986). Time series analysis of motor learning: KR versus no KR. *Human Movement Science, 5,* 59-74.

Stark, H., and Woods, J.W. (1994). *Probability, random processes, and estimation theory for engineers* (2nd Ed.). Englewood Cliffs, NJ: Prentice Hall.

Starkes, J. (2000). The road to expertise: Is practice the only determinant? *International Journal of Sport Psychology, 31,* 431-451.

Starkes, J.L., Deakin, J.M., Allard, F., Hodges, N.J., and Hayes., A. (1996). Deliberate practice in sports: What is it anyway? In K.A. Ericsson (Ed.), *The road to excellence: The acquisition of expert performance in the arts, sciences, sports and games* (pp. 81-106). Mahwah, NJ: Erlbaum.

Starkes, J.L., Helsen, W.F., and Jack, R. (2001). Expert performance in sport and dance. In R.N. Singer, H.A. Hausenblas, and C.M. Janelle (Eds.), *Handbook of sport psychology* (2nd ed., pp. 174-201). New York: Macmillan.

Steenbergen, B., Marteniuk, R.G., and Kalbfleisch, L.E. (1995). Achieving coordination in prehension: Joint freezing and postural contributions. *Journal of Motor Behavior, 27,* 333-348.

Stein, R.B. (1965). *Biophysical Journal, 5,* 173-194.

Stelmach, G.E. (Ed.). (1975). *Motor control: Issues and trends.* New York: Academic Press.

Stergiou, N. (ed.) (2003). *Innovation analyses of human movement.* Champaign, IL: Human Kinetics.

Stergiou, N., and Bates, B.T. (1997). The relationship between subtalar and knee joint function as a possible mechanism for running injuries. *Gait and Posture, 6,* 177-185.

Stergiou, N., Bates, B.T., and James, S.L. (1999). Asynchrony between subtalar and knee joint function during running. *Medicine and Science in Sports and Exercise, 31,* 1645-55.

Stergiou, N., Jensen, J.L., Bates, B.T., Scholten, S.D., and Tzetzis, G. (2001). A dynamical systems investigation of lower extremity coordination during running over obstacles. *Clinical Biomechanics, 16,* 213-221.

Stergiou, N., Scholten, S.D, Jenson, J.L., and Blanke, D. (2001). Intra-limb coordination following obstacle clearance during running: The effect of obstacle height. *Gait and Posture, 13,* 210-220.

Sternad, D., Dean, W.J., and Newell, K.M. (2000). Force and timing variability in rhythmic unimanual tapping. *J. Motor Behav., 32,* 249-267.

Sternberg, R.J. (1996). Costs of expertise. In K.A. Ericsson (Ed.), *The road to excellence: The acquisition of expert performance in the arts and sciences, sports and games* (pp. 347-353). Mahwah, NJ: Erlbaum.

Stienen, G.J., Kiers, J.L., Bottinelli, R., and Reggiani, C. (1996). Myofibrillar ATPase activity in skinned human skeletal muscle fibres: Fibre type and temperature dependence. *J. Physiol. (Lond.), 493,* 299-307.

Stoffregen, T.A. (1985). Flow structure versus retinal location in the optical control of stance. *Journal of Experimental Psychology: Human Perception and Performance, 11,* 554-565.

Stoffregen, T.A., Adolph, K.E., Thelen, E., Gorday, K.M., and Sheng, Y.Y. (1997). Toddler's postural adaptations to different support surfaces. *Motor Control, 1,* 119-137.

Stoffregen, T.A., Bardy, B.G., Merhi, O., and Oullier, O. (2004). Postural responses to real and virtual optic flow. *Presence: Teleoperators and Virtual Environment, 13*(5), 601-615.

Stoffregen, T.A., and Riccio, G.E. (1988). An ecological theory of orientation and the vestibular system. *Psychological Review, 95,* 3-14.

Stoffregen, T.A., Smart Jr., L.J., Bardy, B.G., and Pagulayan, R.J. (1999). Postural stabilization of looking. *Journal of Experimental Psychology: Human Perception and Performance, 25,* 1641-1658.

Strogatz, S.H. (1994). *Nonlinear dynamics and chaos.* New York: Addison-Wesley.

Strogatz, S.H. (2000). From Kuramoto to Crawford: Exploring the onset of synchronization in populations of coupled oscillators. *Physica D, 143,* 1-20.

Strogatz, S.H., and Stewart, I. (1993). Coupled oscillators and biological synchronization. *Scientific American, 269*(6), 68-75.

Subotnick, S.I. (1975). Orthotic foot control and the overuse syndrome. *Physician and Sports Medicine, 3,* 32-38.

Szafran, J. (1968). "Neural noise" as a factor limiting "channel capacity." *Biomedical Science Instrumentation, 4,* 171-178.

Takeuchi, A.H., and Hulse, S.H. (1993). Absolute pitch. *Psychological Bulletin, 113,* 345-361.

Tass, P., Rosenblum, M.G., Weule, J., Kurths, J., Pikovsky, A., Volkmann, J., Schnitzler, A., Freund, H.J. (1998). Detection of n:m phase locking from noisy data: Application to magnetoencephalography. *Phys. Rev. Lett., 81,* 3291-3294.

Tass, P.A. (1999). *Phase resetting in medicine and biology—Stochastic modelling and data analysis.* Berlin: Springer-Verlag.

Tass, P.A. (2000). Stochastic phase resetting: A theory for deep brain stimulation. *Prog. Theor. Phys. Suppl., 139,* 301-313.

Taylor, A., Steege, J., and Enoka, R. (2000). Increased variability of motor unit discharge rate decreases the steadiness of simulated isometric contractions. *The Physiologist, 43*(4), 321.

Taylor, C.R. (1985). Force development during sustained locomotion: a determinant of gait, speed and metabolic power. *Journal of Experimental Biology, 115,* 253-262.

Taylor, R.R., Mamotte, C.D.S., Fallon, K., and van Bockxmeer, F.M. (1999). Elite athletes and the gene for angiotensin-converting enzyme. *Journal of Applied Physiology, 87,* 1035-1037.

Temprado, J.J., Della-Grast, M., Farrell, M., and Laurent, M. (1997). A novice-expert comparison of (intra-limb) coordination subserving the volleyball serve. *Human Movement Science, 16,* 653-676.

Temprado, J.J., Swinnen, S. P., Carson, R.G., Tourment, A., and Laurent, M. (2003). Interaction of directional, neuromuscular and egocentric constraints on the stability of preferred bimanual coordination patterns. *Human Movement Science, 22,* 339-63.

Tepavac, D., and Field-Fote, E.C. (2001). Vector coding: A technique for quantification of intersegmental coupling in multicyclic behaviors. *Journal of Applied Biomechanics, 17,* 259-270.

Thelen, E. (1979). Rhythmical stereotypes in normal human infants. *Animal Behaviour, 27,* 699-715.

Thelen, E. (1986). Development of coordinated movement: Implications for early human development. In M.G. Wade and H.T.A. Whiting (Eds.), *Motor development in children: Aspects of coordination and control* (pp. 107-124). Dordrecht, Netherlands: Martinus Nijhoff.

Thelen, E. (1995). Motor development: A new synthesis. *American Psychologist, 50,* 79-95.

Thelen, E. (1998). Bernstein's legacy for motor development: How infants learn to reach. In M.L. Latash (Ed.), *Progress in motor control—Volume 1: Bernstein's traditions in movement studies* (pp. 267-288). Champaign, IL: Human Kinetics.

Thelen, E., Corbetta, D., Kamm, K., Spencer, J., Schneider, K., and Zernicke, R.F. (1993). The transition to reaching: Mapping intention and intrinsic dynamics. *Child Development, 64,* 1058-1098.

Thelen, E., Corbetta, D., and Spencer, J.P. (1996). The development of reaching during the first year: The role of movement speed. *Journal of Experimental Psychology: Human Perception and Performance, 22,* 1059-1076.

Thelen, E., Fisher, D., Ridley Johnson, R. (1984). The relationship between physical growth and a newborn reflex. *Infant Behavior and Development, 7,* 479-493.

Thelen, E., and Smith, L.B. (1994). *A dynamic systems approach to the development of cognition and action.* Cambridge, MA: MIT Press.

Thelen, E., Zernicke, R.F., Schneider, K., Jensen, J.L., Kamm, K., and Corbetta, D. (1992). The role of intersegmental dynamics in infant neuromotor development. In G.E. Stelmach and J. Requin (Eds.), *Tutorials in motor behavior II* (pp. 533-548). Amsterdam: North-Holland.

Thomas, J.R., and Nelson, J.K. (2001). *Research methods in physical activity* (4th Ed.). Champaign, IL: Human Kinetics.

Thomas, J.S., Schmidt, E.M., and Hambrecht, F.T. (1978). Facility of motor unit control during tasks defined directly in terms of unit behaviors. *Exp. Neurol., 59,* 384-397.

Thompson, J.M.T., and Stewart, H.B. (2002). *Nonlinear dynamics and chaos* (2nd Ed.). New York: Wiley.

Todorov, E., and Jordan, M.I. (2002). Optimal feedback control as a theory of motor coordination. *Nature Neuroscience, 5,* 1226-1235.

Tolman, E.C. (1948). Cognitive maps in rats and men. *Psychological Review, 55,* 189-208.

Tracy, B.L., and Enoka, R.M. (2002). Older adults are less steady during submaximal isometric contractions with the knee extensor muscles. *Journal of Applied Physiology, 92*(3), 1004-1012.

Tracy, B.L., Kern, D.S., Mehoudar, P.D., Sehnert, S.M, Byrnes, W.C., and Enoka, R.M. (2001). Strength training does not improve the steadiness of muscle contractions in the knee extensors of older adults. *Medicine and Science in Sports and Exercise, 33*(5), S254.

Tracy, B.L., Mehoudar, P.D., Ortega, J.D., and Enoka, R.M. (2002). The steadiness of isometric contractions is similar between upper and lower extremity muscle groups. *Medicine and Science in Sports and Exercise, 34*(Suppl. 5), S19.

Tuller, B., Fitch, H.L., and Turvey, M.T. (1982). The Bernstein perspective: II. The concept of muscle linkage or coordinative structure. In J.A.S. Kelso (Ed.), *Human motor behavior: An introduction* (pp. 253-270). Hillsdale, NJ: Erlbaum.

Turvey, M.T. (1990). Coordination. *American Psychologist, 45,* 938-953.

Turvey, M.T., and Fitzpatrick, P. (1993). Commentary: Development of perception-action systems and general principles of pattern formation. *Child Development, 64,* 1175-1190.

Uhl, C. (1999). *Analysis of neurophysiological brain functioning.* Berlin: Springer-Verlag.

Ulrich, B. D., Ulrich, D. A., Angulo-Kinzler, R., and Chapman, D. D. (1997). Sensitivity of infants with and without down syndrome to intrinsic dynamics. *Research Quarterly for Exercise and Sport, 68*(1), 10-19.

Vaday, M. and Nemessuri, M. (1971). Motor pattern of free-style swimming. In *Biomechanics and Swimming I* (edited by L. Lewillie and J.P. Clarys), pp. 167-173. Brussels: The Free University of Brussels.

Vaillancourt, D., and Newell, K.M. (2000). The dynamics of resting and postural tremor in Parkinson's disease. *Clinical Neurophysiology, 111,* 2046-2056.

Vaillancourt, D.E., Larsson, L., and Newell, K.M. (2002). Time-dependent structure in the discharge rate of human motor units. *Clinical Neurophysiology, 113,* 1325-1328.

Vaillancourt, D.E., Larsson, L., and Newell, K.M. (2003). Effects of aging on force variability, motor unit discharge patterns, and the structure of 10, 20 and 40 Hz EMG activity. *Neurobiology of Aging: Experimental and Clinical Research, 24,* 25-35.

Vaillancourt, D.E., and Newell, K.M. (2002). Changing complexity in human behavior and physiology through aging and disease. *Neurobiology of Aging, 23,* 1-11.

Vaillancourt, D.E., and Newell, K.M. (2003). Aging and the time and frequency structure of force output variability. *Journal of Applied Physiology, 94,* 903-912.

Vaillancourt, D.E., Slifkin, A.B., and Newell, K.M. (2002). Inter-digit individuation and force variability in precision grip. *Motor Control, 6,* 113-128.

van Asten, W.N.J.C., Gielen, C.C.A.M., and Denier van der Gon, J.J. (1988). Postural adjustments induced by simulated motion of differently structured environments. *Experimental Brain Research, 73,* 371-383.

Van der Kamp, J., and Savelsbergh, G.J.P. (1994). Exploring exploration in the development of action. *Clinical Center for Child Development, Annual Report 1993-94.* (pp.43-46).

Van der Kamp, J., Savelsbergh, G.J.P., and Davis, W.E. (1998). Body-scaled ratio as control parameter for prehension of 5-9 year old children. *Developmental Psychobiology, 33,* 351-361.

Van der Kamp, J., Savelsbergh, G.J.P., and Smeets, J.B. (1997). Multiple information sources in interceptive timing. *Human Movement Science, 16,* 787-822.

Van der Kamp, J., Vereijken, B., and Savelsbergh, G. J.P. (1996). Physical and informational constraints in the coordination and control of human movement. *Corpus, Psyche and Societas,* 3(2), 102-118.

Van der Maas, H.L.J., Molenaar, P.C.M. (1992). Stagewise cognitive development: An application of catastrophe theory. *Psychological Review, 99,* 395-417.

Van der Meer, A., Van der Weel, F., Lee, D., Laing, I., and Lin, J. (1995). Development of prospective control of catching in premature at risk infants. *Developmental Medicine and Child Neurology, 37,* 145-158.

Van Emmerik, R.E.A., and van Wegen, E.E.H. (2000). On variability and stability in human movement. *Journal of Applied Biomechanics, 16,* 394-406.

Van Emmerik, R.E.A., and van Wegen, E.E.H. (2002). On the functional aspects of variability in postural control. *Exercise and Sport Science Reviews, 30,* 177-193.

Van Emmerik, R.E.A., and Wagenaar, R.C. (1995). The functional role of movement variability: Implications for learning and relearning processes. *Corpus, Psyche et Societas, 2,* 56-70.

Van Emmerik, R.E.A., and Wagenaar, R.C. (1996). Effects of walking velocity on relative phase dynamics in the trunk in human walking. *Journal of Biomechanics, 29,* 1175-1184.

Van Emmerik, R.E.A., Wagenaar, R.C., Winogrodzka, A., and Wolters, E.C. (1999). Identification of axial rigidity during locomotion in Parkinson's disease. *Archives of Physical Medicine and Rehabilitation, 80,* 186-191.

Van Galen, G.P., and De Jong, W.P. (1995). Fitts' law as the outcome of a dynamic noise filtering model of motor control. *Human Movement Science, 14,* 539-571.

van Geert, P. (1994). *Dynamic systems of development: Change between complexity and chaos.* New York: Harvester Wheatsheaf.

Van Hof, P., van der Kamp, J. and Savelsbergh, G.J.P. (2002). The relation of unimanual and bimanual reaching to crossing the midline. *Child Development 73,* 1353-1362.

van Uden, C.J.T., Bloo, J.K.C., Kooloos, J.G.M., van Kampen, A., de Witte, J., and Wagenaar, R.C. (2003). Coordination and stability of one-legged hopping patterns in patients with anterior cruciate ligament reconstruction: Preliminary results. *Clinical Biomechanics, 18,* 84-87.

Van Vliet, K.M. (1981). Classification of noise phenomena. In P.H.E. Meijer, R.D. Mountain, and R.J. Soulen, Jr. (Eds.), *Sixth International Conference On Noise in Physical Systems* (pp. 3-11). Washington, DC: U.S. Department of Commerce and National Bureau of Standards.

van Wegen, E.E.H., Van Emmerik, R.E.A, and Riccio, G.E. (2002). Postural orientation: Age-related changes in variability and time-to-boundary. *Human Movement Science, 21,* 61-84.

Vandermeulen Luyt, D.M. (2002). *Variability in force magnitude and direction in a two-joint lower extremity discrete isometric task.* Unpublished master's thesis, University of Illinois, Urbana-Champaign.

Vandervoort, A.A. (2002). Aging of the human neuromuscular system. *Muscle and Nerve, 25(1),* 17-25.

Vaughan, C.L. (1984). Computer simulation of human motion in sports biomechanics. In R.L. Terjung (Ed.), *Exercise and sport sciences reviews—Volume 12* (pp. 373-416). Baltimore: Lippincott, Williams and Wilkins.

Vereijken, B., Van Emmerik, R.A.E., Whiting, H.T.A., and Newell, K.M. (1992). Free(z)ing degrees of freedom in skill acquisition. *Journal of Motor Behavior, 24*, 133-142.

Vereijken, B., Whiting, H.T.A., and Beek, W.J. (1992). A dynamical systems approach towards skill acquisition. *Quarterly Journal of Experimental Psychology, 45A*, 323-344.

von Holst, E., and Mittelstaedt, H. (1950), Das reafferenzprinzip. Wechselwirkung zwischen zentralnervensystem und peripherie [The Reafference principle. Exchanges between central and peripheral nervous systems]. *Naturwissenschaften, 37*, 464-476.

Vuillerme, N., Danion, F., Marin, L., Boyadjian, A., Prieur, J. M., Weise, I., and Nougier, V. (2001). The effect of expertise in gymnastics on postural control. *Neuroscience Letters, 303*, 83-86.

Vuillerme, N., Nougier, V., and Prieur, J.M. (2001). Can vision compensate for a lower limbs muscular fatigue for controlling posture in humans? *Neuroscience Letters, 308*, 103-106.

Wagenaar, R.C., and Van Emmerik, R.E.A. (1994). Dynamics of pathological gait. *Human Movement Science, 13*, 441-471.

Wagenaar, W.A. (1972). Generation of random sequences by human participants: A critical survey of literature. *Psychological Bulletin, 77*, 65-72.

Wallace, S.A. (1996). Dynamic pattern perspective of rhythmic movement: An introduction. In H.N. Zelaznik (Ed.), *Advances in motor learning and control* (pp.155-194). Champaign, IL: Human Kinetics.

Wallace, S.A., Stevenson, E., Spear, A., and Weeks, D.L. (1994). Scanning the dynamics of reaching and grasping movements. *Human Movement Science, 13*, 255-289.

Wallenstein, G.V., Kelso, J.A.S., and Bressler, S.L. (1995). Phase transitions in spatiotemporal patterns of brain activity and behavior. *Physica D, 84*, 626-634.

Wallingford, R. (1975). Long distance running. In A.W. Tayler and F. Landry (Eds.), *The scientific aspects of sport training* (pp. 118-130). Springfield, IL: Charles C Thomas.

Ward, L.M. (2002). *Dynamical cognitive science.* Cambridge, MA: MIT Press.

Warren, W.H. (1984). Perceiving affordance: Visual guidance of stair climbing. *Journal of Experimental Psychology: Human Perception and Performance, 10*, 683-703.

Warren, W.H., Kay, B.A., and Yilmaz, E.H. (1996). Visual control of posture during walking: Functional specificity. *Journal of Experimental Psychology: Human Perception and Performance, 22*, 818-838.

Welford, A.T. (1965). Performance, biological mechanisms and age: A theoretical sketch. In A.T. Welford and J.E. Birren (Eds.), *Ageing and the nervous system* (pp. 3-20). Springfield, IL: Charles C Thomas.

Welford, A.T. (1968). *Fundamentals of skill.* London: Methuen.

Welford, A.T. (1981). Signal, noise, performance, and age. *Human Factors, 23*, 97-109.

West, B.J., and Deering, B. (1995). *The lure of modern science: Fractal thinking.* Singapore: World Scientific.

Westerblad, H., Allen, D.G., Bruton, J.D., Andrade, F.H., and Lannergren, J. (1998). Mechanisms underlying the reduction of isometric force in skeletal muscle fatigue. *Acta Physiol. Scand., 162*(3), 253-260.

Wheat, J.S., Bartlett, R.M., and Milner, C.E. (2003). Continuous relative phase calculation: Phase angle definition. *Journal of Sports Sciences, 21*, 253-254.

Wheat, J.S., Mullineaux, D.R., Bartlett, R.M., and Milner, C.E. (2002). Quantifying variability in coordination during running. In K.E. Gianikellis (Ed.), *Scientific Proceedings of the XXth International Symposium on Biomechanics in Sports* (pp. 519-523). Caceres, Spain: Universidad de Extremadura.

Whiting, H.T.A., and Cockerill, I.M. (1972). Eyes on hand—Eyes on target? *Journal of Motor Behavior, 4,* 155-162.

Whiting, H.T.A., and Vereijken, B. (1993). The acquisition of coordination in skill learning. *International Journal of Sport Psychology, 24,* 343-357.

Whiting, W.C., and Zernicke, R.F. (1982). Correlation of movement patterns via pattern recognition. *Journal of Motor Behavior, 14,* 135-142.

Whiting, W.C., and Zernicke, R.F. (1998). *Biomechanics of Musculoskeletal Injury.* Champaign, IL: Human Kinetics.

Wickens, C.D. (1984). *Engineering psychology and human performance.* Columbus, OH: Merrill.

Widrick, J.J., Knuth, S.T., Norenberg, K.M., Romatowski, J.G., Bain, J.L., Riley, D.A., Karhanek, M., Trappe, S.W., Trappe, T.A., Costill, D.L., and Fitts, R.H. (1999). Effect of a 17 day spaceflight on contractile properties of human soleus muscle fibres. *J. Physiol. (Lond.), 516,* 915-930.

Wiesendanger, M. (1986). Initiation of voluntary movements and the supplementary motor area. In H. Heurer and C. Fromm (Eds.), *Generation and modulation of action patterns* (pp. 3-13). Berlin: Springer-Verlag.

Wiesenfeld, K., and Moss, F. (1995). Stochastic resonance and the benefits of noise: From ice ages to crayfish and SQUIDS. *Nature, 373,* 33-36.

Williams, A.G., Dhamrait, S.S., Wootton, P.T., Day, S.H., Hawe, E., Payne, J.R., Myerson, S.G., World, M., Budgett, R., Humphries, S.E., Montgomery, H.E.. (2004). Bradykinin receptor gene variant and human physical performance. *Journal of Applied Physiology 96,* 938-942.

Williams, A.G., Rayson, M.P., Jubb, M., World, M., Woods, D.R., Hayward, M., Martin, J., Humphries, S.E. and Montgomery, H.E. (2000). Physiology—The ACE gene and muscle performance. *Nature, 403,* 614.

Williams, A.M. (2000). Perceptual skill in soccer: Implications for talent identification and development. *Journal of Sports Sciences, 18,* 737-750.

Williams, A.M., Davids, K., and Williams, J.G. (1999). *Visual perception and action in sport.* London: Routledge, Taylor and Francis.

Williams, K. (1998). Intralimb coordination of older adults during locomotion: Stair descend. *Journal of Human Movement Studies, 34,* 95-117.

Williams, K.R. (1993). Biomechanics of distance running. In M.D. Grabiner (Ed.), *Current issues in biomechanics* (pp. 3-31). Champaign, IL: Human Kinetics.

Williams, L.R., and Gross, J.B. (1980). Heritability of motor skill. *Acta Genetica Medica, 29*(2), 127-136.

Willis, T. (1664/1964) *The anatomy of the brain and nerves (cerebri anatome)* - Tercentenary Edition. Montreal, QB: McGill University Press.

Willis, T. (1971). *Two discourses concerning the soul of brutes, which is that of the vital and sensitive of man.* (S. Diamond, Introduction). Gainesville, FL: Scholars' Facsimilies and Reprints. (Original work published 1683).

Willott, J.F. (1999). Movement and the production of behavior. In J.F. Willott (Ed.), *Neurogerontology. Aging and the nervous system* (pp. 203-224). New York: Springer-Verlag.

Wilson, M.A., and McNaughton, B.L. (1993). Dynamics of the hippocampal ensemble code for space. *Science, 261,* 1055-1058.

Wimmers, R.H., Beek, P.J., Savelsbergh, G.J.P., and Hopkins, B. (1998). Transition in the development of prehension. *The British Journal of Developmental Psychology, 16,* 45-63.

Wimmers, R.H., and Savelsbergh, G.J.P. (2001). Variability in the emergence of early reaching. *Journal of Human Movement Studies, 40,* 65-81.

Wimmers, R.H., Savelsbergh, G.J.P., Beek, P.J., and Hopkins, B. (1998). Evidence for a phase transition in the early development of prehension. *Developmental Psychobiology, 32,* 235-248.

Wimmers, R.H., Savelsbergh, G.J.P., van der Kamp, J., and Hartelman, P. (1998). A cusp catastrophe model as a model for transition in the development of prehension. *Developmental Psychobiology, 32,* 23-35.

Wing, A.M., and Kristofferson, A.B. (1973). Response delays and the timing of discrete motor responses. *Perception and Psychophysics, 14,* 5-12.

Winter, D.A. (1989). Future directions in biomechanics research of human movement. In J.S. Skinner, C.B. Corbin, D.M. Landers, P.E. Martin, and C.L. Wells (Eds.), *Future directions in exercise and sport science research* (pp. 201-207). Champaign, IL: Human Kinetics.

Winter, D.A. (1990). *Biomechanics and motor control of human movement.* New York: Wiley.

Winter, D.A. (1995). Human balance and posture control during standing and walking. *Gait and Posture, 3,* 193-214.

Winter, D.A., and Bishop, P.J. (1992). Lower extremity injury: Biomechanical factors associated with chronic injury to the lower extremity. *Sports Medicine, 14,* 149-156.

Winters, J.M., and Stark, L. (1985). Analysis of fundamental human movement patterns through the use of in-depth antagonistic muscle models. *IEEE Transactions of Biomedical Engineering BME, 32*(10), 826-839.

Woledge, R.C., Curtin, N.A., and Homsher, E. (1985). Energetic aspects of muscle contraction. *Monogr. Physiol. Soc., 41,* 1-357.

Wood, D.S., Sorenson, M.M., Eastwood, A.B., Charash, W.E., and Reuben, J.P. (1978). Duchenne dystrophy: Abnormal generation of tension and Ca++ regulation in single skinned fibres. *Neurology, 28,* 447-457.

Wood, G.A. (1982). Data smoothing and differentiation procedures in biomechanics. *Exercise and Sports Sciences Reviews, 10,* 308-362.

Woods, D.R., Hickman, M., Jamshidi, Y., Brull, D., Vassiliou, V., Jones, A., Humphries S., and Montgomery H. (2001). Elite swimmers and the D allele of the ACE I/D polymorphism. *Human Genetics, 108,* 230-232.

Woods, D.R., Humphries, S.E., and Montgomery, H.E. (2000). The ACE I/D polymorphism and human physical performance. *Trends in Endocrinology and Metabolism, 11,* 416-420.

Woods, D.R., World, M., Rayson, M.P., Williams, A.G., Jubb, M., Jamshidi, Y., Hayward M., Mary D.A., Humphries S.E., and Montgomery H.E. (2002). Endurance enhancement related to the human angiotensin I-converting enzyme I-D polymorphism is not due to differences in the cardiorespiratory response to training. *European Journal of Applied Physiology, 86,* 240-244.

Woodworth, R.S. (1899). The accuracy of voluntary movement. *Psychological Review, 3*(Suppl. 13), 1-119.

Woollacott, M.H., and Jensen, J.L. (1996). Posture and locomotion. In H. Heuer and S. Keele (Eds.), *Handbook of perception and action; Vol. 2: Motor Skills* (pp. 333-403). London: Academic Press.

Woollacott, M.H., Shumway-Cook, A., Nashner, L. (1986). Aging and postural control: Changes in sensory organization and muscular coordination. *International Journal of Aging and Human Development, 23,* 97-114.

Wright, C.E., and Meyer, D.E. (1983). Conditions for a linear speed-accuracy trade-off in aimed movements. *Quarterly Journal of Experimental Psychology, 35A,* 279-296.

Wright, J.J., Liley, D.T.J. (1996). Dynamics of the brain at global and microscopic scales: Neural networks and the EEG. *Behav. Brain Sci., 19,* 285-320.

Yan, J.H. (1999). Tai chi practice reduces movement force variability for seniors. *Journal of Gerontology A Biological Science Medical Science, 54*(12), M629-634.

Yan, J.H. (2000). Effects of aging on linear and curvilinear aiming arm movements. *Experimental Aging Research, 26*(4), 393-407.

Yan, J.H., Thomas, J.R., and Stelmach, G.E. (1998). Aging and rapid aiming arm movement control. *Experimental Aging Research, 24*(2), 155-168.

Yang, J.F., Winter, D.A., and Wells, R.P. (1990). Postural dynamics in the standing human. *Biological Cybernetics, 62,* 309-320.

Yao, W., Fuglevand, R.J., and Enoka, R.M. (2000). Motor-unit synchronization increases EMG amplitude and decreases force steadiness of simulated contractions. *Journal of Neurophysiology, 83*(1), 441-452.

Yates, F.E. (1993). Self-organizing systems. In C. Boyd and D. Noble (Eds.), *Logic of life* (pp. 189-218). Oxford, UK: Oxford University Press.

Yeadon, M.R., and Challis, J.H. (1994). The future of performance-related sports biomechanics research. *Journal of Sports Sciences, 12,* 3-32.

Yin, R.K. (1988). *Case study research.* Newbury Park, CA: Sage Publications.

Yoneda, S., and Tokumasu, K. (1986). Frequency analysis of body sway in the upright posture. *Acta Otolaryngology, 102,* 87-92.

Young B.W., and Salmela, J.H. (2002). Perceptions of training and deliberate practice of middle distance runners. *International Journal of Sport Psychology, 33,* 167-181.

Young, D.S. (1988). Describing the information for action. In O.G. Meijer and K. Roth (Eds.), *Complex movement behaviour: "The" motor-action controversy* (pp. 419-437). Amsterdam: North-Holland.

Zanone, P.G., and Kelso, J.A.S. (1992). Evolution of behavioural attractors with learning: Nonequilibrium phase transitions. *Journal of Experimental Psychology: Human Perception and Performance, 18,* 403-421.

Zatsiorsky, V.M. (Ed.). (2000). *Biomechanics in sport: Performance enhancement and injury prevention—Volume 9 of the IOC Encyclopaedia of Sports Medicine.* Oxford, UK: Blackwell Scientific.

Zatsiorsky, V.M., and Fortney, V.L. (1993). Sport biomechanics 2000. *Journal of Sports Sciences, 11,* 279-283.

Zelaznik, H.N., Mone, S., McCabe, G.P., and Thaman, C. (1988). Role of temporal and spatial precision in determining the nature of the speed-accuracy trade-off in aimed-hand movements. *Journal of Experimental Psychology: Human Perception and Performance, 14,* 221-230.

Zelaznik, H.N., Shapiro, D.C., and McClosky, D. (1981). Effects of a secondary task on the accuracy of single aiming movements. *Journal of Experimental Psychology: Human Perception and Performance, 7,* 1007-1018.

Zernicke, R.F., and Schneider, K. (1993). Biomechanics and developmental neuromotor control. *Child Development, 64,* 982-1004.

Zernicke, R.F., and Whiting, W.C. (2000). Mechanisms of musculoskeletal injury. In V.M. Zatsiorsky (Ed.), *Biomechanics in sport: Performance enhancement and injury prevention—Volume 9 of the IOC Encyclopaedia of Sports Medicine* (pp. 507-522). Oxford, UK: Blackwell Scientific.

Index

Note: The italicized *f* and *t* following page numbers refer to figures and tables, respectively.

About the Editors

Keith Davids, PhD, is dean of the School of Physical Education at the University of Otago in New Zealand. For 25 years he has taught and conducted research in the field of motor learning and control. In addition, he has produced three books in this area and written numerous chapters and articles for journals.

Davids has worked in higher education in both Europe and New Zealand. He is currently a coeditor of the *International Journal of Sport Psychology* and received a PhD in motor control from Leeds University, UK, in 1986.

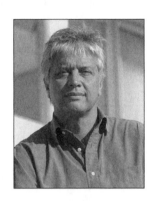

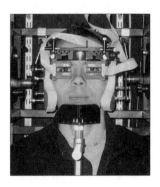

Simon Bennett, PhD, has taught and conducted research in the field of motor control for over 10 years. He is a senior lecturer in motor control at Manchester Metropolitan University, UK, where he also serves as research team leader and laboratory director. Bennett received his PhD from Manchester Metropolitan University.

Bennett's research interests include specificity of learning, coordination dynamics, information sources for interceptive actions, intermittent vision, ventral and dorsal processing, and observational learning. He has coauthored several chapters and articles for journals in this field.

Karl Newell, PhD, is associate dean for research and graduate education in the College of Health and Human Development at Penn State University. He has conducted a longstanding research program on the role of movement variability in motor control and has helped create a new way to think about movement variability.

Newell is former editor of the *Journal of Motor Behavior* and served as president of the North American Society for Psychology of Sport and Physical Activity.

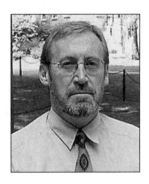

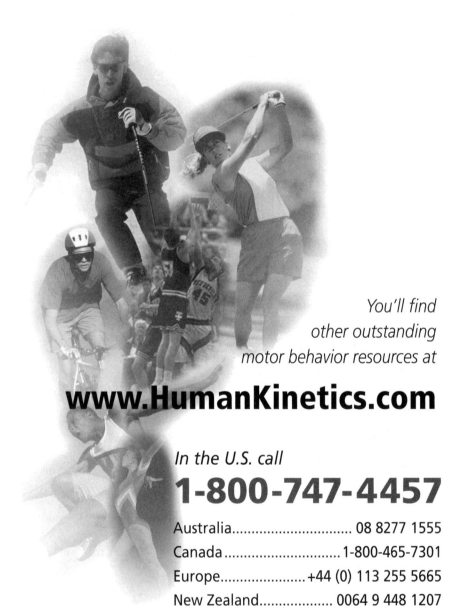

*You'll find
other outstanding
motor behavior resources at*

www.HumanKinetics.com

In the U.S. call

1-800-747-4457

Australia............................. 08 8277 1555
Canada 1-800-465-7301
Europe.....................+44 (0) 113 255 5665
New Zealand................... 0064 9 448 1207

HUMAN KINETICS
The Information Leader in Physical Activity
P.O. Box 5076 • Champaign, IL 61825-5076 USA